21

Update in Intensive Care and Emergency Medicine

Edited by J.-L. Vincent

Springer

Berlin
Heidelberg
New York
Barcelona
Budapest
Hong Kong
London
Milan
Paris
Santa Clara
Singapore
Tokyo

A. Revhaug (Editor)

Acute
Catabolic State

With 46 Figures

Springer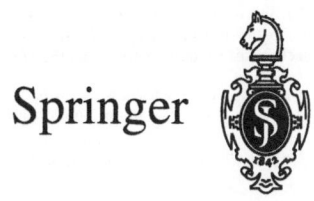

Series Editor

Prof. Dr. Jean-Louis Vincent
Clinical Director, Department of Intensive Care
Erasme University Hospital
Route de Lennik 808, 1070 Brussels, Belgium

Volume Editor

Professor Arthur Revhaug
University of Tromsø
School of Medicine
Department of Surgery
9038 Tromsø, Norway

Library of Congress Cataloging-in-Publication Data

Acute catabolic state / A. Revhaug (editor).
       p.   cm. -- (Update intensive care and emergency medicine ; 21)
    Includes index.
    Includes bibliographical references and index.
    1. Clinical biochemistry. 2. Metabolism--Disorders. 3. Acute
phase reaction. 4. Stress (Physiology) 5. Physiology,
Pathological.   I. Revhaug, A. (Arthur), 1950-   . II. Series.
    [DNLM: 1. Acute-Phase Reaction--metabolism. 2. Wounds and
Injuries--metabolism. 3. Stress--metabolism.   W1 UP66H v.21 1995 /
QZ 150 A188 1995]
RB112.5.A28   1995
616.07--dc20
DNLM/DLC
for Library of Congress   95-10442
                                                              CIP

ISBN-13: 978-3-642-48803-0   e-ISBN-13: 978-3-642-48801-6
DOI: 10.1007/ 978-3-642-48801-6

© Springer-Verlag Berlin Heidelberg 1996
Softcover reprint of the hardcover 1st edition 1996

Production: PRODUserv Springer Produktions-Gesellschaft, Berlin
Typesetting, Printing and Binding: Brühlsche Universitätsdruckerei, Gießen

SPIN 10478491   19/3020-543210   Printed on acid-free paper

Preface

This aim of this book is to focus on a very common situation seen in medical practice, the acute catabolic state. This pathophysiological situation is rarely discussed as a separate entity, possibly because it is seen in all specialties of medicine and results from a great diversity of agents, insults, and diseases. It thus seemed to be high time to gather the most important and up-to-date knowledge on this entity, and the primary aim of the book is to offer a collection of updated information on the acute catabolic state.

Another objective of the book is to make clear that, apart from the general response of the whole organism during the acute catabolic state, a series of organ-specific responses will also take place, which must also be considered during treatment. It has become very clear from working on this book that current knowledge of these organ-specific responses is very sparse and in some areas almost nonexistent; this book thus also focuses on the responses and changes which take place in different organs during the acute catabolic state and the interaction between these organs and their responses.

Acute catabolic situations have one common feature, namely, the changes are the results of some acutely ocurring destructive causes such as trauma or infection. The changes which take place during the first minutes or hours are crucial and will determine the outcome and changes observed during the following days and weeks. Accordingly, there is a need for an increased focus on understanding the pathophysiological changes that occur during the first early instances after the organism has been offended.

The second part of the book focuses on some of the many ways in which the acute catabolic state can be ameliorated, dampened, inhibited, or modified. The intention has not been to treat all its aspects or possible methods of intervention, either in diversity or in depth, as this would obviously require us to cover the entire scope of modern biochemical and biomedical literature. Rather, we have sought to focus on some of the main strategies and ways of interfering with the acute catabolic state in order to stimulate further studies and research in the field.

This volume provides all those who deal with these patients in some way with a general introduction to this fascinating and extremely rapidly changing field of medicine. The authors come from a wide range of specialities in international medicine. Their different backgrounds and focuses give the reader an excellent opportunity of understanding the complexity and challenges which the acute catabolic state imposes on scientists and practitioners alike. Research in this particular field is still at an early stage. The final and overall objective of this book is, therefore, to stimulate further research which will give us a more comprehensive understanding of general physiology and pathophysiology within this field.

The book is dedicated to all the young doctors and scientists who would like to further their research on the acute catabolic state.

October 1995   A. Revhaug

Contents

List of Contributors

N. N. Abumrad
Department of Surgery
HSC T-19 Rm 020
SUNY Stony Brook
Stony Brook, NY 11794-8191
USA

B. P. Bode
Division of Surgical Oncology
Massachusetts General Hospital
Harvard Medical School
100 Blossom Street, Cox 626
Boston, MA 02114-2617
USA

J. R. Bradley
Department of Medicine
Addenbrooke's Hospital
Hills Road
Cambridge CB2 2QQ
UK

A. M. Cotterill
Department of Endocrinology
St. Bartholomew's Hospital
London EC1A 7BE
UK

A. Foster
University of Maryland
Baltimore School of Medicine
Division of Thoracic and
Cardiovascular Surgery
22 South Greene Street
N4W94
Baltimore, MD 21201
USA

K.-E. Giercksky
Department of Surgical Oncology
The Norwegian Radium
Hospital and
Institute of Cancer Research
University of Oslo
0130 Oslo
Norway

D. A. Gilpin
Shriners Burns Institute
Department of Surgery
University of Texas Medical Branch
815 Market Street
Galveston, TX 77550
USA

D. N. Herndon
Shriners Burns Institute
Department of Surgery
University of Texas Medical Branch
815 Market Street
Galveston, TX 77550
USA

A. G. Hill
Laboratory of Nutrition and
Metabolism
Brigham and Women's Hospital
75 Francis Street
Boston, MA 02115
USA

Ø. Irtun
Department of Surgery
P.O. Box 2
Tromsø University Hospital
9038 Tromsø
Norway

T. G. Jenssen
Department of Medicine
Division of Nephrology
Tromsø University Hospital
9038 Tromsø
Norway

H. Kehlet
Department of Surgical
Gastroenterology
Hvidovre University Hospital
2650 Hvidovre
Denmark

J. Kjæve
Department of Surgery
P.O. Box 2
Tromsø University Hospital
9038 Tromsø
Norway

C. Meijer
Department of Surgery
Free University Hospital
De Boelelaan 1117
1081 HV Amsterdam
The Netherlands

H. R. Michie
City Hospital
Dudley Road
Birmingham B18 7QH
UK

M. Mjaaland
Department of Surgery
P.O. Box 2
Tromsø University Hospital
9038 Tromsø
Norway

P. E. Molina
Department of Surgery
HSC T-19 Rm 020
SUNY Stony Brook
Stony Brook, NY 11794
USA

T. Myrmel
Department of Surgery
P.O. Box 2
Tromsø University Hospital
9038 Tromsø
Norway

M. Pan
Division of Surgical Oncology
Massachusetts General Hospital
Harvard Medical School
100 Blossom Street, Cox 626
Boston, MA 02114-2617
USA

B. Plytycz
Department of Experimental
Pathology
Institute of Medical Biology
9037 Tromsø
Norway

H. Qvist
Department of Surgical Oncology
The Norwegian Radium
Hospital and
Institute of Cancer Research
University of Oslo
0130 Oslo
Norway

O. Reikerås
National Orthopedic Centre
Sophies Minde
0570 Oslo
Norway

A. Revhaug
Department of Surgery
P.O. Box 2
Tromsø University Hospital
9038 Tromsø
Norway

R. J. M. Ross
Department of Endocrinology
St. Bartholomew's Hospital
London EC1A 7BE
UK

D. Rubenstein
Department of Medicine
Addenbrooke's Hospital
Hills Road
Cambridge CB2 2QQ
UK

R. Slejelid
Department of Experimental
Pathology
Institute of Medical Biology
9037 Tromsø
Norway

D. Sørlie
Department of Surgery
P.O. Box 2
Tromsø University Hospital
9038 Tromsø
Norway

W. W. Souba
Division of Surgical Oncology
Massachusetts General Hospital
Harvard Medical School
100 Blossom Street, Cox 626
Boston, MA 02114-2617
USA

M. G. Statius Muller
Department of Surgery
Free University Hospital
De Boelelaan 1117
1081 HV Amsterdam
The Netherlands

K. Unneberg
Department of Surgery
P.O. Box 2
Tromsø University Hospital
9038 Tromsø
Norway

P. A. M. van Leeuwen
Department of Surgery
Free University Hospital
De Boelelaan 1117
1081 HV Amsterdam
The Netherlands

B. Vonen
Department of Surgery
P.O. Box 2
Tromsø University Hospital
9038 Tromsø
Norway

J. Wernerman
Department of Anesthesiology
and Intensive Care
Huddinge University Hospital
Karolinska Institute
Stockholm
Sweden

D. W. Wilmore
Laboratory of Nutrition and
Metabolism
Brigham and Women's Hospital
75 Francis Street
Boston, MA 02115
USA

The Acute Catabolic State:
Do We Have to Get Worse to Get Better?

A. Revhaug

Whenever an acute injury or disease takes place, the phenomenon of catabolism occurs. The word "catabolism" derives from the Greek word *katabole* ("to throw down") and implies a generalized phenomenon of destructive metabolism in which living tissue is changed into products of a simpler chemical composition.

As the catabolic state which occurs in the traumatized and diseased patient may last from minutes to months, it is necessary to describe and understand the different responses that occur at the different stages.

The intention behind this book is to organize and clarify the present knowledge of the very early phase of the catabolic state. The reason for the interst in this first phase, or flow phase, of catabolism is that the changes which take place in the first few minutes and hours after injury or acute disease determine how the organism reacts as a result of the actual challenge.

Additionally, the possibilities of modifying the catabolic state are greatest in the very initial phase. Important examples of how the acute catabolic phase can be modified are therefore also included in this book.

As all progress in patient care must be preceded by systematic research, a main purpose of this book is also to challenge medical truths in order to illustrate the vast lack of knowledge in this field of medicine. It is therefore important to acknowledge the need for and to stimulate further research in this field. As the acute catabolic state has been recognized for a such long time, we must ask why the body reacts in this way to injury and acute disease and how this complex reaction takes place. The fundamental question, then, is whether we actually have to go through a phase of acute destruction before we get better?

Disease and trauma are a constant threat to all living organisms, including man. Originally, organisms were created or developed to survive a great diversity of diseases and insults without relying upon any support other than that which the body itself could provide.

Ever since modern medicine developed in ancient Egypt and Greece, the main theory has been that an organism's defense system is a beneficial and necessary factor in survival. The idea held by Hippocrates that disease is cured by natural powers (by the vis medicatrix naturae) implies the existence of agents ready to function correctly when the normal state of the organism is disturbed. This formed the first definition of physiological homeostasis, which was later analyzed by Claude Bernard in 1878 [1] and by physiologists in our own century. The dynamic phases of homeostasis following severe injury and infection have been investigated and described extensively during the last decade. Common features are seen in a diversity of such disease states, all ending with common patterns, i.e., severe destruction of the cells in all vital organs and the destruction of any possible reserve tissue (muscle, fat).

If the body has to cope with an insult by itself in the natural way, it is undoubtedly true that the defense systems are beneficial and necessary. Thus, modern medicine generally regards an organism's defense systems (e.g., fever, release of stress hormones, acute phase response, etc.) as beneficial in combating and surviving injury and disease.

Is this defense theory really valid? Could it be that the defense systems are beneficial only when the organism suffers an insult which can be remedied without the assistance of modern medicine? Could it be that the defense systems are in fact deleterious and antiquated when the body is exposed to an insult which requires modern intensive care? When trying to anser this question, one must consider some fundamental facts. First, the defense systems have probably not changed significantly during the last few thousand years. Descriptions of diseases, at least as judged by history from ancient times up to today, are basically the same. The same defense systems are present in pylogenetically old species and have probably been conserved for a very long time through developmental history from the older to the youngest species. Second, the defense systems are only adequate because they were meant to help the individual to survive a corresponding insult. However, in this context such an insult would be of the type which the individual could manage to survive left to itself in nature (e.g., fractured leg, loss of fingers, local infections, etc.). However, today's medicine has changed the outcome dramatically; man is able to survive insults of a magnitude which is far beyond the capacity of the natural defense systems left alone to take care of the organism.

In discussing what history has taught us about the defense systems, we must look at the way in which medicine and technology have developed in order to assist the main defense systems. Throughout history, man has tried to assist nature in the healing processes. Active drainage of abscesses, primitive hemostatic procedures that have evolved into today's use of sutures, and other techniques have helped nature's own resources to enable countless patients to survive. Until a very short time ago, induced hemorrhage was regarded as an important and beneficial medical remedy. Blood-letting was used in a diversity of disease states. When Travers suggested blood transfusions instead of blood-letting as a treatment for severe gun wounds in 1826 [2], the entire established medical society rose up in anger. Modern transfusion and volume therapy have totally changed the prognosis of severe hemorrhages in a way that nature's own defense systems could never have managed.

The results and further development of Lister's, Semmelweiss', and Fleming's work changed medical theory and practice completely. Human ingenuity places the natural defense systems against infections in a totally different situation [3].

The demonstration to the Viennese surgical society early in our century of an experimental organ transplantation provoked such strong feelings that the surgeon involved was never accepted in the medical society again, yet some 70 years later there is almost no organ that cannot be transplanted. The main problem is that the defense systems induce important reactions towards foreign materials, causing them to be rejected.

In the developed world, patients whose lives depend on organ substitutes such as an artificial kidney have become more common than patients suffering from diphtheria and poliomyelitis. Mechanical ventilators keep millions of people alive for the time required to restore normal body functions, and the heart has essentially become a very advanced pump that can be substituted with a man-made machine made of steel and plastic. Biochemistry has created substances which are able to keep man alive for 10–20 years without ever eating anything. Major surgical procedures which only a century ago would have been totally lethal can be performed today almost without morbidity, provided that anesthesia, pain control, surgery, and nutrition are adequate.

The question arises as to whether there is a magnitude of insult beyond which the organism responds inadequately. After injury and trauma, several defense systems are stimulated to such a degree that almost all the cells in the body are injured by the very same systems. Thus, shortly after a severe trauma, the neurohumoral, leukocyte, complement, coagulation, and other defense systems damage the organism. In this state, tissue destruction is massive, and the lean body mass is dramatically reduced. This is probably due to the interaction of the neurohormonal responses with cellular release of free radicals, prostaglandins, lymphokines and/or monokines, and possibly other systems. The muscle is broken down to give glutamine and alanine, which are used as primary fuels in the injury and post-injury phase [4–6].

Is this destructive process necessary? If a healthy youngster suffers a fracture of the femur and the pelvis, the described events will take place; if treated conservatively, he or she will be in great danger of dying, and at best the total healing process will last for a long time. If a similar procedure (e.g., rotational osteotomy and crista bone transplantation) is performed under modern anesthesia with the proper surgical technique, the total body response will be almost undetectable and the bone heals at least as quickly as in the first case. This is also the case in injured and bleeding patients if volume is replaced and the injury surgically treated immediately after the trauma. In this case the defense systems have not been allowed "to run the show", but the healing is nevertheless good.

As far as the threat posed by bacteria is concerned, there is no evidence that even a thousand bacteria in the circulation are dangerous. Bacteria become dangerous because they liberate toxic substances when confronted with our defence systems, which destroy not only the bacteria but also a great part of the organism's normal cell mass.

What good does fever do in these cases? An increase of 2° C induced by infection increases oxygen consumption and the metabolic rate by some 20%–30% and the release of toxic substances, such as free radicals and lysozymes, takes place faster than it does at normal temperature.

These observations lead to the following hypothesis of bodily overreaction: the organism responds in an uncontrolled and devastating way when challenged by an insult of such proportions that survival is impossible without the intervention of man. A less energetic endogenous response would allow modern medicine to handle the major part of the insult with exogenously provided defense and healing systems in a better way.

Major systems can now be blocked, e.g., the stress hormones with alpha and beta blockade, the cyclooxygenase and lipooxygenase systems with inhibitors. The necessary substrate generated from the lean body mass can be supplied and the energy needs thus easily supplied without having to use up the organism's own resources. The development of recombinant gene technology will soon provide substances with specific stimulating or inhibiting properties on a diversity of cell and organ systems.

If all these described modalities were used in an integrated and controlled way together with established therapy, would it not then be possible to avoid some of the morbidity and mortality due to the body's overreaction seen as a result of the changes taking place in the early catabolic phase? Are we not just in the very early phases of understanding how the body's overreaction can be modified and controlled? The future will show the way, provided controlled and systematic investigations are carried out.

References

1. Bernard C (1878) Les phänomanes de la vie. Ballière, Paris
2. Travers B (1826) An inquiry concerning the disturbed state of the vital functions usually denominated constitutional irritation. In: Stevenson H (ed) New York
3. Smith TE (1985) From artifacts to antisepsis: a brief history of pre-modern surgery. Am Coll Surg Bull 70:3–7
4. Cannon W, Bayliss W (1919) Note on muscle injury in relation to shock. Rep Med Res Council 26:1
5. Moore FD (1958) Systemic mediators of surgical injury. Can Med Assoc J 78:85–91
6. Schoemaker WC (1985) Critical care. Surg Clin North Am 65:4

The History of the Metabolic Response to Injury

A. G. Hill and D. W. Wilmore

Introduction

It was 200 years ago that Hunter [1] made the observation that: *"... there is a circumstance attending accidental injury which does not belong to disease – viz. that the injury done has in all cases a tendency to produce both the disposition and the means of cure."*

It was another 140 years until this phenomenon was more clearly described by Sir David Cuthbertson in Scotland. Work since then has more clearly characterized the metabolic responses to injury and aided our understanding of the mechanisms involved. Pivotal to the recent growth in knowledge was clarification of the neuro-endocrine changes following injury, the development of parenteral nutrition for its use in the critically ill, and the discovery and characterization of cytokines and other cell signaling factors.

While initial work was based on the premise that the metabolic response to injury was harmful, more recent data suggest that this response is a useful mechanism and beneficial to the host. Efforts have now been directed toward diminishing the harmful aspects of the response and enhancing the positive effects through the use of biological response modifiers, nutritional manipulation, and the use of growth factors.

In 1932, Cuthbertson [2] described a group of patients who had either undergone bone surgery or who had sustained long-bone fractures; he noted an enhanced loss of nitrogen from the body. This negative nitrogen balance was maximal from day 2 through to day 8 after the injury and lasted for up to 1 month. He was then able to divide the metabolic response to injury into two phases, the ebb phase and the flow phase [3]. The ebb phase was so called because of a decrease in metabolic activity and was followed by the flow phase, a hypermetabolic state in which metabolic rate, temperature, and urinary nitrogen excretion all increased (Table 1). These observations have influenced thought on the metabolic response to injury for over 60 years.

Moore [4] and others further clarified the early neuroendocrine changes associated with injury, demonstrating that during the ebb phase elevations in the counter-regulatory hormones and a decrease in insulin occur. Following resuscitation and during the flow phase, when nitrogen losses are greatest, insulin rises and the counterregulatory hormones return toward baseline levels. Nitrogen is lost from gut and skeletal muscle and the liver accelerates its uptake of these compounds to make

Table 1. The ebb and the flow phases described by Cuthbertson [3]

Ebb phase	Flow phase
Hypometabolic	Hypermetabolic
Low core temperature	Elevated core temperature
Decreased energy expenditure	Increased energy expenditure
Normal glucose production	Increased glucose production
Mild protein catabolism	Profound protein catabolism
Elevated blood glucose	Elevated or normal blood glucose
Elevated catecholamines	Elevated or normal catecholamines
Elevated glucocorticoids	Elevated or normal glucocorticoids
Low insulin	Elevated insulin
Elevated glucagon	Elevated or normal glucagon
Poor tissue perfusion	Normal tissue perfusion

new glucose and acute phase proteins. During this time there is profound insulin resistance [5].

Although suggested by Hunter, Cuthbertson [3] was the first to recognize that the purpose of breakdown of muscle was *"to meet the exigencies of the metabolism of the recuperative process,"* a concept later developed by Moore [4]: *"it is our conviction that the destruction of lean tissue mass has as its purpose the provision of raw materials for wound healing."*

Additional efforts were directed towards understanding the fluxes of substrates between organs and characterizing the metabolism of protein and carbohydrates. In prolonged critical illness, the initial response was the breakdown of liver and muscle glycogen stores. Following rapid exhaustion of glycogen, the new glucose was derived from gluconeogenic precursors which arose primarily from skeletal muscle. This was accompanied by a blunting of the normal adaptive ketonemic response to starvation.

With simple elective surgery, protein synthesis was found to be inhibited, while catabolism was unchanged; with more extensive injury, both synthesis and catabolism were increased but the rate of degradation clearly outstripped that of synthesis [6].

Other work has been directed at clarifying the body's compositional changes and the cellular energetic changes occurring in critical illness [7, 8].

Early Investigations

The first efforts to understand the etiology of the profound changes in protein metabolism focused on the role of the neuroendocrine response to injury.

Campbell and Ingle investigated the role of glucocorticoids in protein metabolism. In adrenalectomized rats, the loss of nitrogen observed following femoral shaft fracture was obliterated [9, 10]. However, when glucocorticoids were replaced at physiological levels nitrogen loss was still observed, suggesting a "permissive" effect of these steroids.

Egdahl convincingly demonstrated the importance of the peripheral nervous system in the early endocrine response to injury. He disconnected a limb from the body of an anesthetized dog, leaving only the sciatic nerve and femoral artery and vein. Trauma to the innervated portion of this limb evoked glucocorticoid secretion. The nerve was then divided and repeated trauma failed to produce a rise in glucocorticoids [11].

In addition to afferent nervous signals, circulating factors also initiated the metabolic response to injury. Drucker et al. [12] studied paraplegics with chronic decubitus ulcers; he noted that an operation on a denervated area resulted in alterations in glucose metabolism. Wilmore et al. [13] later showed that patients with burn injury and spinal transection maintain a hypermetabolic response, as do similar patients in whom the afferent nervous signals are interrupted by local, regional, or general anesthesia. Wilmore also showed that only in patients with brain death was the hypermetabolic response to burn injury diminished.

Role of the Neuroendocrine Response

The evidence available at the end of the 1970s led investigators to conclude that stress evoked by a wide variety of stimuli resulted in a similar set of central nervous system (CNS) responses and that the neuroendocrine response represented a final common pathway directed at maintaining the integrity of the body cell mass and protecting against potentially harmful events [14].

Significant objections to the role of the neuroendocrine axis as the mediator of the postinjury metabolic derangement had previously been voiced by Cuthbertson [15], his principle arguments being:

1. The neuroendocrine response to surgery was limited to 24 h, whereas the increased nitrogen output attained its maximum several days later.
2. The response of protein metabolism to injury was almost completely obliterated by prior protein depletion, whereas the nitrogen loss provoked by glucocorticoids remained unchanged in protein-depleted animals.
3. Urinary nitrogen output did not rise after trauma to adrenalectomized rats. However, an increase in nitrogen loss did occur in adrenalectomized rats maintained on low levels of glucocorticoids, not themselves sufficient to provoke such a response.

However, strong arguments were made for an important role for the neuroendocrine response, especially in the ebb phase. Infusion of the counterregulatory hormones (as a "triple-hormone infusion") into normal human volunteers, in concentrations seen in the ebb phase, resulted in metabolic alterations similar to those observed in septic or injured patients [16]. The nitrogen loss seen with this combination of hormones was modest, however, and was not associated with net skeletal muscle protein breakdown.

Bessey and Lowe [17] showed that by using somatostatin to block insulin secretion, as observed in the ebb phase of injury, a triple-hormone infusion resulted in much larger nitrogen losses. This study also showed that excessive nitrogen loss in the first 48 h of an insulin-suppressive triple-hormone infusion, compared to a stan-

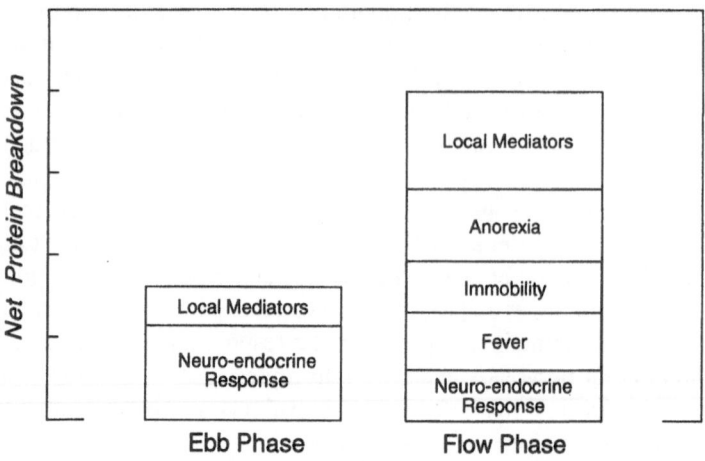

Fig. 1. Contributions to protein catabolism in injury. The relative contribution of the ebb phase to protein catabolism is small and is largely mediated by the neuroendocrine response. These hormonal responses, associated with poor tissue perfusion and oxygenation, and the generation of mediators, such as oxygen free radicals and cytokines, set the stage for the hypermetabolic flow phase, in which anorexia, immobility, fever, and humoral mediators all play a part in the exaggerated nitrogen loss

dard triple-hormone infusion, was not associated with increases in forearm amino acid nitrogen efflux, suggesting that the nitrogen originated from elsewhere, splanchnic tissues being the most likely, as the gut has one of the highest protein turnover rates in the body.

These data suggest that the role of the ebb phase is to set the stage for the more profound metabolic alterations seen the flow phase. This is accomplished by the secretion of the counterregulatory hormones, a decrease in insulin, and the generation of mediators such as oxygen free radicals and cytokines, released during the conditions of poor tissue perfusion and oxygenation of the ebb phase. With the restoration of tissue perfusion, especially in extreme injury involving contaminated and damaged tissue, these mediators, in association with anorexia, pyrexia, and immobility, act to cause the skeletal muscle protein breakdown so characteristic of the flow phase (Fig. 1).

Role of Humoral Mediators

In 1893, Coley [18] first demonstrated the regression of tumors injected with bacterial toxins. This work was largely ignored until later work was carried out by Cerami's group, who purified the cytokine tumor necrosis factor (TNF) cachectin. Independent work by other groups purified interleukin-1 (IL-1), a key mediator of the hepatic acute phase response and an endogenous pyrogen.

TNF has been infused into humans and animals and induces a net catabolic state in the host by mediating increased catabolism at the level of the specific tissues, by causing anorexia, and by activating the hypothalamic–pituitary–adrenal axis (HPA) [19–22]. In increasing amounts, the metabolic effects after TNF administration are dose related and include enhanced energy expenditure, increased hepatic gluconeogenesis, increased whole body protein breakdown, activation of the HPA, and increased whole body lipolysis [21, 23–26). In even larger doses, TNF triggers potentially catastrophic tissue injury and lethal shock [27, 28].

Like TNF, in lower concentrations IL-1 is beneficial to the host and stimulates defense mechanisms [29]. However, in higher concentrations, it stimulates the production of a number of mediators which cause its biological effects, including fever, hypotension, inflammation, and proteolysis [30, 31].

IL-1 and TNF may have a synergistic effect in producing the metabolic manifestations seen after injury or infection, as infusing the two cytokines together in rabbits has more effect than the two individual cytokines on energy substrate metabolism [32].

However, a number of pieces of evidence argue against systemic cytokine release accounting for all of the metabolic changes seen after injury. First, cytokines have not been consistently found in the blood stream of injured patients (with the exception of IL-6). Second, the effects of peripherally administered cytokines, although profound in the short term, are not sustained and tend to diminish quickly. Third, cytokines do not appear to have direct effects on muscle protein breakdown.

Attention therefore has recently turned to the role of cytokines at the tissue level, such as the liver and the CNS. IL-1 and IL-6 have been detected in the cerebrospinal fluid (CSF) of head-injured patients, and IL-1 may be able to cross the blood–brain barrier [33–35]. TNF receptors are present in the murine brain and TNF is produced by rat astrocytes in vitro [36, 37]. TNF and IL-1 are found in the CSF of children with meningitis and, in experimental meningitis, TNF is found in the CSF without being found in the serum, suggesting that in vivo TNF is produced in the brain [38–41]. There is an extensive network of IL-1 nerve fibers innervating the hypothalamus, and recent work has demonstrated that chronic CNS exposure to IL-1 produces catabolism in the rat [42, 43]. It has recently been demonstrated that after thermal injury a very early rise in liver and lung IL-1 is observed [44].

Some cytokines exhibit polymorphism in that several biologically active forms, including cell membrane-associated species, may exist. This polymorphism permits direct cell–cell signaling to occur in the absence of detectable activity in the systemic circulation [45]. It is also possible that the problem lies in the assays currently available, as more sensitive assays have recently demonstrated IL-1 in very low concentrations in the plasma after trauma [46]. These concentrations are still probably too low to produce significant metabolic effects, however, and may represent overspill of IL-1 produced at the tissue level, where the concentrations are most likely much higher.

The role of IL-6, which may be an important mediator in the ebb phase, is probably to stimulate the liver to produce the acute phase proteins. Although very high levels of IL-6 correlate with mortality in trauma, IL-6 is probably a marker of severity of injury (such as C-reactive protein) rather than the major causal agent [46, 47].

Although the relative contributions of cytokines and the counterregulatory hormones are unclear, they appear to have synergistic effects when they act together. When IL-1 was induced by etiocholanolone injection and counterregulatory hormones were simultaneously infused, there was a substantial increase in protein breakdown compared with either stimulus given alone [48].

Others have found small circulating peptides in humans and animals which cause skeletal muscle proteolysis after injury or infection [49, 50]. After extensive work, Goldberg et al. [51] concluded that there is still an unidentified proteolytic factor produced by activated macrophages. The contribution of these, and other factors, to postinjury metabolism remains to be determined.

Interventions and Related Research

Hand in hand with investigations into the metabolic response to injury came attempts to attenuate the response. The first successful intervention was performed by Cuthbertson et al. [52], who utilized pituitary extract and optimized nutrition to improve nitrogen balance after injury in rats. He also noted a protein-sparing effect of carbohydrate in the form of cane sugar in rats with femoral shaft fractures [53].

With the identification of the active agent in the pituitary extract as growth hormone (GH), investigators began to use GH therapeutically. In 1974 it was shown that in the catabolic phase in burn patients, associated with high-caloric feedings, GH improved nitrogen balance [54]. Interest in the therapeutic use of GH has increased since 1985, when recombinant gene technology enabled its manufacture on a large-scale basis.

Kinney and Elwyn [55] noted in 1985 that *"... the initial observations of nitrogen loss after injury were followed by nearly 40 years of minimal research activity in search of a basic explanation. It is of interest that the rapid increase in research activity of the past decade has coincided with the commercial availability of crystalline amino acids for intravenous therapy."*

Although parenteral nutrition has been of inestimable benefit in the management of the injured patient, the provision of an adequate diet is unable to prevent substantial body protein loss during severe catabolic illness. However, feeding the patient greatly attenuates the negative nitrogen balance [56].

With the demonstration that standard parenteral nutrition was incapable of replenishing body protein during catabolism, attention turned to the role of individual nutrients and the altered requirements that occurred following injury.

Glutamine is the most abundant free amino acid, but during catabolic illness demand may exceed supply. In several studies postoperative administration of glutamine has improved nitrogen balance [57]. Other efforts at dietary manipulation have been largely disappointing. Work, however, is progressing with the administration of the antioxidant vitamins to attenuate tissue injury and with the use of other amino acids and fats to modify immunological responses.

With the increase understanding of the role of cytokines, and other mediators, efforts have been made to attenuate protein loss with the use of anticytokine monoclonal antibodies, nonsteroidal anti-inflammatory drugs, and glucocorticoids. At this point in time, the role for these therapies still remains ill-defined.

Kehlet has pioneered the use of neural blockade to prevent afferent information from reaching the CNS and so breaking the neurophysiological reflex arc. This has lead to measurable improvements in nitrogen losses in elective surgical patients [58]. Although this technique decreases the neuroendocrine response to injury, it is also possible that the blockade of neural efferent signals may directly reduce the breakdown of skeletal muscle protein.

The most recent development in this field has been the introduction of laparoscopic surgery. Minimally invasive surgery has been associated with improvements in postoperative fatigue and outcome, but no change has been observed in the early neuroendocrine response to surgery [59, 60]. However, few formal metabolic studies have been performed in patients undergoing these procedures, and further understanding of the mechanisms underlying the obvious improvements in outcome holds potential benefit for the chronically ill hypermetabolic patient.

Conclusion

The response to injury is conveniently divided into an ebb phase and a flow phase. The metabolic perturbations of the ebb phase are best understood as a reflex arc

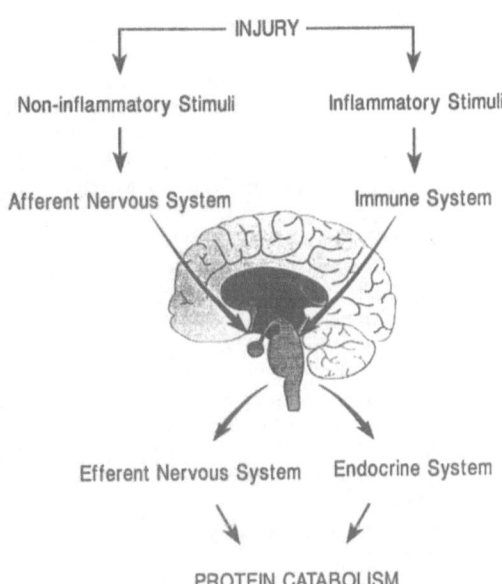

Fig. 2. Nervous, immune, and endocrine system interactions in injury. Injury sets up a reflex arc with the peripheral nervous system conveying information regarding noninflammatory stimuli, such as hypotension and pain, and the immune system conveying information regarding inflammatory stimuli, via cytokines, to the central nervous system. In the central nervous system, this information is processed and a stereotypical response occurs with the efferent nervous system, including sympathetic efferents, and the endocrine system acting together with locally generated mediators to produce protein catabolism

with the peripheral nervous system and the immune system, via cytokines, as the afferent limb, the CNS as the coordinator, and the counterregulatory hormones acting as the efferent effectors. These, along with alterations in tissue oxygenation, free radical generation, cytokine production, and other mediators set the stage for the profound metabolic changes seen in the flow phase.

Cytokines are produced in injury states and are capable of stimulating neuroendocrine activity, hepatic acute phase protein production, anorexia, and fever, all features of the metabolic response to injury. Thus it is likely that they are key players in the metabolic response to injury and that this effect is mediated via the hypothalamus. Also important may be efferent CNS activity in mediating muscle breakdown.

Therapeutic intervention with anticytokines, epidural anesthesia, growth hormone, and nutritional modification have shown some promise and have led to better understanding of the underlying mechanisms involved. Further research into the modification of the metabolic response by laparoscopic surgery may provide further insights leading to more rational modification of these highly conserved responses.

References

1. Hunter J (1794) A treatise on the blood, inflammation and gunshot wounds. George Nicol, London, p 190
2. Cuthbertson DP (1932) Observations on the disturbance of metabolism produced by injury to the limbs. Q J Med 25:233–246
3. Cuthbertson DP (1942) Post-shock metabolic response. Lancet 1:433–437
4. Moore FD (1953) Bodily changes in surgical convalescence. Ann Surg 137:289–315
5. Black PR, Brooks DC, Bessey PQ, Wolfe RR, Wilmore DW (1982) Mechanisms of insulin resistance following injury. Ann Surg 196:420–435
6. Douglas RG, Shaw JHF (1989) Metabolic response to sepsis and trauma. Br J Surg 76:115–122
7. Jacobs DO, Robinson MK (1993) Applications of magnetic resonance spectroscopy to nutrition and metabolism. In: Wilmore DW, Carpentier YA (eds) Metabolic support of the critically ill patient. Springer, Berlin Heidelberg New York, pp 19–45
8. Hill GL, Monk D, Plank LD (1993) Measuring body compositional changes and biochemical functions. In: Wilmore DW, Carpentier YA (eds) Metabolic support of the critically ill patient. Springer, Berlin Heidelberg New York, pp 3–18
9. Campbell RM, Sharp G, Boyne AW, Cuthbertson DP (1954) Cortisone and the metabolic response to injury. Br J Exp Pathol 35:566–576
10. Ingle DJ, Ward EO, Kuizenga MH (1947) The relationship of the adrenal glands to changes in urinary non-protein nitrogen following multiple fractures in the force-red rat. Am J Physiol 149:510–515
11. Egdahl RH (1959) Pituitary-adrenal response following trauma to the isolated leg. Surgery 46:9–21
12. Drucker WH, Craig JW, Hubray CA, Davis JH, Woodward H (1961) The metabolic effects of trauma to denervated tissue in man. J Trauma 1:306–321
13. Wilmore DW, Taylor JW, Hander EW, Mason AD, Pruitt BA (1976) Central nervous system function following thermal injury. In: Wilkinson AW, Cuthbertson D (eds) Metabolism and the response to injury. Pitman, London, pp 274–286
14. Wilmore DW, Long JM, Mason AD, Pruitt BA (1976) Stress in surgical patients as a neurophysiologic reflex response. Surg Gynecol Obstet 142:257–269
15. Cuthbertson DP (1964) Physical injury and its effects on protein metabolism. In: Munro HN, Allison JB (eds) Mammalian protein metabolism, vol 3. Academic, New York, pp 373–414

16. Bessey PQ, Watters JM, Aoki TT, Wilmore DW (1984) Combined hormonal infusion stimulates the metabolic response to injury. Ann Surg. 200:264–281
17. Bessey PQ, Lowe KA (1993) Early hormonal changes affect the catabolic response to trauma. Ann Surg 218:476–489
18. Coley WB (1893) The treatment of malignant tumors by repeated inoculations of erysipelas: with a report of ten original cases. Am J Med Sci 150:487–511
19. Oliff A, Defeo-Jones D, Boyer M et al. (1987) Tumors secreting human TNF/cachectin induce cachexia in mice. Cell 50:555–563
20. Michie HR, Sherman ML, Spriggs DR, Rounds J, Christie M, Wilmore DW (1989) Chronic TNF infusion causes anorexia but not accelerated nitrogen loss. Ann Surg 209:19–24
21. Starnes HF, Warren RS, Jeevanandam M et al. (1988) Tumor necrosis factor and the acute metabolic response to injury in man. J Clin Invest 82:1321–1325
22. Tracey KJ, Wei H, Manogue KR et al. (1988) Cachectin/tumor necrosis factor induces cachexia, anemia, and inflammation. J Exp Med 167:1211–1227
23. Kawakami M, Cerami A (1981) Studies of endotoxin-induced decrease in lipoprotein lipase activity. J Exp Med 154:631–639
24. Warren RS, Starnes HF, Alcock N, Calvano S, Brennan MF (1988) Hormonal and metabolic response to recombinant tumor necrosis factor in rat: in vitro and in vivo. Am J Physiol 255:E206–E212
25. Zamir O, Hasselgren PO, Kunkel SL, Frederick J, Higashiguchi T, Fischer JE (1992) Evidence that tumor necrosis factor participates in the regulation of muscle proteolysis during sepsis. Arch Surg 127:170–174
26. Beutler B, Mahoney J, Trang NL, Pekala P, Cerami A (1985) Purification of cachectin, a lipoprotein lipase suppressing hormone secreted by endotoxin-induced RAW 264. 7 cells. J Exp Med 161:984–995
27. Tracey KJ, Beutler B, Lowry SJ et al. (1986) Shock and tissue injury induced by recombinant human cachectin. Science 234:470–474
28. Tracey KJ, Lowry SF, Fahey TJ et al. (1987) Cachectin/tumor necrosis factor induces lethal shock and stress hormone responses in the dog. Surg Gynecol Obstet 164:415–422
29. Dinarello CA, Wolff S (1993) The role of interleukin-1 in disease. N Engl J Med 328:106–113
30. Baracos V, Rodemann HP, Dinarello CA, Goldberg AL (1983) Stimulation of muscle protein degradation and prostaglandin E2 release by leukocytic pyrogen (interleukin-1). N Engl J Med 308:553–558
31. Zamir O, Hasselgren PO, von Allmen D, Fischer JE (1991) The effect of interleukin-1α and the glucocorticoid receptor blocker RU 38486 on total and myofibrillar protein breakdown in skeletal muscle. J Surg Res 50:579–583
32. Tredget EE, Zu YM, Zhong S et al. (1988) Role of interleukin 1 and tumor necrosis factor on energy metabolism in rabbits. Am J Physiol 255:E760–E768
33. Banks WA, Kastin AJ, Durham DJ (1989) Bidirectional transport of interleukin-1 across the blood-brain barrier. Br Res Bll 23:433–437
34. McClain CJ, Cohen D, Ott L, Dinarello CA, Young B (1987) Ventricular fluid interleukin-1 activity in patients with head injury. J Lab Clin Med 110:48–54
35. McClain C, Cohen D, Phillips R, Ott L, Young B (1991) Increased plasma and ventricular fluid interleukin-6 levels in patients with head injury. J Lab Clin Med 118:225–231
36. Kinouchi K, Brown G, Pasternak G, Donner DB (1991) Identification and characterization of receptors for tumor necrosis factor-α in the brain. Biochem Biophys Res Commun 181:1532–1538
37. Lieberman AP, Pitha PM, Shin HS, Shin ML (1989) Production of tumor necrosis factor and other cytokines by astrocytes stimulated with lipopolysaccharide or a neurotropic virus. Proc Natl Acad Sci USA 86:6348–6352
38. Mustafa MM, Lebel MH, Ramilo O et al. (1989) Correlation of interleukin-1β and cachectin concentrations in cerebrospinal fluid and outcome from bacterial meningitis. J Pediatr 115:208–213
39. Mustafa M, Ramilo O, Olsen KD et al. (1989) Tumor necrosis factor in mediating experimental *Haemophilus influenzae* type B meningitis. J Clin Invest 84:1253–1259

40. Mustafa MM, Ramilo O, Saez-Llorens X, Mertsola J, McCracken GH (1989) Role of tumor necrosis factor alpha (cachectin) in experimental and clinical bacterial meningitis. Pediatr Infect Dis J 8:907–908
41. Leist TP, Frei K, Kam-Hansen S, Zinkernagel RM, Fontana A (1988) Tumor necrosis factor α in cerebrospinal fluid during bacterial, but not viral, meningitis. J Exp Med 167:1743–1748
42. Hill AG, Gonzalez J, Rounds J, Wilmore DW (1994) Chronic central nervous system exposure to interleukin-1, but not interleukin-6, mediates catabolism in the rat. Surg Forum 45:38–41, 1994
43. Breder CD, Dinarello CA, Saper CB (1988) Interleukin-1 immunoreactive innervation of the human hypothalamus. Science 240:321–324
44. Mester M, Carter EA, Tompkins RG et al. (1994) Thermal injury induces very early production of interleukin-1α in the rat by mechanisms other than endotoxemia. Surgery 115:588–596
45. Lowry S (1990) The route of feeding influences injury responses. J Trauma 30:S10–S15
46. Svoboda P, Kantorova I, Ochmann J (1994) Dynamics of interleukin 1, 2, and 6 and tumor necrosis factor alpha in multiple trauma patients. J Trauma 36:336–340
47. Ayala A, Perrin MM, Wang P, Chaudry IH (1992) Sepsis induces an early increased spontaneous release of hepatocellular stimulatory factor (interleukin-6) by Kupffer cells in both endotoxin tolerant and intolerant mice. J Surg Res 52:635–641
48. Watters JM, Bessey PQ, Dinarello CA, Wolff SM, Wilmore DW (1986) Both inflammatory and endocrine mediators stimulate host responses to sepsis. Arch Surg 121:179–190
49. Clowes GHA, George BC, Villee CA, Saravis CA (1983) Muscle proteolysis induced by a circulating peptide in patients with sepsis or trauma. N Engl J Med 308:546–552
50. Warner BW, Hasselgren PO, James JH, Hummel RP, Riegel DF, Fischer JE (1990) Reduced amino acid transport in skeletal muscle caused by a circulating factor during endotoxemia. Ann Surg 211:918–923
51. Goldberg AL, Kettelhut IC, Furuno K, Fagan JM, Baracos V (1988) Activation of protein breakdown and prostaglandin E$_2$ production in rat skeletal muscle in fever is signaled by a macrophage product distinct from interleukin 1 or other known monokines. J Clin Invest 81:1378–1383
52. Cuthbertson DP, Shaw GB, Young FG (1941) The anterior pituitary gland and protein metabolism. II. The influence of anterior pituitary extract on the metabolic response of the rat to injury. J Endocrinol 2:468–474
53. Cuthbertson DP, McGirr JL, Robertson JSM (1939) The effect of fracture of bone on the metabolism of the rat. Q J Physiol 29:13–25
54. Wilmore DW, Moylan JA, Bristow BF, Mason AD, Pruitt BA (1974) Anabolic effects of human growth hormone and high caloric feedings following thermal injury. Surg Gynecol Obstet 138:875–884
55. Kinney JM, Elwyn DH (1985) Protein metabolism in the traumatized patient. Acta Chir Scand Suppl 522:45–56
56. Streat SJ, Beddoe AH, Hill GL (1987) Aggressive nutritional support does not prevent protein loss despite fat gain in septic intensive care patients. J Trauma 27:262–266
57. Hammarqvist F, Wernerman J, Ali R, von der Decken A, Vinnars E (1989) Addition of glutamine to total parenteral nutrition after elective abdominal surgery spares free glutamine in muscle, counteracts the fall in muscle protein synthesis, and improves nitrogen balance. Ann Surg 209:455–461
58. Brandt MR, Fernandes A, Mordhorst R, Kehlet H (1978) Epidural analgesia improves postoperative nitrogen balance. Br Med J 1:1106–1108
59. Hill AG, Finn P, Schroeder D (1993) Postoperative fatigue after laparoscopic surgery. Aust N Z J Surg 63:946–951
60. Mealy K, Gallagher H, Barry M, Lennon F, Traynor O, Hyland J (1992) Physiological and metabolic responses to open and laparoscopic cholecystectomy. Br J Surg 79:1061–1064

Substrate Handling in the Stress-Induced Catabolic State – Where is the Challenge?

M. Mjaaland

Introduction

Sir David Cuthbertson was the first to interpret the whole body net loss of nitrogen after injury as a generalized response to the organism's "urgent needs ... of repair and maintenance", the net loss far exceeding the loss due to immobilization [1] and being too extensive to come from the local area of damaged tissue alone [2]. From the relationship between the losses of nitrogen, sulfur, and phosphorus Cuthbertson postulated that the catabolized tissue was mainly skeletal muscle [1]. The nitrogen loss was generally related to the extent of the injury and was also associated with an increased oxygen consumption and elevated body temperature [2]. Later, he was also the first to demonstrate that injection of pituitary extracts after trauma could diminish the nitrogen loss [3].

Substrate Storage and Interactions

In humans, fat is the principal storage form of energy [4]. This is the most efficient form of energy on a weight basis (yields 9.4 kcal per g pure triglycerides), and therefore lipid synthesis and storage are important for survival in species in which mobility is critical. In humans, lipid expansion occurs in abundance and is depleted during deprivation [4]. Although the lipid tissue has other functions as well, such as insulation and mechanical padding, these are minor functions compared to its importance as energy reserves [5].

Carbohydrate and protein also serve as substrate reserves. The storage form of carbohydrate in animals is glycogen, which is stored in skeletal muscle and liver. Glycogen yields 4 kcal per g dry carbohydrate, but the need to keep each gram of glycogen in a solution of 1–2 g water and electrolytes to keep the environment isotonic reduces the weight efficiency of glycogen as an energy source [6]. However, glucose is a more flexible substrate than lipids and is an essential substrate for several tissues. In normal humans, most of the glucose is metabolized in the brain, which oxidizes it completely to carbon dioxide and water [7–9]. Other obligate glycolytic tissues, i.e., erythrocytes, leukocytes, bone marrow, renal medulla, peripheral nerve, and to some degree skeletal muscle, primarily convert glucose to lactate and pyruvate, which are carried with the blood stream to the liver and kidney, where glucose can be resynthesized. The energy for this process is derived from the oxidation of fat in the liver [10].

Despite the role of glucose as an essential substrate for several important organs, the total reserves of glycogen amount to only 1000–1500 kcal in an adult, representing a very small part of the total energy storage. Most of this is degraded after a night's fasting. Thereafter, the organism has to rely on gluconeogenesis to cover its glucose needs. Glucose is readily converted to lipids when present in abundance, but this process is not reversible. Only the glycerol skeleton of the triglycerides can be converted to glucose.

In terms of energy reserve, muscle is the most important substrate reserve besides fat tissue. However, each protein molecule also serves an important nonfuel function; it may serve as an enzyme or a contractile or structural protein, or it may serve several functions. The bulk of protein is in skeletal muscle. Visceral proteins have been subject to less study, mainly because of the limited availability of this protein compartment. The turnover rate of visceral proteins apparently is higher than in skeletal muscle, however [11, 12], and this protein compartment may therefore represent a more dynamic protein source.

In catabolic states, there is net proteolysis with release of amino acids from skeletal muscles. The amino acids released from skeletal muscle are mainly glutamine and alanine [13], which are synthesized de novo from the branch-chained amino acids [14, 15], the carbon skeleton coming from pyruvate in the case of alanine and form α-ketoglutarate via glutamate in the case of glutamine [16, 17]. The released amino acids serve several functions. One is to participate in the acute phase protein synthesis in the liver [18] and protein synthesis in the healing wound. Degradation of proteins also yields energy locally in the muscle. Another important function is the delivery of precursors for gluconeogenesis. Both the alanine and the glutamine released from skeletal muscle enter the gluconeogenesis in the liver [16, 19]. This process is fuelled by the combustion of fat.

Thus, proteins form the necessary link between the flexible substrate (glucose) and the efficient storage substrate (lipids). In spite of the protein's obvious functional significance, it is sacrificed when the organism is unable to supply sufficient exogenous substrate. In terms of survival, these processes are beneficial, but they do have a price.

Substrate Handling During Starvation

In brief fasting, there is a general shift to fat oxidation for energy needs [4, 5, 7, 20]. Tissue that can also metabolize glucose when available, such as heart, kidney cortex, and skeletal muscle, turns to oxidation of fatty acids and ketones. Gluconeogenesis from glycerol, lactate, pyruvate, and gluconeogenic amino acids, primarily alanine, takes place in the liver. The nitrogen from the amino acids enters ureagenesis and is mainly excreted in the urine, resulting in a net nitrogen loss. Subsequently, acetoacetate and β-hydroxybutyrate (ketone bodies) from the oxidation of fatty acids are also produced in the liver [7].

In prolonged starvation, excretion of urinary nitrogen diminishes progressively [8], reflecting attentuation of net protein breakdown. Oxidation of the ketone bodies acetoacetate and β-hydroxybutyrate gradually displaces the oxidation of glucose in the brain [7, 9], thereby diminishing the need for gluconeogenesis from amino acids. This adaptive mechanism enables survival for months instead of weeks. Increasingly, the kidney takes over the gluconeogenesis from the liver [8]. Central in the adaptive process is also a generally diminished energy expenditure, preserving all energy resources.

Substrate Handling During Stress

Principally, the metabolic response to injury, sepsis, and major operations follows the same pattern [20–22]. Cuthbertson divided the response to trauma into the immediately post-traumatic "ebb" phase, characterized by low flow and lowered metabolic activity, and the hyperdynamic, hypermetabolic "flow" phase following successful resuscitation [23]. The magnitude of the response is generally related to the extent of the injury [22, 24, 25]. In some ways the metabolic changes resemble the response seen in starvation. There is a shift to fat oxidation for energy requirements [24] and a net protein breakdown, resulting in a negative nitrogen balance in both situations. However, in spite of these similarities, substrate handling during surgical stress is basically different from what occurs during starvation [26]. All the processes occur at a higher speed after surgical stress. The energy expenditure is increased [27] with increased body temperature and heart rate, and there is a higher rate of fat oxidation to deliver energy. However, carbohydrate oxidation is also increased in an absolute sense, and gluconeogenesis occurs at a higher rate. The rate of nitrogen loss is also elevated. The level of energy consumption and nitrogen losses are both associated with the extent of the injury [28]. After major challenges, this is caused by increased rates of both protein synthesis and breakdown, the breakdown increasing most [28–31]. In contrast, reduced rates of protein synthesis and eventually also of protein breakdown compared to the normal state are observed in starvation. Reduced protein synthesis and breakdown is found after smaller catabolic insults, such as operations [32]. The released amino acids are partly used for acute phase protein synthesis, but also for the increased gluconeogenesis and in the healing process in the wound [31, 33–35]. Glucose serves as primary fuel for granulation tissue in the healing wound [35]. In stress-induced catabolic states, ketogenesis occurs to a very small degree, and the adaptation with time seen in starvation, including sparing of proteins, does not occur in the same fashion after stress [26].

However, the most striking difference between the two catabolic states may be the response to exogenous substrates. If nutrition is given to a starving person, energy expenditure and nitrogen balance are normalized, and a weight gain occurs within short time. In contrast, exogenous nutrition has to date not been able to prevent the breakdown of the organism's own tissue during surgical stress [36–40]. Rowlands et al. showed that even if energy levels were increased and the amount of nitrogen adequate, patients did not obtain protein equilibrium after surgery when

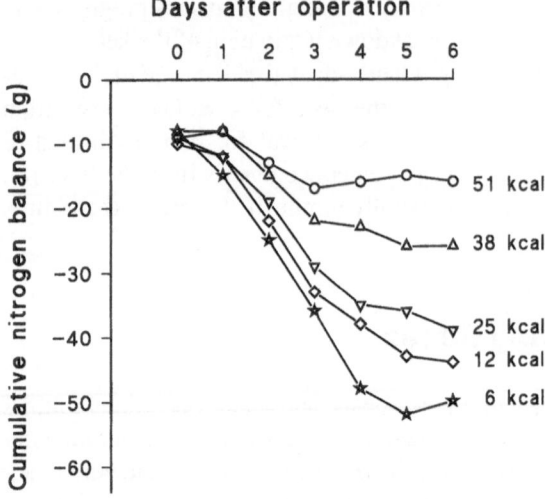

Fig. 1. Effect of increasing parenteral calorie intake with a constant nitrogen intake of 0.23 g/kg per day on cumulative nitrogen balance in patients after abdominal surgery. (Adapted from [39])

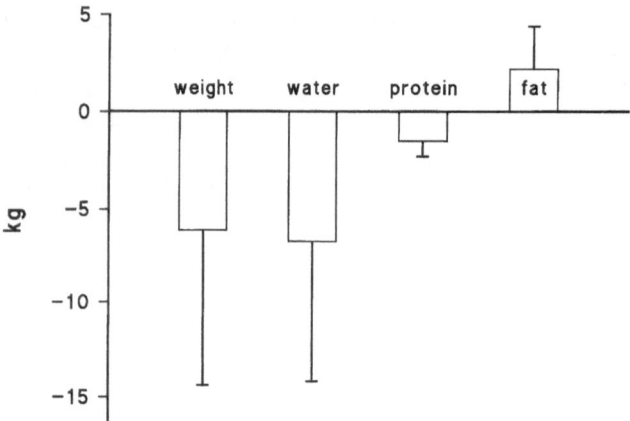

Fig. 2. Changes in weight and body composition in intensive care patients after 10 days of total parenteral nutrition. (Adapted from [40])

given parenteral nutrition (Fig. 1) [39]. Streat et al. studied the changes in body composition in intensive care patients after 10 days of total parenteral nutrition. They found that in spite of the nutritional support, the patients lost weight and lost proteins. Their only gain was an increase in fat tissue (Fig. 2) [40].

From a clinical point of view, this way of handling substrates seems futile. Why does the organism continue to break down the organism's own tissue when the exogenous supply appears to be abundant? Is there some sort of metabolic block which prevents the organism from utilizing exogenous substrate in an efficient way, and if so, what causes it? The inability to handle substrates efficiently continues after the classical stress hormones are normalized. It seems that, once initiated, the length and extent of the post-traumatic course is already determined and is to some extent independent of medical interventions. This suggests that if we want to modulate this process, we should focus on the trauma and the very early post-traumatic phase, i.e., the first few minutes and hours after the trauma occurs.

Inefficient Substrate Utilization During Surgical Stress – A Clinical Problem?

The question arises as to whether it is desirable to modulate the metabolic response to trauma and infection. Minor injuries and elective operations appear to be well handled by the body in this fashion; the tissue lost in the stress phase is eventually resynthesized and replaced during convalescence without complications. However, in severe cases such as multiple trauma, particularly if it is complicated by infection, it may be that the wasting of functionally important tissue in itself threatens survival. Lack of muscular strength may prevent a patient being taken off the respirator, and persistent catabolism may compromise the heart muscle as well as other muscular tissue. In addition, wound healing may be deteriorated and the immune defense impaired. The mortality rate in this patient group is high. This may be interpreted as an overshoot phenomenon; a response which is beneficial in minor and moderate trauma becomes life-threatening when the initiating trauma is too extensive.

The role that the metabolic response as such plays in this complicated scenario is largely unknown. However, we believe that if we can preserve tissue in general without compromising substrate supply to the vital organs, this will protect the patient in crisis. To be able to do that, it seems vital to focus on inefficient substrate utilization during surgical stress.

References

1. Cuthbertson DP (1930) The disturbance of metabolism produced by bony and nonbony injury, with notes on certain abnormal conditions of bone. Biochem J 24:1244–1263
2. Cuthbertson DP (1932) Observations on the disturbance of metabolism produced by injury to the limbs. Q J Med 1:233–246
3. Cuthbertson DP, Shaw GB, Young FG (1941) The anterior pituitary gland and protein metabolism. II. The influence of anterior pituitary extract on the metabolic response of the rat to injury. J Endocrinol 2:468–474
4. Benedict FG (1915) A study of prolonged fasting. Carnegie Institute of Washington, publication 203
5. Cahill GF (1970) Starvation in man. N Engl J Med 12:668:–675
6. Fenn WO, Haege LF (1940) The deposition of glycogen in water in the livers of cats. J Biol Chem 136:87–101
7. Cahill GF, Herrera MG, Morgan AP et al. (1966) Hormone-fuel interrelationships during fasting. J Clin Invest 45:1751–1769
8. Cahill GF, Owen OE, Morgan AP (1968) The consumption of fuels during prolonged starvation. Adv Enzyme Regul 6:143–150
9. Owen OE, Morgan AP, Kemp HG, Sullivan JM, Herrera MG, Cahill GF (1967) Brain metabolism during fasting. J Clin Invest 46:1589–1595

10. Randle PJ, Garland PB, Hales CN, Newsholme EA (1963) The glucose fatty-acid cycle. Its role in insulin sensitivity and the metabolic disturbances of diabetes mellitus. Lancet 1:785–789
11. Rennie MJ, Edwards RHT, Halliday D, Matthews DE, Wolman SL, Millward DJ (1982) Muscle protein synthesis measured by stable isotope techniques in man: the effects of feeding and fasting. Clin Sci 63:519–523
12. Nair KS, Halliday D, Griggs RC (1988) Leucine incorporation into mixed skeletal muscle protein in humans. Am J Physiol 254:E208–E213
13. Ruderman NB, Berger M (1974) The formation of glutamine and alanine in skeletal muscle. J Biol Chem 249:5500–5506
14. Oddyssey R, Khairrallah EA, Goldberg AL (1974) Origin and possible significance of alanine production by skeletal muscle. J Biol Chem 249:7623–7629
15. Garber AJ, Karl IE, Kipnis DM (1976) Alanine and glutamine synthesis and release from skeletal muscle. J Biol Chem 251:836–843
16. Chang TW, Goldberg AL (1978) The metabolic fates of amino acids and the formation of glutamine in skeletal muscle. J Biol Chem 253:3685–3695
17. Goldberg AL, Chang TW (1978) Regulation and significance of amino acid metabolism in skeletal muscle. Fed Proc 37:2301–2307
18. Neuhaus OW, Balegno HF, Chandler AM (1966) Induction of plasma protein synthesis in response to trauma. Am J Physiol 211:151–156
19. Felig P, Pozefsky T, Marliss E, Cahill GF (1970) Alanine: key role in gluconeogenesis. Science 167:1003–1004
20. Moore FD (1953) Bodily changes in surgical convalescence. Ann Surg 137:289–315
21. Beisel WR (1977) Magnitude of the host nutritional responses to infection. Am J Clin Nutr 30:1236–1247
22. Kinney JM, Duke JH, Long CL, Gump FE (1970) Tissue fuel and weight loss after injury. J Clin Path 23:65–72
23. Cuthbertson DP (1942) Post-shock metabolic response. Lancet 6189:433–337
24. Megiud MM, Brennan MF, Aoki TT, Muller WA, Ball MR, Moore FD (1974) Hormone-substrate interrelationship following trauma. Arch Surg 109:776–783
25. Dahn M, Kirkpatrick JR, Bouwman D (1980) Sepsis, glucose intolerance, and protein malnutrition. Arch Surg 115:1415–1418
26. Beisel WR, Wannemacher RW (1980) Gluconeogenesis, ureagenesis, and ketogenesis during sepsis. JPEN J Parenter Enteral Nutr 4:277–285
27. Kien CL, Young VR, Rohrbaugh DK, Burke JF (1978) Increases rats of whole body protein synthesis and breakdown in children recovering from burns. Ann Surg 187:393–391
28. Long CL, Schiller WR, Blakemore WS, Geiger JW, D'Dell M, Henderson K (1977) Muscle protein catabolism in the septic patient as measured by 3-methylhistidine excretion. Am J Clin Nutr 30:1349–1352
29. Arnold J, Campell IT, Samuels TA, Devlin JC, Green CJ, Hipkin LJ, MacDonald IA, Scrimgour CM, Smith K, Rennie MJ (1993) Increased whole body protein breakdown predomiantes over increased whole body protein synthesis in multiple organ failure. Clin Sci 84:655–661
30. Clowes GHA, Randall HT, Cha C-J (1980) Amino acid and energy metabolism in septic and traumatized patients. JPEN J Parenter Enteral Nutr 4:195–205
31. O'Keefe SJD, Sender PM, James WPT (1974) "Catabolic" loss of body nitrogen in response to surgery. Lancet 2:1035–1039
32. Wilmore DW, Goodwin CW, Aulick LH, Powanda MC, Mason AD, Pruitt BA (1980) Effect of injury and infection on visceral metabolism and circulation. Ann Surg 192:491–504
33. Wolfe RR, Durkot MJ, Allsop JR, Burke JF (1979) Glucose metabolism in severely burned patients. Metabolism 28:1031–1039
34. Wilmore DW, Aulick LH, Mason AD, Pruitt BA (1977) Influece of the burn wound on local and systemic influences to injury. Ann Surg 186:444–458
35. Carli F, Webster J, Ramachandra V et al. (1990) Aspects of protein metabolism after elective surgery in patients recieving constant nutritional support. Clin Sci 78:621–628
36. Finley RJ, Inculet RI, Pace R et al. (1986) Major operative trauma increases peripheral amino acid release during the steady state infusion of total parenteral nutrition in man. Surgery 99:491–500

37. Shaw JHF (1988) Influence of stress, depletion, and/or malignant desease on the responsiveness of surgical patients to total parenteral nutrition. Am J Clin Nutr 48:144–147
38. Wilmore DW (1990) Pathophysiology of the hypermetabolic response to burn injury. J Trauma 30:S4–S6
39. Rowlands BJ, Giddings AEB, Johnston AOB, Hindmarsh JT, Clark RG (1977) Nitrogen-sparing effect of different feeding regimes in patients after operations. Br J Anaesth 49:781–787
40. Streat SJ, Beddoe AH, Hill GL (1987) Aggressive nutritional support does not prevent protein loss despite fat gain in septic intensive care patients. J Trauma 27:262–266

The Role of the Nervous System in Modulating the Catabolic State

N. N. Abumrad and P. E. Molina

Central Nervous System as an Integrator

The control of substrate mobilization by the classical hormones, i.e., glucagon, catecholamines, insulin, and growth hormone, has been well established [1], but for over 100 years neurochemical and physiological evidence supporting the role of the brain as the integrative station for neural and hormonal regulation of peripheral metabolism has been reported by several studies [2–9]. Primarily, the hypothalamus is considered as one of the main structures involved in integrating afferent and efferent signals [2, 10], and their activities appear to be modulated by the continuous fluctuations in plasma glucose concentrations [7]. This, in turn, forms the basis of the mechanism by which the brain is thought to modulate fuel mobilization.

The hypothalamus is made up of several nuclei, and each appears to respond differently to the fluctuations in plasma glucose. The lateral and medial hypothalamic nuclei are considered to act reciprocally in modulating the neurometabolic influences in the liver and pancreas [4]. Glucose-sensitive neurons, defined as those whose activity is decreased by direct application of glucose, are present in the lateral hypothalamus (LHA), while glucoreceptors of the ventromedial hypothalamus (VMH) enhance their firing rates in response to glucose [10]. In addition, stimulation of the ventral part of the LHA increases activity in the pancreatic vagus, which results in increased insulin release. The VMH contains glucoreceptor neurons whose activity is enhanced by the direct application of glucose and that increase their discharge when glucose is applied to them. Electrical stimulation of this area (VMH) is followed by a rapid rise in plasma glucose levels and is not abolished by adrenalectomy, suggesting that this is a direct neural pathway for increasing hepatic glucose production [11]. The axons extending from the VMH neurons project to the locus ceruleus, central gray, and parabrachial nuclei. These last two areas project to the sympathetic motor neurons in the intermediolateral cell column of the spinal cord. The locus ceruleus and the parabrachial nucleus project to the nucleus tractus solitarius (NTS) and the dorsal motor nucleus of the vagus. The NTS has direct connections with other nuclei within the hypothalamus which also contain glucose-sensitive neurons located predominantly adjacent to the fourth ventricle [12].

Glucosensors, however, do not appear to be located in a single brain structure. Differences in hypophyseal hormone release have been reported under conditions in which fructose is administered during generalized hypoglycemia. Because the ability of fructose to cross the blood–brain barrier (BBB) is limited, a differentiation has been proposed between the areas that are protected by the BBB versus those that are not. For example, it has been proposed that stimuli for the release of growth hormone arise from areas protected by the BBB and that those for adreno-corticotropic hormone (ACTH) are located both inside and outside the BBB [13]. Alternatively, this could indicate the presence in the central nervous system (CNS) of other glucosensitive areas besides the VMH. Thus, the involvement of multiple areas in the CNS during glucoregulation cannot be ruled out and exclusivity of the VMH is not justified [14–16].

The glucose responsiveness described above is not unique to the cells in the hypothalamic nuclei. For example, glucose sensors of the small intestine, portal vein, and liver also decrease firing when glucose is infused directly into the portal circulation or when glucose is applied directly [3]. Vagal intestinal glucoreceptors have been linked to the splanchnic nerve [17]. Thus, an increase in glucose concentration in the portal blood is relayed as a decrease in the rate of signal from the hepatoportal area to the hypothalamus via the vagus and the NTS in the medulla oblongata [18]. These glucoreceptors, connected to the vagus and the caudal portions of the NTS in the medulla, constitute a major afferent tract to the paraventricular, dorsomedial, and arcuate nuclei of the hypothalamus [12]. The fibers from the lateral hypothalamus (LH) descend via the forebrain bundle and connect with the vagus of the medulla and form the LH–vagal circuit, which innervates several visceral organs mediating neural control of metabolism.

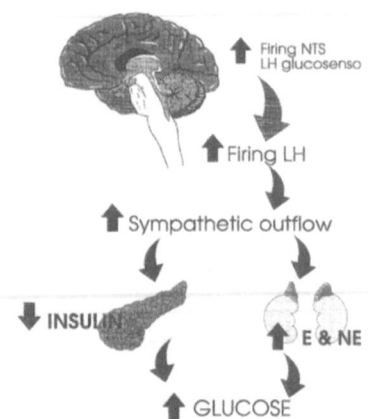

Fig. 1. An integrated feedback loop of glucose control in neuroglucopenia can be speculatively derived from the information presented (see text). The lack of glucose in the periphery or in the central nervous system (CNS) results in an increase in firing in the nucleus tractus solitarius *(NTS)* and lateral hypothalamus *(LH)* glucosensors. This results in increased firing from the LH, which increases sympathetic outflow through the splanchnic nerve and decreased parasympathetic activity. The CNS has sympathetic inhibitory tone upon insulin secretion, most probably to protect the CNS from hypoglycemia. During hyperglycemia, the glucoreceptors in the VMH increase firing and release the inhibitory sympathetic tone on the pancreas, permitting an increase in insulin release. Glucose seems to provide a negative feedback signal sensed by the hypothalamic noradrenergic systems, which in turn appear to stimulate glucose output by a neural mechanism. *E*, epinephrine; *NE*, norepinephrine

Modulation of splanchnic viscera is not limited to vagus tone, but is also influenced by sympathetic tone as well [18]. Thus, it is speculated that the decreased activity of the glucose-sensitive neurons in the LH releases the inhibitory sympathetic tone on pancreatic insulin release. Figure 1 illustrates a simplified version of the flow of stimuli from the brain as it perceives glucopenia and commands the counterregulatory response to return plasma glucose levels to normal.

Neurotransmitter, Hormones, or Peptides

Over the past decade our laboratory has been active in examining the role that the CNS plays in regulating glucose and amino acid metabolism in the body. For this we have chosen to examine in detail the various hormonal changes that occur during insulin-induced hypoglycemia. We and others have shown that insulin-induced hypoglycemia evokes elevations in plasma levels of glucagon, epinephrine, norepinephrine, cortisol, growth hormone, and ACTH [19]. The exact mechanism, however, for the neurochemical basis for the CNS glucose counterregulation remains only vaguely defined. Though the activation of hypothalamic noradrenaline activity was shown to be associated with concurrent increases in plasma glucose concentration, it does not appear to be the sole player. Several other candidates have also been considered to play important roles (Table 1).

Table 1. Candidate mediators of central nervous system (CNS) control of metabolism

Mediator	Localization	Route	Effects[a]
Bombesin [6]	Hypothalamus Brains stem	VMH LH	↑ Glucose ↑ Catechols ↑ Glucagon
Somatostatin [6, 45]	Not clear	VMH LH	↓ CNS-sympathetic out- flow
Neuropeptide Y [46–48]	Arcuate nucleus of hypothalamus PVN	ICV	↑ ACTH ↑ cortisol
Histamine [49–52]	Hypothalamus	ICV	↑ Sympathoadreno-med. ullary axis ↑ CRF release
Opioids/opiates [21, 23, 25]	Hypothalamus	ICV	↑ Catechols ↑ Glucose
CRF [45]	Median eminence, posterior pituitary, - hypothalamus	ICV	↑ NE/E ↑ glucagon ↑ glucose
Thyrotropin-releasing hormone [53–56]	Widely distributed in CNS	LH VMH AH	↑ Catechols ↑ glucose ↑ noradrenergic output

VMH, ventromedial hypothalamus; LH, lateral hypothalamus; ACTH, adrenocorticotropic hormone; CRF, corticotropin releasing factor; NE, norepinephrine; E, epinephrine; PVN, periventricular nuclei; ICV, intracerebroventricular; AH, anterior hypothalamus
[a] Summary of demonstrated metabolic effects of central administration of peptides, hormones, and opioids into the CNS.

In addition to the traditional elevations in plasma epinephrine and norepinephrine described during glucopenia, we have provided evidence for additional elevations in plasma and CSF levels of ir-β-endorphins [20]. In the CNS, β-endorphin with its opiate-like activity has been demonstrated to have similar hyperglycemic effects to morphine [21, 22]. The site of action in the brain of β-endorphin-induced hyperglycemia is not clear, since the direct administration of β-endorphins into the LH and VMH has not been shown to produce significant changes in glucose concentration. Nevertheless, the involvement of the central endorphinergic system in the control of fuel mobilization during glucopenia has been supported by our studies. Intracerebroventricular (ICV) administration of β-endorphin in dogs resulted in significant elevations of plasma glucose, with concomitant rises in plasma insulin. The mechanism of the hyperglycemia is thought to be the result of both an increase in glucose production by the liver and a later inhibition of glucose utilization by "peripheral tissues"; both of these effects are the result of stimulation of the sympathoadrenal axis as supported by 30-fold elevations in circulating plasma epinephrine and sixfold elevations in norepinephrine. Because no rise in plasma glucagon was detected by the administration of ICV β-endorphin, it appears that the hypothalamo–pancreatic axis was not directly stimulated and that the observed rises in plasma insulin were most probably secondary to the hyperglycemia. ACTH and cortisol were also increased by the ICV administration of β-endorphin, but these appear to play lesser, though important, roles in the acute regulation of hepatic glucose production or in altering glucose clearance.

In contrast to the findings with ICV administration of β-endorphin, we demonstrated that the peripheral administration (IV) of β-endorphin resulted in a direct inhibition of hepatic glucose production, without producing any changes in hormone concentrations. These effects appear to be independent of those produced in the CNS.

Additional confirmation for the role of β-endorphin in modulating glucose homeostasis was obtained from our studies in which we injected ICV naloxone prior to the induction of insulin-induced hypoglycemia. ICV naloxone, an effective central opiate blocker, prior to induction of hypoglycemia in dogs, blunted the rise in plasma β-endorphin, epinephrine, and norepinephrine without affecting the responses of glucagon and cortisol [23]. Paradoxically, although pretreatment with naloxone has not been found to affect the hypoglycemic nadir, it did increase the rates of glucose utilization and production, which could well be the result of a diminished glucose-resistante state due to the lower epinephrine concentrations in dogs pretreated with naloxone [24].

More recently, we have shown that plasma and CSF levels of endogenous opiates (specifically, the levels of endogenous opiate alkaloids, morphine, and codeine) increased in response to insulin-induced hypoglycemia. Ongoing preliminary studies in our laboratory are suggestive of a regulatory role of these opiates in both glucose homeostasis as well as regulating protein turnover. Their exact mechanisms are as yet not understood, but appear to involve the activation of CNS μ-receptors. Support for a modulatory role in glucose homeostasis is also evident from our work, which showed that the hyperglycemic effects of morphine result from both a stimulation of hepatic glucose production and an inhibition of glucose clearance [22, 25]. These effects are mediated at the levels of the CNS, since they can be reproduced by the ICV administration of small amounts of morphine that are not detected in the peripheral circulation. Furthermore, the presence of endogenous morphine in mammalian tissues as well as the presence of receptors that specifically bind these substances in the CNS suggest their modulatory functions under basal conditions as well as in situations of stress-induced hypercatabolism [26–28]. Opiate-like substances and endogenous opioid peptides have been shown to exert indirect effects on pituitary secretory activity. The most probable area of action is the hypothalamus, since this is an area in which both the peptides and receptors are found [27].

Neural Control of Counterregulatory Hormones

Glucose counterregulation involves a complex interaction between hormonal and nonhormonal factors [1, 29, 30]. The hormonal contribution to the restoration of plasma glucose concentrations during glucopenia is crucial and indispensable [31–34]. As already stated, insulin-induced hypoglycemia is associated with significant elevations in plasma levels of glucagon, epinephrine, norepinephrine, ACTH, cortisol, and β-endorphin. We and others have reported that the magnitude of the rise in counterregulatory hormones is greater in dogs with generalized hypoglycemia than in those in whom the CNS was kept euglycemic [8]. The relative importance of each of the rises, however, remains unclear. It has been considered that glucagon plays a primary role and epinephrine plays a secondary role in glucose recovery from acute insulin-induced hypoglycemia in man [31]. A role for the immediate action of growth hormone, cortisol, or neurally released norepinephrine in acute hypoglycemic spells has not been supported, even though the long-term excess or deficiency of these factors may influence glucose counterregulation [32, 19].

Work from our laboratory [8] as well as from other laboratories [35] indicates that the observed increments in plasma glucagon and epinephrine seen during hypoglycemia could only account for nearly 50% of the observed rise in hepatic glucose production [35, 36]. The other 50% appears to be a result of a direct CNS activation of hepatic glucose production [35]. The nature and significance of this direct pathway remain unclear and deserve further examination.

Glycogenolysis and Gluconeogenesis

The initial rise in hepatic glucose production during counterregulation to hypoglycemia is mainly derived from glycogenolysis, however, as glucopenia persists, the percentage contribution from gluconeogenesis increases [34]. The increased availability of gluconeogenic precursors as well as the increasing concentrations of counterregulatory hormones result in the predominance of gluconeogenesis during the latter parts of glucoregulation and account for nearly 80% of overall hepatic glucose output; this is considered the predominant factor preventing further development of glucopenia [33, 34].

Of the three main gluconeogenic substrates, lactate derived from the periphery, most likely as the result of increased muscle glycogenolysis, appears to account for most of the gluconeogenic precursor supply [37]. Although the increase in glycerol uptake by the liver in response to glucopenia is significant, the total amount of three carbon precursors that lactate contributes is significantly greater. Although it could be argued that the efficiency with which the liver converts glycerol and alanine into glucose is greater than that for lactate, we have provided evidence for a critical contribution of lactate as a gluconeogenic precursor. Our studies have provided evidence that during prolonged periods of hypoglycemia, the overall contribution of lactate-derived carbons cannot be substituted by those of glycerol and/or alanine [38]. An inhibition of net hepatic lactate uptake results in an inability to sustain the increased rates of hepatic glucose production observed during prolonged hypoglycemia.

There is increasing evidence that the stimulation of hepatic glucose production is not only affected by the counterregulatory hormones and substrate availability [37, 35], but by direct hepatic neural stimulation as well [39, 40]. Three mechanisms have been described through which the sympathetic nervous system activates glycogenolysis: (1) directly through hepatic innervation, (2) secondary to the release of catecholamines from the adrenals, and (3) in response to release of glucagen from the pancreas. Electrical stimulation of portal perivascular nerve bundles increases glucose and lactate release and stimulates *phosphorylase a* activity, suggesting that hepatic glucose production is modulated predominantly by its own sympathetic nerve supply rather than by catecholamines and glucagon. It is probable that these effects are synergistic with that of glucagon and catecholamines on the liver and complement each other in the glycogenolytic and gluconeogenic effect on the liver during hypoglycemia.

Proteolysis

Although the role of the CNS in the control and regulation of carbohydrate metabolism was described as early as 1958 by Bernard [41], control of protein and amino acid metabolism by the brain has not been extensively addressed. Little is known about the hypothalamic control of protein metabolism. However there is some evidence that direct neural input into the liver may modify the activity of enzymes involved in amino acid metabolism. Activity of tyrosine aminotransferase in rat liver is suppressed by sympathetic–adrenergic mechanisms and is induced by the vagal–cholinergic system and after spinal cord transection. Furthermore, cholinergic stimulation of the LH results in activation of tyrosine aminotransferase, an effect which can be blocked by vagotomy.

The effects of glucopenia on protein and amino acid metabolism have been of special interest to our laboratory. Traditionally, increased fuel mobilization from the periphery to provide the liver with gluconeogenic substrates has been proposed to include mobilization of gluconeogenic amino acids from muscle to be shuttled to the liver and into gluconeogenesis. Alanine is the primary amino acid released by muscle and the primary gluconeogenic amino acid extracted by the liver during hypoglycemia [42]. The efficiency of alanine incorporation into glucose has been utilized as an assessment of the gluconeogenic conversion rate, and the proportion of injected alanine recovered as glucose is similar to that of lactate, suggesting prompt incorporation of this amino acid into glucose [36].

Our laboratory has demonstrated that insulin-induced hypoglycemia is characterized not only by the classically described glucose counterregulation of increased glycogenolysis, lipolysis, and gluconeogenesis but also by enhanced protein breakdown [43]. Estimations of whole body proteolysis using the isotopic dilution of leucine showed a marked increase in the rate of leucine appearance in the plasma compartment followed by enhanced rates of amino acid oxidation, both suggestive of increased proteolysis. An initial drop in plasma leucine and leucine rate of appearance (44% and 23%, respectively) was observed within 1 h, but this is followed by a gradual increase to 20% higher than basal values at 3 h. Leucine oxidation increased twofold and nonoxidative disposal remained near basal levels. Interestingly, although the rate of protein synthesis remained near basal, this was not sufficient to offset the increased rates of protein breakdown, with the overall result being a net loss of nitrogen by the body. The primary site of this proteolytic response is not skeletal muscle but primarily the gastrointestinal tract, resulting in an increased net release of both essential and nonessential amino acids across the extrahepatic splanchnic tissues. This increase in leucine release from the splanchnic bed was not limited to this amino acid, but was significant for isoleucine, valine, phenylalanine, and tyrosine. During this process, the majority of amino acids released by the gut were taken up by the liver, but a significant component, specifically that of branched-chain amino acids, was released into the systemic circulation and taken up by other organs, mainly skeletal muscle. Contrary to what would be expected, net balance of leucine across the hindlimb tissues during hypoglycemia switched from neutral balance to a net uptake. The increase in net hindlimb uptake of branched-chain amino acids may help provide amino groups for pyruvate transamination and thus increased alanine release.

The role of the central nervous system in eliciting the proteolytic response to hypoglycemia has been demonstrated in dogs that have been subjected to peripheral hypoglycemia by intravenous infusions of insulin and allowed to either develop neuroglucopenia or infused with glucose through the carotids and the vertebral arteries in order to maintain CNS euglycemia [8]. Prevention of severe CNS glucopenia was associated with marked suppression of proteolysis and its rate of oxidation, in sharp contrast to what was observed in the group in which generalized hypoglycemia was allowed to occur. This was the result of a near complete inhibition of proteolysis across the gastrointestinal tract, as represented by gut leucine balance. We hypothesized that the site of control of the proteolysis associated with hypoglycemia was in the periventricular area. To test this hypothesis, we planned a set of studies in which a cannula was implanted in the third ventricle of the dog to examine the effect of central neuroglucopenia, induced by ICV administration of 2-deoxyglucose (2-DG), on glucose and amino acid kinetics in conscious dogs [44]. As a result of ICV 2-DG administration, plasma glucose levels rose twofold or more by 90 min, blood lactate increased fourfold, and blood alanine did not change from basal levels. The rate of hepatic glucose production, determined isotopically, was increased twofold over basal levels. Significant increases over basal levels were also noted in plasma epinephrine, norepinephrine, insulin, glucagon, and cortisol. Leucine rate of appearance, however, showed a 30% decrease from basal levels to 2.4 ± 0.05 μmol/kg per min with an associated decrease in rates of amino acid oxidation and without an increase in gut amino acid release. These findings suggested that periventricular neuroglucopenia, in the absence of peripheral glucose deprivation, is accompanied by hyperglycemia secondary to enhanced hepatic glucose production with decreased glucose utilization and by increased hepatic uptake of gluconeogenic precursors. These alterations in glucose metabolism, however, were not accompanied by increased whole body proteolysis as was previously seen with generalized glucopenia resulting from insulin-induced hypoglycemia. Therefore, not only is the anatomical location of receptors eliciting such metabolic events still obscure, but the putative mediators involved are also not known.

The gut proteolytic response to glucopenia does not appear to play a major role in restoring glycemia, thus intuitively it can only result in deleterious consequences for the individual. Our results are supportive of a major role for the CNS in controlling this response. However, the determination of the contribution of hormonal, neural, opiate, and peptidergic changes accompanying glucopenia has just recently been initiated. Interestingly, it appears that neurocortisolemia prior to the induction of hypoglycemia modulates the proteolytic response. This could indicate a protective role for cortisol in the CNS. Previously we have demonstrated a rise in cortisol levels in CSF during prolonged hypoglycemia. The role of this has been assumed to be that of a negative feedback inhibition of CRF and thus of ACTH. It is possible that it could also inhibit the triggering mechanism for the proteolytic response. The site of this inhibition or the possible neurotransmitter system involved in this response in the focus of future studies from our laboratory and cannot be discerned based on the available information.

Our recent studies have focused on the contribution of opiate alkaloids to the regulation of metabolism during stress. We have been able to demonstrate their enhanced production during hypoglycemia and fasting and after laparotomy. The levels of these opiates are particularly increased in the brain, suggesting a role in modulating the metabolic response. Furthermore, the synthesis of the alkaloids is responsive to increased substrate supply. Our findings suggest that a 3-day course of dopamine injections results in an increase in brain morphine levels.

Conclusions

Using a well-established model of insulin-induced hypoglycemia that does not incur hemodynamic perturbations during the ebb phase, we have been able to characterize the resulting alterations pertaining to both carbohydrate and protein metabolism. Our studies in small animal models have provided further information about the changes in the gastrointestinal tissues. The focus of our investigations has turned over the past few years from the description of the metabolic perturbations associated with insulin-induced hypoglycemia to a more mechanistic approach. We are now actively studying the role of endogenous opiate alkaloids and their synthesis during conditions of stress in an effort to demonstrate that these are temporally to the alterations in nitrogen metabolism observed. This has opened a wide field of research into the neurohormonal regulation of tissue metabolism, the outcome of which should provide further insight, into the sites of regulation of these metabolic alterations. The central and integrative role of the hypothalamus is evident, but the existence of glucose-sensitive and glucoreceptor neurons in other areas not only of the CNS, but also in the periphery, is supported by several studies. It becomes apparent, when comparing the effects of neural and chemical stimulation of different areas of the CNS, that the regulation of glucose and protein metabolism is interrelated and sometimes stimulated in a parallel manner. However, their individual modulation appears to have some selectivity. Thus, the localization, the neurotransmitter system involved, the second messenger system stimulated, and finally the afferent pathway through which the stimulus is conveyed are shared under some conditions but diverge under others. This makes generalizations as to mechanisms of action of an insult such as glucopenia almost impossible, but is intriguing and exciting enough to stimulate speculative and innovative hypotheses.

Acknowledgements. This work has been supported in part by NIDDK 42562 and GM50567-01.

References

1. Gerich J, Davis J, Lorenzi M et al. (1979) Hormonal mechanisms of recovery from insulin-induced hypoglycemia in man. Am J Physiol 236:E380–E385
2. Oomura Y, Ono T, Ooyama H, Wayner MJ (1969) Glucose and osmosensitive neurones of the rat hypothalamus. Nature 222:282–284
3. Shimizu N, Oomura Y, Novin D, Grijalva CV, Cooper PH (1983) Functional correlations between lateral hypothalamic glucose-sensitive neurons and hepatic portal glucose-sensitive units in rat. Brain Res 265:49–54
4. Shimazu T, Fukuda A, Ban T (1966) Reciprocal influences of the ventromedial and lateral hypothalamic nuclei on blood glucose levels and liver glycogen content. Nature 210:1178–1179
5. Smythe GA, Grunstein HS, Bradshaw JE, Nicholson MV, Compton PJ (1985) Relationships between the brain noradrenergic activity and blood glucose. Nature 308:65–67
6. Iguchi A, Matsunaga H, Nomura T, Gotoh M, Sakamoto N (1984) Glucoregulatory effects of intrahypothalamic injections of bombesin and other peptides. Endocrinology 114:2242–2246
7. Himsworth RL (1970) Hypothalamic control of adrenaline secretion in response to insufficient glucose. J Physiol (Lond) 206:411–417
8. Hourani H, Lacy B, Tayeb KE, Abumrad NN (1992) The role of central nervous system in modulating glucose and protein metabolism during insulin-induced hypoglycemia. Brain Res 587:276–284
9. Niijima A (1989) Neural mechanisms in the control of blood glucose concentration. J Nutr 119:833–840
10. Bleir R, Cohn P, Siggelkow IR (1979) A cytoarchitectonic atlas of the hypothalamus and hypothalamic third ventricle of the rat. In: Morgane PJ, Panksepp J (eds) Handbook of the hypothalamus. Dekker, New York, pp 137–220
11. Mizuno Y, Oomura Y (1984) Glucose responding neurons in the nucleus tractus solitarius of the rat: in vitro study. Brain Res 307:109–116
12. Frohman LA, Bernardis LL (1971) Effect of hypothalamic stimulation on plasma glucose, insulin, and glucagon levels. Am J Physiol 221:1596–1603
13. Vigas M, Tatar P, Jurcovicova J, Jezova D (1990) Glucoreceptors located in different areas mediate the hypoglycemia-induced release of growth hormone, prolactin, and adrenocorticotropin in man. Neuroendocrinology 51:365–368

14. DiRocco R, Grill HJ (1979) The forebrain is not essential for sympathoadrenal hyperglycemic response to glucoprivation. Science 204:1112–1114
15. Ritter RC, Slusser PG, Stone S (1981) Glucoreceptors controlling feeding and blood glucose: location in the hindbrain. Science 213:24–27
16. Keller-Wood ME, Wade CE, Shinsako J, Keil LC, Van Loon GR, Dallmann MF (1982) Insulin-induced hypoglycemia in conscious dogs: effect of maintaining carotid arterial glucose levels on the adrenocorticotropin, epinephrine, and vasopressin responses. Endocrinology 112:624–632
17. Schmitt M (1973) Influences of hepatic portal receptors on hypothalamic feeding and satiety centers. Am J Physiol 225:1089–1095
18. Donovan CM, Halter JB, Bergman RN (1991) Importance of hepatic glucoreceptors in sympathoadrenal response to hypoglycemia. Diabetes 40:155–158
19. Fish HR, Chernow B, O'Brien JT (1986) Endocrine and neurophysiologic responses of the pituitary to insulin-induced hypoglycemia: a review. Metabolism 35:763–780
20. Radosevich PM, Laca DB, Brown LL, Williams PE, Abumrad NN (1988) Effects of insulin-induced hypoglycemia on plasma and cerebrospinal fluid levels of ir-β-endorphins, ACTH, cortisol, norepinephrine, insulin and glucose in the conscious dog. Brain Res 458:325–338
21. Radosevich PM, Lacy DB, Brown LL, Williams PE, Abumrad NN (1989) Central effects of β-endorphins on glucose homeostasis in the conscious dog. Am J Physiol 256:E322–E330
22. Radosevich PM, Williams PE, Lacy DB et al. (1984) Effects of morphine on glucose homeostasis in the conscious dog. J Clin Invest 74:1473–1480
23. Nash JA, Radosevich PM, Lacy DB et al. (1989) Effects of naloxone on glucose homeostasis during insulin-induced hypoglycemia. Am J Physiol 257:E367–E373
24. Ipp E, Garberoglio C, Richter H, Moosa AR, Rubenstein AH (1981) Naloxone decreases centrally induced hyperglycemia in dogs. Diabetes 33:619–621
25. Molina PE, Hashiguchi Y, Ajmal M, Mazza M, Abumrad NN (1995) Differential hemodynamic, metabolic and hormonal effects of morphine and morphine-6-glucuronide. Brain Res (in press)
26. Donnerer J, Cardinale G, Coffey J, Lisek CA, Jardine I, Spector S (1987) Chemical characterization and regulation of endogenous morphine and codeine in the rat. J Pharmacol Exp Ther 242:583–587
27. Akil H, Watson SJ, Young E, Lewis ME, Khachaturian H, Walker JM (1984) Endogenous opioids: biology and function. Annu Rev Neurosci 7:223–255
28. Weitz CJ, Lowney LI, Faull KF, Feistner G, Goldstein A (1986) Morphine and codeine from mammalian brain. Proc Natl Acad Sci USA 83:9784–9788
29. Havel PJ, Taborsky GJ (1989) The contribution of the autonomic nervous system to changes of glucagon and insulin secretion during hypoglycemic stress. Endocr Rev 10:332–350
30. Havel PJ, Veith RC, Dunning BE, Taborsky GJ (1991) Role for autonomic nervous system to increase pancreatic glucagon secretion during marked insulin-induced hypoglycemia in dogs. Diabetes 40(9):1107–1114
31. Santiago JV, Clarke WL, Shah SD, Cryer PE (1980) Epinephrine, norepinephrine, glucagon, and release in association with physiological decrements in the plasma glucose concentration in normal and diabetic man. J Clin Endocrinol Metab 51:877–883
32. Garber AJ, Cryer PE, Santiago JV, Haymond MW, Pagliara AS, Kipnis DM (1976) The role of adrenergic mechanisms in the substrate and hormonal response to insulin-induced hypoglycemia in man. J Clin Invest 58:7–15
33. Lecavalier L, Bolli G, Cryer P, Gerich J (1989) Contributions of gluconeogenesis and glycogenolysis during glucose counterregulation in normal humans. Am J Physiol 256:E844–E851
34. Frizzell RT, Campbell PJ, Cherrington AD (1988) Gluconeogenesis and hypoglycemia. Diabetes Metab Rev 4:51–70
35. Frizzell RT, Hendrick GK, Brown LL et al. (1988) Stimulation of glucose production through hormone secretion and other mechanisms during insulin-induced hypoglycemia. Diabetes 37:1531–1541
36. Frizzell RT, Hendrick GK, Biggers DW et al. (1988) Role of gluconeogenesis in sustaining glucose production during hypoglycemia caused by continuous insulin infusion in conscious dogs. Diabetes 37:749–759

37. Jahoor F, Peters EJ, Wolf RR (1990) The relationship between the gluconeogenic substrate supply and glucose production in humans. Am J Physiol 258:E288–E296
38. Molina PE, Jabbour K, Williams PE, Abumrad NN (1994) Ethanol modulates hepatic glucose production during insulin-induced hypoglycemia by inhibiting net hepatic lactate uptake. Am J Physiol (in press)
39. Iguchi A, Kunoh Y, Miura H et al. (1989) Central nervous system control of glycogenolysis and gluconeogenesis in fed and fasted rat liver. Metabolism 38:1216–1221
40. Matsunaga H, Iguchi A, Yatomi A et al. (1989) The relative importance of nervous system and hormones to the 2-deoxy-D-glucose-induced hyperglycemia in fed rats. Endocrinology 124:1259–1264
41. Bernard MC (1958) Leçons surs la physiologie et la pathologie. In: Système nerveux. Baillière, Paris, pp 349–370
42. Felig P (1973) The glucose-alanine cycle. Metabolism 22:179–206
43. Hourani H, Williams PE, Morris JA, May MM, Abumrad NN (1990) Effect of insulin-induced hypoglycemia on protein metabolism in vivo. Am J Physiol 259:E342–E350
44. Molina PE, Tayeb KE, Hourani H, Okamura K, Williams P, Abumrad NN (1993) Hormonal and metabolic effects of neuroglucopenia. Brain Res 614:99–108
45. Brown MR, Fisher L (1984) Brain peptide regulation of adrenal epinephrine secretion. Am J Physiol 247:E41–E46
46. Emson PC (1979) Peptides as neurotransmitter candidates in the mammalian CNS. Prog Neurobiol 13:61–65
47. Inui A, Inoue T, Nakajima M et al. (1990) Brain neuropeptide Y in the control of adrenocorticotropic hormone secretion in the dog. Brain Res 510:211–215
48. Danger JM, Toon MC, Jenks BG et al. (1990) Neuropeptide Y: localization in the central nervous system and neuroendocrine functions. Fundam Clin Pharmacol 4:307–340
49. Wada H, Watanabe T, Yamatodani A et al. (1985) Physiological functions of histamine in the brain. In: Ganellin CR, Schwartz JC (eds) Frontiers in histamine research. Pergamon, Oxford, pp 225–235
50. Knigge U, Matzen S, Warberg J (1990) Histamine as a neuroendocrine regulator of the stress-induced release of peripheral catecholamines. Endocrinology 126:1430–1434
51. Nishibori M, Itoh Y, Oishi R, Saeki K (1990) Effect of microinjection of histamine into the brain on plasma levels of epinephrine and glucose in freely moving rats. Jpn J Pharmacol 54:257–263
52. Bealer SL (1993) Histamine releases norepinephrine from the paraventricular nucleus/anterior hypothalamus region in the conscious rat. J Pharmacol Exp Ther 264(2):734–738
53. Pilotte NS, Sharif NA, Burt DR (1984) Characterization and autoradiographic localization of TRH receptors in sections of rat brain. Brain Res 293:372–376
54. Kabayama Y, Kato Y, Tojo K, Shimatsu A, Ohta H, Imura H (1985) Central effects of DN1417, a novel TRH analog, on plasma glucose and catecholamines in conscious rats. Life Sci 36:1287–1294
55. Shen DC, Lin MT, Shian LR (1985) Thyrotropin-releasing hormone-induced hyperglycemia: possible involvement of cholinergic receptors in the lateral hypothalamus. Neuroendocrinology 41:499–503
56. Amir S, Jackson I (1980) Immunological blockade of endogenous thyrotropin-releasing hormone impairs recovery from hyperglycemia in mice. Brain Res 462:159–162

The Early Endocrine Response to Injury

A. H. Foster

Introduction

The name hormone was originally given to substances that are secreted by glandular tissue and transported by the blood or lymph to perform specific regulatory actions in target cells. The word is derived from the Greek hormaein, meaning "to set in motion" or "spur on" and was first used in 1905 by Starling and Bayliss. Study of the organs whose function is to secrete these substances (the endocrine system) over the subsequent 90 years has allowed the field of integrated physiology to emerge. During this time, dozens of substances that may be termed hormones have been added, and hundreds of cell types have been identified that act as glands and target tissues for these factors. Organs traditionally considered to have simple primary functions, such as the heart, brain, and endothelium are now understood to possess additional and equally important "glandular" or endocrine function. The following discussion of the endocrine response to injury is limited to circulating substances of the classical endocrine system, i.e., those hormones controlled by the hypothalamic-pituitary axis and those hormones controlled by the autonomic nervous system. Mediator substances such as cytokines and endothelial cell products such as prostaglandins, endothelins, and nitric oxide may also spill over into the systemic circulation and thereby act as endocrine substances, but these are beyond the scope of this chapter.

This chapter describes the early endocrine response to injury, i.e., that which occurs during the acute, catabolic phase of the injury response and which Cuthbertson termed the "ebb phase" [1]. It must be emphasized that, although "typical" response patterns have been identified, the response patterns of individual patients are unique because of the complex interplay of pre-existing factors such as age, gender, nutritional status, chronic disease, infection, and multiple and/or repetitive stimuli. In contrast to the traditional concept of homeostasis, defined by Cannon in 1939 as "the coordinated physiological process which maintains most of the steady states in the organisms" [2], modern analytical methods have allowed a more accurate description of the inumerable processes that maintain internal steady state conditions. Constant integration and modulation occurs to maintain biologic stability. Change not stasis is the essential process that characterizes the steady state of health and successful recovery responses after injury. For this reason, homeodynamic stability is a more accurate descriptor than the term homeostasis [3]. A thorough understanding of the temporal nature of these responses, i.e., of the trajectory of each system output over time [4], is essential to achieve ultimate recovery of the patient. Injury, operation, disease, and aging each engage multiple, interacting systems with temporal trajectories that must be anticipated and guided to achieve healing and functional recovery of those who are critically ill or injured.

The Neuroendocrine Response

It is impossible to divorce the neural system from that of the endocrine, since the two systems are, in fact, co-existent: the perturbations that stimulate the efferent limbs of the endocrine system are modulated both peripherally and centrally by the nervous system. The endocrine response is effected primarily via the hypothalamic-pituitary axis and the efferent limb of the autonomic nervous system.

Neuroendocrine reflexes require intact signal receptors, signal transduction, rapid transmembrane potential changes, integration, and modulation, followed by afferent neural transmission to target endocrine organs. This fact is demonstrated by the observation that adrenocortical stimulation from laparotomy or burn injury is absent when the stimulated areas are denervated [5, 6] or when the stimulus arises below the level of cord transection in paraplegic patients [7]. This simple observation is validated on a daily basis by the efficacy of local anesthetic agents to minimize or avoid the pain and stress response during minor operations. The complex effects of general anesthesia in modulating neuroendocrine reflexes in both experimental [8, 9] and clinical circumstances [10] have also been recognized.

The paradigm injury response is that of the simple neuronal reflex arc that passes to the spinal cord level and produces rapid response (withdrawal). However, most stimuli in trauma and critical illness involve multiple, interacting factors and elicit more complex central regulation and control. Specialized peripheral and central receptors transduce the stimulus into discrete afferent neural inputs that are transmitted to the central nervous system (CNS) through specific neural pathways. In the higher-level neural centers, such as the locus ceruleus at the level of the pons, the inputs are integrated and modulated with other signals, resulting in the production of a discrete set of efferent neural outputs that produce multiple and widespread effector signals via hormonal secretion. These effects include potentiation and are characterized by longer response times and greater duration of action. Hormonal effects include nuclear transcription for de novo protein synthesis, immunologic activation, and proliferation of cells. Complex stimuli also affect highest-order cortical neuronal activity, causing conscious and unconscious thoughts with behavioral and other complex responses.

On a cellular level, injurious stimuli provoke rapid secretion of multiple substances such as endothelial cell nitric oxide to maintain vascular tone and allow continued oxygen delivery. The immediate need for energy may deplete constituitive energy depots and shunt to nonoxidative metabolism. Additional responses by multiple cell types involve cytokine secretion, acute phase protein release, abrupt alterations in coagulation proteins, ion shifts, rapid transcription, and protein synthesis. Certain paracrine factors may be released into the general circulation in times of severe or prolonged stress and can be considered as endocrine factors in these circumstances by eliciting actions on distant target organs. In the absence of significant injury, sepsis, or starvation, the physiologic alterations are minor, and the adjustments required to maintain homeostasis are easily and successfully made. In the presence of significant injury, sepsis, or starvation, the stimuli are multiple and intensified, and the responses are directed to preserve oxygen delivery, mobilize energy substrates, and minimize pain. When subsequent compensation becomes inadequate or poorly modulated, the inexorable progression of profound shock or the syndrome of multiple organ dysfunction may follow and result in death.

Stimuli or Neuroendocrine Reflexes

The major stimuli to neuroendocrine reflexes are: (1) alterations in effective circulating fluid volume, (2) changes in blood hydrogen ion concentration and in oxygen or carbon dioxide partial pressure, (3) pain or changes in emotion, (4) altered substrate availability, (5) changes in temperature, and (6) the presence of infection (Fig. 1).

Loss of effective circulating volume occurs as a result of most significant injuries. Hemorrhage, the sequestration of plasma volume (as in dehydration or burn injury), and the inability of blood to circulate (as in cardiac tamponade or pulmonary embolism) are typical scenarios for this stimulus. Hypovolemia is sensed by high-pressure baroreceptors in the aorta, carotid arteries, and kidneys and by low-pressure stretch receptors in the atria [11–13]. Arterial baroreceptors transduce the magnitude and rate of change of arterial pressure [13]. Stretch receptors transduce atrial volume and rate of volume change [14]. Tonic inhibition of hormonal release and of CNS and autonomic nervous system activities result from the afferent signals of high-pressure baroreceptors in the carotid arteries and aorta and from low-pressure stretch receptors of the atria. When effective circulating volume is reduced, baroreceptor and stretch receptor activities decrease, and loss of tonic inhi-

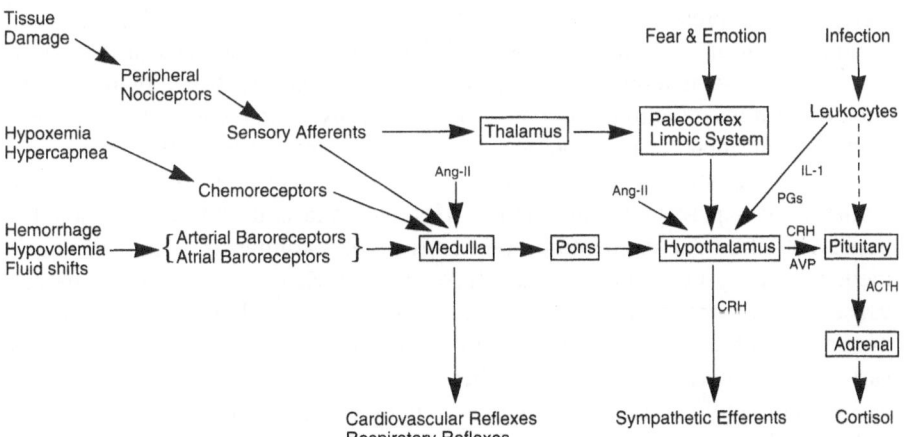

Fig. 1. Schematic representation of the hypothalamic-pituitary-adrenal system showing stimuli (afferent inputs), neural, endocrine and mediator modulation, and simple responses (efferent output). ANG-II, angiotensin II; PGs, protaglandins; IL-1, interleukin 1; CRH, corticotropin-releasing hormone; AVP, arginine vasopressin; ACTH, adrenocorticotropin-releasing hormone. (Reprinted with permission from [37])

bition occurs [12]. Afferent nerves from the baroreceptors are carried by the vagus nerve to the tractus solitarius of the medulla and through the reticular formation of the brainstem and hypothalamus (Fig. 1). This response causes further neuroendocrine stimulation, including secretion of angiotensin II (AII) via renin [15], secretion of aldosterone via AII and adrenocorticotropic hormone (ACTH) [16], secretion of cortisol via ACTH [12], secretion of glucagon via epinephrine [17], and reduced secretion of insulin through the effect of epinephrine [18]. Decreases in the effective circulating volume that are sensed by stretch receptors in the juxtaglomerular complexes of the kidney also lead to the secretion of renin and thereby to the formation of angiotensin and to the secretion of aldosterone [19]. The decrease in baroreceptor and stretch receptor discharge also stimulates heart rate, cardiac contractility, and vasoconstriction via increases in sympathetic and decreases in parasympathetic nervous system output [20]. Maximal sensitivity for the baroreceptor response occurs at approximately 80 mmHg [21].

Alterations in the partial pressure of oxygen and carbon dioxide, and in the concentration of hydrogen ion initiate cardiovascular, pulmonary, and neuroendocrine responses through peripheral chemoreceptor activation. The peripheral chemoreceptors are 1–2 mm in size and are composed of dopamine-containing, richly vascularized tissue (glomus cells) which are located in the carotid bodies at the bifurcation of the common carotid arteries (primary receptors) and in the aortic bodies located above and below the aortic arch [22]. Carotid glomus cells are activated by reductions in oxygen and, to a lesser extent, by increses in carbon dioxide tension and by hydrogen ions [23]. As a result of the extremely high blood flow through the chemoreceptors, the oxygen content of arterial blood, glomus cells, and venous blood is nearly equal. As a consequence of the low arteriovenous difference, decreases in both arterial blood flow and in arterial oxygen tension result in increased extraction of oxygen by the chemoreceptor tissue, cause decreased venous oxygen content, and elicit receptor activation. Chemoreceptors respond most rapidly when oxygen partial pressure falls below 50 torr [23]. Chemoreceptor activation results in stimulation of the hypothalamus and of the vascular component of the sympathetic nervous system that causes increased heart rate and contractility. In addition, chemoreceptor activation stimulates the respiratory center via central receptors, leading to an increase in respiratory rate. Interactions occur, so that increases in chemoreceptor activity that are caused by reduced oxygen tension are further potentiated by hypercapnia and acidosis. Hypovolemia is usually accompanied by hyperventilation due to chemoreceptor activation. A complex interplay of vagally mediated and sympathetic afferent reflexes occurs when chemoreceptors are activated by endogenous substances such as prostaglandin and kinins [22]. The most important central chemoreceptors are those situated just below the ventral medulla surrounded by cerebral spinal fluid. These receptors are sensitive to carbon dioxide tension and to diffusion-related changes in hydrogen ion concentration.

Pain and emotional arousal are characteristic of most injuries and cause neuroendocrine activation. Pain results in stimulation of the thalamus and hypothalamus through projections of peripheral nociceptive fibers [24]. Emotional arousal is produced by the perception or threat of injury and through the limbic areas of the brain evokes anger, fear, or anxiety [25]. Emotion stimulates neuroenderocrine reflexes through projections from the limbic system to hypothalamic and lower brainstem nuclei. Pain and emotional arousal cause secretion of ACTH, cortisol, arginine vasopressin (AVP), aldosterone, catecholamines, and endogenous opioid peptides, and increased activation of the autonomic nervous system (Fig. 1).

A change in plasma glucose concentration is the primary substrate alteration that causes neuroendocrine activation, but amino acid alterations also lead to hormonal secretion [26]. The glucose concentration is sensed by receptors in the ventromedial nucleus of the hypothalamus and in the pancreas [27]. Decreases in plasma glucose concentration stimulate the release of ACTH, cortisol, AVP, growth hormone (GH), catecholamines, and β-endorphin through central pathways (hypothalamus and autonomic nervous system) and stimulate the release of glucagon by autonomic and pancreatic activation [26, 27]. Insulin secretion is inhibited through autonomic nervous system pathways [28] and by direct action at pancreatic cells [18, 29]. The effects of amino acids on hormonal secretion are partially mediated by cell surface receptors and are structure-specific. Arginine, for example is a potent stim-

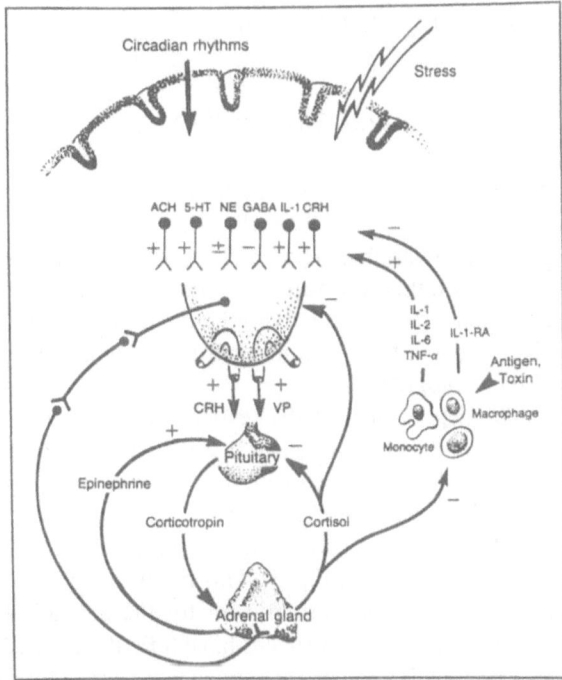

Fig. 2. Bidirectional interactions between hypothalamic, pituitary, and immunocompetent cells. External factors such as circadian rhythm, emotional stress, and injury, and by activated immunocompetent cells that secrete cytokines and other factors modulate the neuronal response. Cyto-kines induce the release of corticotropin-releasing factor (CRF) and arginine vasopressin (VP) from the hypothalamus, thereby stimulating corticotropin secretion. Circulating adrenal epinephrine acts synergistically with CRF and VP. Cortisol inhibits lymphocyte activation and modulates further secretion cytokines and other mediators. ACH, acetylcholine; 5-HT, serotonin; NE, norepinephrine; GABA, gamma-aminobutyric acid; IL, interleukin; IL-1-RA, interleukin 1 receptor antagonist. (Reprinted with permission from [61])

ulus to the secretion of insulin and of glucagon, while leucine, which also stimulates the secretion of insulin, does not stimulate the secretion of glucagon [30]. Increased local concentrations of certain amino acids are known to increase the activity of growth factors in wounds [10]. Amino acids are parent compounds of a number of hormones and of neurotransmitters including thyroxine, peptide hormones, catecholamines, histamine, and serotonin.

Alterations in core body temperature are sensed in the preoptic area of the hypothalamus [31, 32], and alter the secretion of hormones that include ACTH, cortisol, AVP, GH, aldosterone, thyroxine, and catecholamines [33–35]. Core temperature may be affected by changes in ambient temperature, by loss of thermal insulation as in burn injury, by reduced hepatic blood flow as in hypovolemia, by substrate deficiency as in starvation states, and by inadequate vasomotor control as in sepsis.

Circulating endotoxin may stimulate the neuroendocrine system directly [36] or may produce neuroendocrine effects by secondary changes in blood volume, oxygen delivery, substrate concentrations, and the presence of pain. The ubiquitous neuroendocrine interactions of cytokines and other mediators which are released during sepsis are the subject of much intense study and have been recently reviewed (Figs. 1, 2) [37–39].

Integration and Modulation

As a result of the integration of sensory inputs into the CNS and the modulation of efferent signals from the CNS, the neuroendocrine response to a given stimulus is graded and variable. The precise response depends on the magnitude and duration of the stimulus, the timing or presence of simultaneous and sequential stimuli, circadian effects, and overall physiologic conditions that include concomitant diseases, age, nutrition, immunologic competence, and effects of chronic or acute pharmacologic therapy.

The dependence of the response to intensity and duration and the importance of CNS integration is well-described for cardiopulmonary reflexes and for adrenomedullary catecholamine secretion. In contrast to the potent activation of the sympathetic nervous system (SNS) by small nonhypotensive hemorrhages [40, 41], true hormonal adrenomedullary secretion of catecholamines occurs only when hypotension occurs [42, 43]. This finding suggests that inactivation of cardiac stretch receptors alone is not sufficient for the activation of catecholamine release since nonhypotensive hemorrhages have little if any effect on these arterial baroreceptors. Similarly, activation of chemoreceptors alone [44] or inactivation of baroreceptors in isolation [45] have potent effects upon SNS activity but only minor ones on adrenal catecholamine secretion. Catecholamine secretion does, however, occur during hypotensive hemorrhages when both high- and low-pressure baroreceptors are activated.

In addition to stimulus intensity and duration, stimulation rate is important to the integration and modulation of efferent signals. In the case of experimental hemorrhage, for example, plasma epinephrine concentration is significantly greater following rapid blood loss than it is in slow hemorrhage where blood volumes remain constant [46].

Stimulus transduction is influenced by concomitant neuroendocrine input. For example, the setpoint and gain of central hypothalamic osmoreceptors are altered by baroreceptor input and by baroreceptor-mediated secretion of AVP [47, 48]. Similarly, the setpoint and gain of baroreceptors may be altered by the convergence of viscerosomatic and somatosensory afferents with baroreceptor inputs in the cardiovascular areas of the medulla [13, 49, 50] and baroreceptor responsiveness may be increased by AVP, AII, and catecholamines [51–53]. The sensitivity of some receptors such as those of the adrenal cortex may also change as a function of the time of day [54]. Thus a particular stimulus of the same magnitude, rate, and duration may have variable effects under differing circumstances.

In clinical circumstances, the stimuli accompanying injury, sepsis, and starvation rarely occur in isolation. The neuroendocrine response to injury is the summation of each stimulus which is often different from the response to any single stimulus [55, 56]. Injuries may occur in combination with different types of stimuli and may be separated by variable time periods. The response to the second or subsequent stimuli may be unchanged or may be greater than the initial response (the process of potentiation). The mechanism by which potentiation occurs remains poorly understood, but in the case of the hypothalamic-pituitary axis, it requires 60 to 90 minutes to offset cortisol feedback inhibition and persists for approximately 24 hours [57]. Physiologic potentiation for cortisol and catecholamines has been described for the response to sequential hemorrhages, sequential operations [58, 59], and hypoxia [60]. Potentiation of the response to temperature has also been observed for ACTH, cortisol, and AVP secretion [34]. Therefore, the initial neuroendocrine responses to trauma, shock, and sepsis do modify later responses induced by the stimulus of subsequent operation or repeated episodes of shock or sepsis.

Efferent Output

The efferent limb of the reflex neuroendocrine response to injury is comprised of multiple, nested layers than can be broadly classified as the neuroendocrine response, the mediator response, and the intracellular response. The first layer, that of the neuroendocrine response, is described below. The neural reflex response that is mediated predominantly in the brainstem also activates central hypothalamic regions and distal innervated endocrine organs. Similarly, inflammatory and immunologic responses that produce the secretion of endothelial factors and cytokines have systemic physiologic consequences in certain circumstances in addition to localized or paracrine effects and also interact with neuroendocrine reflexes. The bidirectional interactions of neuroendocrine hormones and mediator substances are complex and remain an area of active investigation (Fig. 2) [61].

The neuroendocrine response may be further subdivided into those substances controlled by the hypothalamic-pituitary axis and those by the autonomic regions of the brainstem. Secretion of cortisol, thyroxine, GH, and AVP is primarily under hypothalamic-pituitary control, while that of insulin, glucagon, and catecholamines is primarily under autonomic system control. Injury causes release of all hypothalamic-pituitary hormones and of all hormones mediated by the autonomic nervous

Table 1. Endocrine response to injury during the catabolic phase

Influence on release	Substance
Increased	Adrenocorticotropic hormone
	Cortisol
	Arginine vasopressin
	Oxytocin
	Growth hormone
	Prolactin
	Beta-endorphin
	Enkephalins
	Epinephrine
	Norepinephrine
	Dopamine
	Renin
	Angiotensin II
	Aldosterone
	Atrial natriuretic peptides[a]
	Glucagon
Decreased	Thyroid-stimulating hormone
	Thyroxine
	Triiodothyronine
	Luteinizing hormone
	Testosterone
	Estrogen
	Follicle-stimulating hormone
	Insulin
	Insulin-like growth factors[b]

[a] Increased primarily in response to tachycardia following hemorrhage.
[b] Reduced secretion of insulin-like growth factors appears to correlate with reduced insulin.

system, except for the release of thyroid hormones, gonadotropins, and insulin (Table 1).

Hormones secreted by endocrine organs, mediator substances released by cells, and neurotransmitters released at nerve terminals fall into one of three chemical classes: proteins, fatty acid derivatives, and amino acid derivatives (Table 2). These substances act at receptors that are present on the cell membrane surface or in the cell cytoplasm. The density and affinity of receptors can be modulated by factors which include conformational change at varied sites on either side of the cell membrane [62], by the effects of circulating receptor antagonists, and by post-binding alterations within the target cell [63].

Mechanisms of Hormone Action

The mechanisms by which hormones, mediators, and neurotransmitters cause intracellular change depend on lipid and water solubility. In general, the signalling substance or ligand changes either ion membrane permeability, genomic transcription, or both. Those ligands that directly alter transcription tend to be lipid soluble

Table 2. Chemical classes of hormones

Class	Hormones
Proteins (polypeptides, small peptides and glycoproteins)	Growth hormone Thyroid-stimulating hormone Arginine vasopressin Thyrotropin-releasing hormone Follicle-stimulating hormone Luteinizing hormone Renin Angiotensin II Insulin Glucagon Atrial natriuretic peptides Insulin-like growth factors Somatostatin
Fatty acid derivatives (lipid-soluble, cholesterol)	Cortisol Aldosterone Testosterone
Amino acid derivatives	Thyroxine Epinephrine Norepinephrine Dopamine

and are permeable to the lipid bilayer of cell membranes. Other ligands alter ion transport by attachment to membrane receptors, either directly (at the channel) or indirectly by coupling to G-proteins, intracellular calcium, or other modulators of the cell signal. These hormones act through secondary alterations in the intracellular second messengers such as cyclic adenosine $3'5'$-monophosphate (cAMP), through influx and/or mobilization of calcium, or through hormone-receptor protein kinase activity (Fig. 3) [62, 64].

Nuclear Hormone Signal Transduction

The primary actions of steroids and thyroid hormones are mediated by receptor proteins that bind to specific genes after free diffusion through the lipid bilayer of the cell membrane [63]. After rapid diffusion, steroid hormones bind to cytosolic receptors [65–67] of the steroid receptor superfamily [68] and migrate to the cell nucleus where transcription of messenger RNA (mRNA) for protein synthesis occurs (Fig. 4) [63, 69]. Thyroxine (T3) also acts, in part, through nuclear mechanisms [70] which may account for the 1- to 2-h interval that is observed before detecting the primary actions of this and other membrane-soluble hormones. Some, more rapidly detectable, actions of steroids [71] and of T3 [72] may also result from interaction with the cell membrane. Thyroid hormones do not bind to cytosolic receptors after diffusion through the cell membrane. Binding of thyroid hormones to nonhistone proteins of the nuclear chromatin activates gene expression [70].

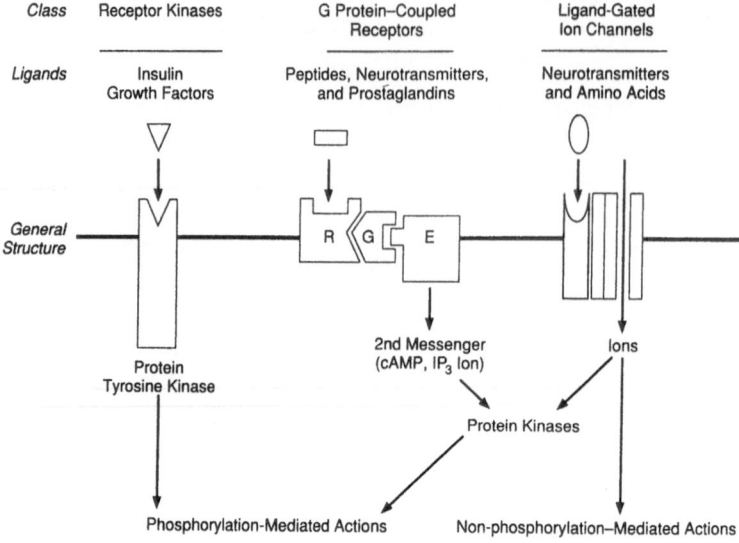

Fig. 3. Three major types of membrane receptors for hormones. Insulin growth factors bind to cell-surface receptors that stimulate the phosphorylation of proteins on tyrosine residues (protein tyrosine kinases). Peptide hormones bind to receptors (R) that are coupled to effector (E) enzymes and produce second messengers that activate distinct proteins (generally serine/threonine kinases). Amino acid derivatives and neurotransmitters bind to ligand-gated ion channels, which may also be coupled to G proteins (G). (Reprinted with permission from [322])

Membrane-Active Hormone Signal Transduction

Protein and amino acid derivative hormones that are water-soluble bind to cell membrane surface receptors. Three major classes of cell membrane receptors are present which include those with intrinsic tyrosine kinase activity, those coupled via G proteins (guanine nucleotide-binding proteins) to adenylate cyclase or phosphatidylinositol turnover, and those associated with ligand-gated ion channels (Fig. 3). After receptor-ligand interaction, the hormone-receptor comples may directly phosphorylate the tyrosine residue of the protein via specific protein kinase (e.g., insulin and growth factors) or may activate protein kinases through G protein regulated pathways [73, 74] that involve intermediate formation of cAMP via membrane adenylate cyclase or via intracellular calcium release (e.g., peptides, neurotransmitters, and prostaglandins). Ion channels that control potassium, sodium, chloride, and calcium fluxes at the membrane may be charge- or ligand-regulated. Ligand-gated channels (e.g., nicotinic cholinergic receptors) may also involve G proteins as signal transducers (e.g., myocardial β-adrenergic calcium channel and cholinergic muscarinic potassium channels) [75]. Actions of water-soluble hormones that utilize second messengers to direct the activity of regulatory proteins and enzymes cause cellular effects to occur more rapidly than those directed by the lipid-soluble, or genomic- or nuclear-acting hormones.

G proteins alter the activity of cell surface hormone receptors via membrane-bound enzymes that include adenylate cyclase, phospholipase A_2 and phospholipase

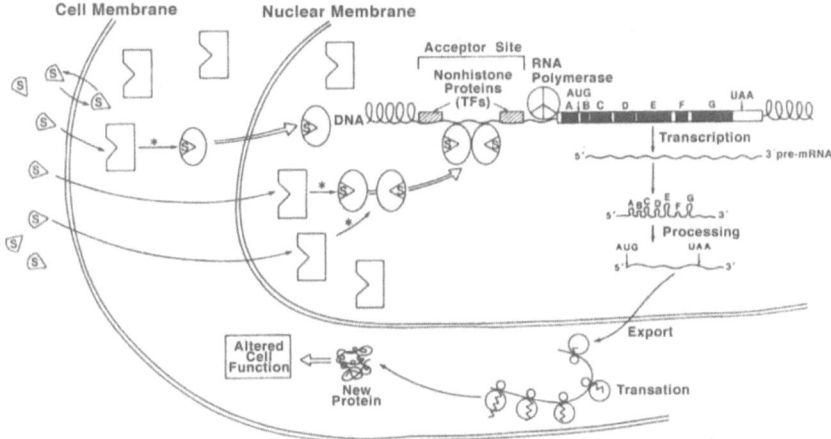

Fig. 4. Pathway for the action of steroid hormones. Steroid diffusion through the cell membrane lipid bilayer to bind to cytosolic or nuclear receptor proteins causes displacement of heat shock protein and activation of the receptor. This allows nonhistone protein binding and DNA transcription by RNA polymers. After RNA processing and export to the cytosol, new proteins are produced that alter cell function. (Reprinted with permission from [63])

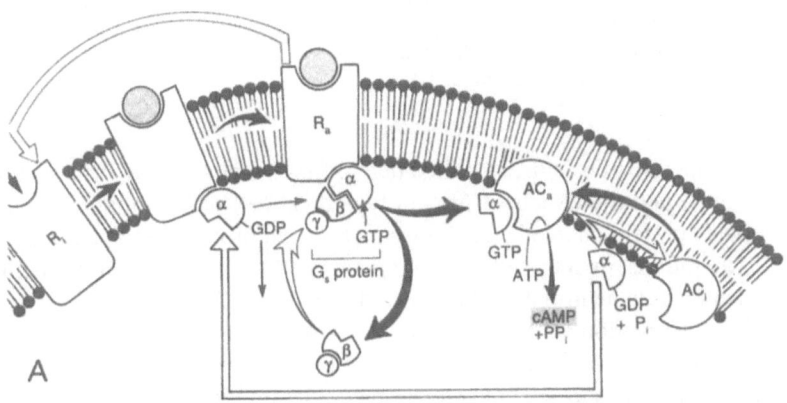

Fig. 5. The activation of adenylate cyclase and cAMP-dependent protein kinases elicited by epinephrine, adrenocorticotropin, and thyrotropin. Ri, inactive receptor; Ra, active receptor; ACi, inactive adenylate cyclase; ACa, active adenylate cyclase. (Reprinted with permission from [321])

C, and ligand-gated potassium and calcium channels [76–78]. G proteins may consequently have stimulatory or inhibitory effects [79]. ACTH, thyroid-stimulating hormone (TSH), β-adrenergic catecholamine, and glucagon receptors are coupled to stimulatory G proteins and affect adenylate cyclase and calcium channels (Fig. 5). α-Adrenergic catecholamine, muscarinic, somatostatin, and perhaps insulin receptors are coupled to inhibitory G proteins that reduce the activity of adenylate cyclase or probability of potassium or calcium channel opening [62]. Oncogene

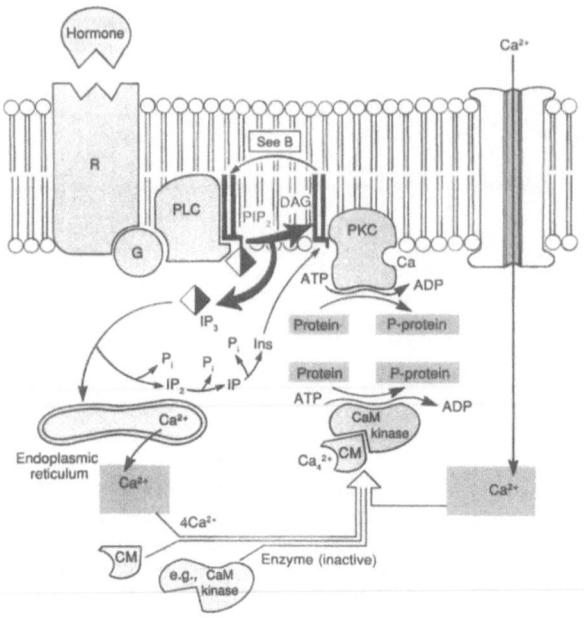

Fig. 6. Ca2+-mediated signal transduction. Arginine vasopressin, angiotensin, and α_1-adrenergic receptors function by this mechanism. CaM kinase, calcium/calmodulin dependent kinase; CM, calmodulin; IP, IP2, IP3, inositol monophosphate, diphosphate, and triphosphate, respectively; DAG, diacylglycerol; PIP, phosphatidylinositol; PKC, protein kinase C; PLC, phospholipase C. (Reprinted with permission from [321])

transcripts (*ras* proteins, so-called due to first isolation from viruses that caused rat sarcoma) and the effects of growth factors on cell proliferation are believed to involve G protein coupled signal transduction and protein tyrosine kinase action [80].

Alterations in intracellular calcium (Fig. 6) cause ubiquitous cellular effects which include neuronal, endocrine and exocrine cell exocytosis, cell motility, excitation–contraction coupling, neuronal transport, smooth muscle contraction, platelet aggregation, and a host of biochemical effects that include regulatory binding to calmodulin and subsequent activation of calcium kinases. These alterations are critical to many cellular functions, may be transduced by G protein coupled membrane receptors via the inositol trisphosphate ($InsP_3$) receptor pathways and via voltage-activated mechanisms (Fig. 6) [81, 82]. The bifurcating messenger inositol lipid system produces $InsP_3$ that mobilizes calcium from internal stores and produces diacylglycerol (DAG) that activates protein kinase C [83]. The range of $InsP_3$ action may be quite extensive and involves calcium ions and cyclic ADP ribose (cADPR) as second messengers for AVP, AII, α_1-adenergic receptors, and insulin [84, 85].

Intracellular alterations in cAMP (Fig. 5) activate protein kinase A and mediate, at least in part, the actions of several hormones that include ACTH, AVP, TSH, catecholamines, insulin, glucagon, and parathyroid hormone. Intracellular alterations in cGMP are produced by factors which include atrial natriuretic peptides (ANP).

Hormones Under Hypothalamic-Pituitary Control [86]

Corticotropin-Releasing Factor, Adrenocorticotropic Hormone, and Cortisol

The synthesis and release of cortisol from the adrenal zona fasiculata is primarily regulated by ACTH, which is controlled by pituitary secretion of corticotropin releasing factor (CRF), also called corticotropin releasing hormone (CRH) [87]. The effector hormone, cortisol, is secreted following injury to establish the metabolic availability of glucose from liver, skeletal muscle, and adipose tissue. In addition, cortisol has permissive effects in combination with other hormones [88, 89] that are essential to blood volume restitution [90]. Cortisol also has immunologic effects that are incompletely characterized [61, 91]. The hypothalamic-pituitary-adrenal system contains multiple afferent pathways, neural inputs, neuroendocrine, and neuroimmune interactions (Figs. 1, 2).

CRF is a 41-amino-acid polypeptide that is synthesized primarily in hypothalamic cells of the paraventricular nucleus and is located near cells that secrete AVP (formerly called antidiuretic hormone or ADH). The release of CRF into the hypophyseal-portal venous system is induced by neurogenic hypothalamic input and is potentiated by AVP [92].

ACTH is synthesized, stored and released by chromophobe cells of the anterior pituitary as a fragment of a larger, precursor molecule, proopiomelanocortin (POMC). POMC also contains γ- and β-lipotropin, α-melanocyte stimulating hormone, and β-endorphin. ACTH binds to cell surface receptors and signals for cortisol release through intracellular changes in cAMP within 2–3 min following receptor activation. Pituitary ACTH release is stimulated by CRF and modulated by AVP [93], and possibly by oxytocin [94]. Mediator cytokines such as interleukin-1 (IL-1) [96, 96] and interleukin-2 (IL-2) [97] also stimulate pituitary ACTH release [98, 99]. Additional evidence for central neuro-immunomodulation via the hypothalamic-pituitary axis includes identification of a protein released by the pituitary, called macrophage inhibitory factor (MIF), that potentiates lethal endotoxemia in experimental circumstances [100]. The release of ACTH is inhibited by cortisol and by ACTH itself, by long and short feedback loops, respectively [87]. ACTH stimulates lipolysis in fat cells and stimulates amino acid and glucose uptake in skeletal muscle cells [101].

Cortisol has widespread effects on carbohydrate, amino acid, and fatty acid metabolism. In the liver, cortisol inhibits the pentose phosphate shunt, the action of insulin, and regulatory glycolytic enzymes, that include glucokinase, phosphofructokinase, and pyruvate kinase. Cortisol stimulates the activity of glycogen synthetase. Cortisol stimulates amino acid uptake, amino acid transaminase activities, and the activities and de novo synthesis of several regulatory gluconeogenic enzymes, including pyruvate carboxylase, phosphoenolpyruvate carboxylase (PEPCK), and glucose 6-phosphatase [102–106]. In conjunction with epinephrine and ACTH, pyruvate dehydrogenase activity is reduced and, as a consequence, the availability of pyruvate to be used for gluconeogenesis increases. Cortisol also potentiates the actions of glucagon and epinephrine on the liver [89].

Despite these major effects upon hepatic carbohydrate metabolism, adrenalecto-mized animals do not exhibit marked alterations in carbohydrate metabolism if food is constantly available [107]. However, in the presence of injury or of starva-tion, adrenalectomized animals do exhibit marked alterations in hepatic carbohy-drate metabolism that result in rapid hypoglycemia and a reduction in the release of nonglucose solute from the liver [108]. The absence of cortisol-mediated induction of de novo synthesis of hepatic enzymes is not sufficient to explain the reduction in serum glucose because enzyme synthesis requires several hours [102]. Fur-thermore, perfusion of the livers of adrenalectomized animals in the absence of any gluconeogenic hormones, such as epinephrine or glucagon, reveals no difference in the gluconeogenic conversion of lactate or alanine to glucose when compared with control animals [109]. However, total glucose release is impaired and glycogen stores are virtually absent [110]. Furthermore, in the presence of glucagon or epinephrine, the perfused livers of adrenalectomized animals do exhibit a marked impairment of gluconeogenesis [109]. Thus, stress-induced hypoglycemia in adrenalectomized animals appears to be partially the result of the inability to store glycogen and the absence of the permissive action of corticosteroids on glucagon- and epinephrine-mediated gluconeogenesis.

In skeletal muscle tissue, cortisol has no direct effect on glucose uptake or gluco-neogenesis, but does inhibit insulin-mediated glucose uptake [88, 111]. Cortisol reduces the uptake and increases the release of amino acids by skeletal muscle [111]. The release of amino acids from skeletal muscle that is mediated by cyto-kines such as tumor necrosis factor (TNF), IL-1, γ-interferon (γ-IFN), and prosta-glandin E appears to be mediated by cortisol in various degrees [112]. In the absence of cortisol, amino acid release is decreased. Consequently, cortisol main-tains euglycemia during stress by the release of gluconeogenic substrates from skeletal muscle and by increasing the activities of gluconeogenesic pathways in the liver. In adipose tissue, cortisol decreases glucose uptake and potentiates the lipolytic actions of ACTH, GH, epinephrine, and glucagon [113–115]. Free fatty acid and glycerol concentrations increase.

Cortisol impairs lymphocyte, monocyte, and polymorphonuclear cell function when administered in supraphysiologic amounts [116, 117]. Administration of corticosteroids increases the circulating concentrations of lymphocytes and neutro-phils and decreases the circulating concentrations of monocytes and eosinophils. Corticosteroids markedly reduce accumulation of polymorphonuclear cells, mono-cytes, macrophages, and lymphocytes at inflammatory sites. At physiologic concen-trations, cortisol decreases lymphocyte glucose uptake and amino acid release, decre-ases prostaglandin and leukotriene synthesis via phospholipase A inhibition, and sup-presses leukocyte production of IL-1, IL-2, γ-IFN, β-endorphin, kinins, and prote-ases associated with inflammation [61, 118]. Recent appreciation of the roles of cytokines in the pathogenesis of the multiple organ dysfunction syndrome [119] is re-flected by recent use of the term systemic inflammatory response syndrome [120] in describing therapeutic modalities directed at pituitary–mediator interactions [121].

Injury acutely stimulates secretion of CRF, ACTH, and cortisol. ACTH secre-tion is stimulated by several mechanisms which include nociceptors, baroreceptors, hypothalamic receptors that tranduce alterations in glucose concentration, and carotid and aortic body receptors that sense oxygen tension. Mixed stimuli, such as the combination of pain and hemorrhage, interact such that ACTH secretion is minimal on tooth pulp stimulation or thermal stimulation alone, but is markedly potentiated when hemorrhage accompanies either stimulus [56, 122].

Cortisol and mineralocorticoid secretion influence plasma volume, electrolyte balance, and regulation of the renin-angiotensin system. An absence of glucocorticoid secretion results in hypotension that persists until the hormone is replaced. Catecholamine release is greatly increased in association with Addisonian hypotension, but steroid replacement remains essential. The mechanism for this requirement is unclear, but may be related to the sensitization of vascular smooth muscle to catecholamines that is caused by cortisol [123] and to the increased synthesis of the vasodilator prostaglandin I_2 that occurs in the absence of cortisol [86]. The restitution of blood volume also requires cortisol. During the first of the two phases of volume restitution that occur following many types of injury, fluid from the intracellular space shifts to the interstitial compartment following a transient increase in plasma osmolality. The increase in extracellular osmolality observed during this phase requires cortisol [12, 124, 125]. The second phase occurs when protein rich fluid from the expanded interstitium replenishes plasma volume.

Cortisol may remain elevated for up to 4 weeks following thermal injury, for less than 1 week following soft tissue trauma, and for several days following hemorrhage. In pure hypovolemia, plasma cortisol normalizes when blood volume is restored. Infection prolongs the duration of the cortisol response to injury. The circadian rhythm, well-described in the case of adrenal activity and the hypothalamic-pituitary axis, is disrupted in critically ill or postoperative patients in proportion to the length of operation [126] and to the magnitude of injury [127]. Persistent elevations of serum cortisol are associated with reduced survival.

Other Posterior Pituitary Hormones

Arginine Vasopressin

Certain hormones, such as AVP and oxytocin, are synthesized by hypothalamic cells prior to storage in cells of the posterior pituitary or neurohypophysis. AVP is synthesized by cells of the supraoptic and paraventricular nuclei before transport to the posterior pituitary (Fig. 2) [87, 128]. The biologic half-life of AVP is 5 min. The primary stimulus to AVP secretion is an increase in plasma osmolality [13, 14, 87]. Alteration in plasma osmolality are sensed by sodium-sensitive osmoreceptors located in the hypothalamus near the third ventricles and by extracerebral osmoreceptors located in the liver or portal circulation [13, 129, 130]. Hyperglycemia stimulates AVP secretion but does so through a nonosmotic pathway [131]. Changes in effective circulating volume also stimulate AVP release via baroreceptor, atrial stretch receptor, and chemoreceptor reflexes [14, 132]. Two- to three-fold increases in AVP result from as little as 10% reduction in the effective circulating volume (equivalent to a change from the supine to the upright position) [132].

AVP interacts with many hormones [133, 134]. The control of pituitary ACTH secretion exerted by AVP has received much attention [92]. AII potentiates AVP release by means of central action [134, 135]. Cortisol, catecholamines, opioid peptides, insulin, and histamine affect AVP secretion through alterations in blood volume, plasma osmolality, and blood glucose concentration [87, 136]. Numerous additional agents enhance release of AVP that include β-adrenergic agents, prostaglandin E_2, hypoxia, hypercapnia, histamine, morphine, anesthetic agents, pain, emotional arousal, and exercise [14, 128, 137].

The actions of AVP relate to osmoregulation, vasoregulation, and glucose metabolism. The solute-free water resorption action of AVP on renal distal tubules and collecting ducts is mediated via cell surface receptor signal transduction through G protein activation of adenylate cyclase [138] and protein kinase that cause microtubule-dependent insertion of membrane patches containing water channels and/or ion-specific transport channels in apical cell membranes [139, 140]. AVP causes peripheral vasoconstriction, especially in the splanchnic bed [51]. Physiologic concentrations of AVP stimulate hepatic glycogenolysis through a calcium-dependent, cAMP-independent mechanism [141], enhance hepatic gluconeogenesis [105], and inhibit hepatic ketogenesis [142].

Secretion of AVP increases following major operation, trauma, hemorrhage, sepsis, dehydration [143], and burns [144–146]. Early AVP release is mediated by reflexes related to changes in blood volume reductions. In the absence of osmolality or blood volume alterations, the prolonged (5- to 7-day) elevation of AVP following major operation is believed secondary to emotional arousal, narcotics, and incisional pain. The increased secretion of AVP that is observed following thermal injury is related to the significant reductions in blood volume observed in burn patients [147]. The secretion of AVP that occurs following hemorrhage is important in blood pressure control and, as in the case of AII [148], has been implicated in the pathophysiology of splanchnic vasoconstriction that predisposes to intestinal ischemia and bacterial translocation in the gut [149]. Increases in AVP are also implicated in paralytic ileus that can follow celiotomy [150]. The metabolic actions of AVP contribute to the hyperglycemia that follows injury; on a molar basis, AVP is more active than glucagon in this action [103, 105]. The osmotic effects of post-injury hyperglycemia act to restore effective circulating blood volume via Starling forces.

Oxytocin

Oxytocin is a nonapeptide synthesized in the supraoptic and paraventricular nucleus of the hypothalamus. Oxytocin is transported with a neurophysin substance to the posterior pituitary. Oxytocin is normally released in response to vaginal distension and suckling, but may also be released in response to increased concentration of AII or in association with emotional stimuli. Oxytoxin release is also stimulated by hypotension and reduction in plasma osmolality, but a well-defined role in the neuroendocrine response to injury has not been established.

Other Anterior Pituitary Hormones

Growth Hormone

Growth hormone (GH) is synthesized and released by acidophilic cells of the anterior pituitary. Release of GH is stimulated primarily by hypothalamic growth hormone releasing hormone (GHRH) and inhibited by somatostatin and cortisol. Release of GH is also stimulated by ACTH, AVP, thyroxine, α-melanocyte-stimulating hormone (α-MSH), testosterone, estrogens, α-adrenergic stimulation, and increasing amino acid concentrations. GH release is inhibited by β-adrenergic stimulation, hyperglycemia, and increasing plasma fatty acid concentrations. The half-life of GH is 20 min. In addition to direct effects of GH, secondary release of insulin-like growth factors (IGF I) also mediate the effects of GH. These peptides, formerly called somatomedins, are released primarily in the liver and have important metabolic effects on hepatic and skeletal muscle cells [151].

GH increases hepatocyte and skeletal muscle cell amino acid uptake and protein synthesis and inhibits hepatocyte ureagenesis [152]. GH also inhibits glucose transport, in part from inhibition of insulin action and from reduced activity of glucokinase [26]. In adipose tissue, GH stimulates lipolysis and potentiates the actions of catecholamines. GH promotes hepatic ketogenesis. IGF I mediates much, but not all, of the hepatic suppression of proteolysis [153], increased amino acid uptake, and cellular proliferation in liver and skeletal muscle and, with other growth factors, has profound effects on wound healing [154]. Interestingly, recent work suggests that growth factors such as GH and peptide mediators such as IL-6 share structural similarity in cell receptors, together constituting a hematopoietic receptor superfamily [155].

GH secretion increases following hemorrhage, injury, and anesthesia [156, 157]. Paradoxically, IGF I levels decrease following injury, correlating with injury-induced reduction in insulin secretion and observed negative nitrogen balance [158]. GH infusion will increase IGF I levels and can cause upregulation of IGF I receptors. Recent clinical studies using recombinant GH and IGF I infusions indicate that complex interactions occur among hepatocyte membrane transport mechanisms [159], skeletal muscle protein catabolism, and levels of GH, IGF I, and insulin in patients following operation as well as in those receiving hyperalimentation [160], those with sepsis [161], and those with cancer [162].

Thyroid Hormones

Hypothalamic thyrotropin releasing hormone (TRH) stimulates the release of TSH, a tripeptide that is released by basophilic anterior pituitary cells. TSH stimulates the release of thyroxine (T_4) from thyroid T_4, is converted to the most biologically potent form, triiodothyronine (T_3), in peripheral tissues. Hypothalamic TRH release and pituitary TSH release are inhibited by T_3 and T_4 [163, 164]. Pituitary TSH release is stimulated by estrogens and inhibited by T_3, cortisol, GH, somatostatin, and by fasting [70, 165, 166]. T_3 and T_4 have acute cellular effects that may be mediated by extranuclear receptors [72]. The primary actions of T_3 and T_4 are mediated by genomic signal transduction mechanisms via T_3 binding to nonhistone proteins of the nuclear chromatin to activate gene expression. The cellular effects that are thereby exerted are long-lasting (several days to a week of duration) [70]. Thyroid hormones increase oxygen consumption, heat production [167], and sympathetic nervous system activity [67]. Thyroid hormone excess, as in thyrotoxicosis, stimulates glycolysis, gluconeogenesis, glycogenolysis, proteolysis, lipolysis, and ketogenesis [70].

Even though the plasma concentrations of free and total T_3 are frequently decreased after injury or surgery, TSH secretion is not increased. This is caused by rapid conversion of T_4 to T_3 in thyrotrophic cells of the anterior pituitary [168] and the fact that T_4 and T_3 become equipotent inhibitors of TSH secretion following injury [169]. Reductions in serum TSH concentration that have been observed in burn patients are paradoxically associated with low serum concentrations of both free T_4 and free T_3 [170]. The typical net changes following injury (overall reduction in thyroid hormone activity) may persist for several weeks. This situation is similar to the euthyroid sick syndrome observed in critically ill nonsurgical patients and may be the result of an impairment in hypothalamic or pituitary secretion by corticosteroids or alterations in binding of thyroid hormones in the periphery.

Following injury, burns, and major operations, the peripheral conversion of T_4 to T_3 is impaired, resulting in reduced circulating concentrations of both free and total T_3 [171, 172]. In part, this is the result of a cortisol-mediated block of the conversion of T_4 to T_3 [172] and the result of an increased conversion of T_4 to the biologically inactive molecule reverse T_3 [173]. An increase in reverse T_3 is also characteristic of injury. Plasma total T_4 may be reduced after injury, but free T_4 concentrations usually remain normal. In fact, depressed concentrations of free T_4 are associated with poor outcomes in injured, burned, and critically ill patients.

Gonadotropins

Follicle-stimulating hormone (FSH) and luteinizing hormone (LH) are glycoproteins composed of similar α-chains and dissimilar β-chains that are synthesized and secreted by basophilic cells of the adenohypophysis. The release of these hormones is under the stimulatory influence of luteinizing hormone-releasing hormone (LHRH) and estrogens and the inhibitory influence of estrogens, progestins, prolactin, and androgens [174].

Secretion of FSH and LH is suppressed following operation, emotional stress, and burns [169, 175–178]. Gonadotropin inhibition is mediated by CRF release [179]. Decreased serum testosterone levels have also been observed after injury [175, 176]. Alterations in gonadotropin secretion may account for the menstrual dysfunction that is common following stress and trauma. Pharmacologic administration of testosterone or conjugated estrogens shortly before induced shock has been demonstrated to improve survival [180], but the significance of this finding is not fully understood. There is also evidence for interactions of the gonadal and immunologic systems that implicate cytokine-induced gonadotropin-releasing hormone (GnRH) release and gonadotropin-mediated alterations in immune competence [181, 182].

Prolactin

Prolactin is synthesized and secreted by acidophilic cells of the anterior pituitary gland in response to various emotional and physical stressors. The control of prolactin release, like that of GH, is under stimulatory and inhibitory influences. Secretion is stimulated by CRF, TRH, GHRH, and vasoactive intestinal peptide. Secretion is inhibited by GnRH and gonadotropin-associated peptide. A specific prolactin-stimulating hormone appears to operate through a serotonergic mechanism. Inhibition is mediated by a dopaminergic pathway. After section of the pituitary stalk, prolactin secretion increases, which contrasts with the decreased release observed for ACTH, TSH, GH, and the gonadotropins.

Although prolactin appears to act primarily on the breast to induce lactation and mammary development, prolactin receptors have also been identified in the kidney and liver [101]. The presence of these receptors may explain the alterations produced by prolactin on fluid, electrolyte, carbohydrate, and nitrogen metabolism. Prolactin stimulates the retention of salt, water, and potassium [101, 183]. In addition, the administration of prolactin or induction of hyperprolactinemia produces metabolic effects similar to those produced by GH. These effects include increased retention of nitrogen, increased mobilization of lipids, and carbohydrate intolerance [101]. Stimulatory effects of prolactin on lymphocyte function have been reported recently [184].

Trauma stimulates increased prolactin secretion [169]. Increases in serum prolactin levels follow exposure to ether [185], restraint [186], and hemorrhage [187], and correlate in magnitude with the extent of injury [188]. The response can vary, as in the case of severe closed head injury when prolactin secretion may diminish [189]. The increase in prolactin appears to be the result of direct stimulation, rather than suppression of tonic inhibition.

Opioid Peptides

Endogenous opioids are secreted by many cells including those located in the CNS, hypothalamus, intermediate lobe of the pituitary gland, spinal cord, sympathetic autonomic neurons, intestinal wall, and adrenal medulla [87]. These opioids derive from three precursor molecules: preproopiomelanocortin, preproenkephalin A, and preprodynorphin [190, 191]. Preproopiomelanocortin is found primarily in the anterior pituitary and is also present in other cell types [192]. Preproopiomelanocortin contains the amino acid sequences for ACTH and γ-melanocyte-stimulating hormone as well as those for the opioids, β-lipotropin, and β- and γ-endorphin [191]. Consequently, ACTH and β-endorphin are co-secreted by the pituitary gland in response to a variety of stressors [91, 193]. At least nine opiate-like substances have been found in the nervous system [194]. Anesthesia with fentanyl, a potent opiate agonist, suppresses the ACTH response to operation [195]. Elevated plasma concentrations of β-endorphin have been documented after surgery, sepsis, trauma, and hemorrhagic and septic shock [196–199].

Preproenkephalin A is found in the adrenal gland, brain, gut, and sympathetic ganglia [191]. It is a polyenkephalin from which the pentapeptides methionine-enkephalial (met-enkephalin) and leucine-enkephalin (leu-enkephalin) derive in a 4 : 1 ratio [200, 201]. The concentrations of both of these hormones have been noted to increase after acute hypotension of hemorrhage [202, 203]. Met- and leu-enkephalin and β-endorphin are found in the chromaffin granules of the adrenal medulla are released with catecholamines. Preprodynorphin is found primarily in the brain, spinal cord, and gut [191]. Preprodynorphin cleavage yields neo-β-endorphin and dynorphin, which has 200 times the analgesic potency of morphine. The physiologic significance of these compounds remains unresolved.

Receptor subtypes for opioids have been identified, namely μ, δ, and κ [204]. Morphine and fentanyl bind primarily to μ-receptors; met-enkephalin and leu-enkephalin bind to δ-receptors; and dynorphin binds to κ-receptors. Overlap in receptor binding for opiates occurs, as in the case of β-endorphin, which acts at both μ- and δ-receptors [204]. Endogenous opiates affect sensory perception, cardiovascular function, intermediary metabolism, neuroendocrine modulation, and immunologic function [91, 197, 205]. Analgesic activity is found at both μ- and δ-receptors but not at κ-receptors [204].

Opiates have been shown to cause diminished spinal cord blood flow following local trauma by central mechanisms [206]. Therapeutic potential for opioid peptides is suggested by the observation that μ-receptor blockade by naloxone improves hemodynamics and survival following hemorrhage [207], sepsis [208], and spinal shock [209–211]. Endorphins, enkephalins, and morphine (via μ- and δ-receptors) have significant cardiovascular activity: β-endorphin produces hypotension that is mediated through serotoninergic pathways [212]. Enkephalins produce hypertension and tachycardia that appears to be mediated through sympathetic reflexes [213]. Morphine produces hypotension but is not as potent as β-endorphin [214].

Centrally administered β-endorphin, like morphine, causes hyperglycemia [215]. β-Endorphin stimulates pancreatic release of insulin and glucagon [216, 217] and appears to alter glucose kinetics by central mechanisms [26]. Nonspecific opioid receptor blockade with naloxone increases glucose uptake in skeletal muscle [218], decreases gluconeogenesis in the liver and blunts the hyperglycemic response to injury [219, 220]. The fact that β-endorphin lacks any apparent effects on glucose uptake by skeletal muscle and hepatic gluconeogenesis in physiologic concentrations [221] suggests the presence of complex interactions by central, peripheral, and intermediary metabolic mechanisms.

Endogenous opiates affect several arms of neuroendocrine activity [38, 91]. β-Endorphin potentiates the release of GH, AVP, and prolactin and inhibits the release of ACTH [205]. Receptor blockade with naloxone suppresses hypoglycemia-induced elevations of GH and prolactin and potentiates ACTH release. Endogenous opioids increase adrenal catecholamine release and adrenal cortical cortisol secretion [215, 222]. Administration of morphine or its analogs stimulates release of GH [223] and AVP [224] and inhibits release of gonadotropins and TSH [87]. Administration of TRH has been proposed as an adjunct in patients with spinal shock because of antagonist effects at opiate receptors [225].

The immunologic effects of opioids are not fully clarified. In vivo suppression of lymphocyte cytotoxicity may be due to centrally mediated effects, since the actions of opioids on peripheral leukocytes demonstrate enhancement of many immunologic functions [226]. Opioid peptides are believed to influence the suppression of cytotoxicity that can accompany trauma [227] and septic shock [208]. Plasma elevation of circulating opioid levels may influence leukocyte function following trauma [199] and thermal injury [228]. On a cellular level, the intriguing possibility of a vitronectin-endorphin complex feedback loop that induces cytokine release has been recently postulated [226]. β-Endorphin binds in a highly specific manner through nonopioid sites to vitronectin after the latter, a monocyte-secreted coagulation and complement system protein (S protein), is activated by glycosaminoglycans or terminal complement factor complexes [229, 230]. Since the N-terminus of endorphin exerts chemotactic effects [231] and since vitronectin enhances monocyte phagocytosis [232], this complex may activate leukocytes to secrete cytokines that, in turn, might stimulate additional pituitary or leukocyte β-endorphin release [226]. The complex actions of these ubiquitous peptides are clinically relevant to the treatment of immunological depression and to the frequent occurrence of traumatic injury in individuals who are addicted to exogenously administered opioids.

Hormones Under Autonomic Nervous System Control

Catecholamines

The arbitrary nature of the division between the nervous system and the endocrine system is exemplified by the interchangeable and overlapping functions of the catecholamines [233, 234]. Epinephrine, produced almost exclusively by the adrenal medulla, functions primarily as a hormone. The adrenal medulla, which may be viewed as a collection of postganglionic sympathetic neurons without axons, release neurotransmitters stored in chromaffin granules into the general circulation [234]. When adrenal chromaffin cells are stimulated, the chromaffin granules are released into the extracellular fluid through calcium-medited fusion with the plasma membrane [240]. As a result, adrenomedullary catecholamine release occurs in a quantum fashion as granule packets are released. In addition to catecholamines, chromaffin granules contain dopamine, β-hydroxylase, ascorbic acid, met-enkephalin and leu-enkephalin, adenosine triphosphate, and chromogranins [241].

Norepinephrine, dopamine, and to a lesser extent, epinephrine, are released at sympathetic nerve terminals to function as neurotransmitters and are present in the plasma by spillover from the synaptic cleft [235, 236]. The SNS exerts rapid effects, particularly on the cardiovascular system, whereas catecholamine secretion from the adrenal medulla tends to occur more slowly and exerts more lasting effects on metabolic processes. These distinctions are generalizations, however, and the interactions of SNS, adrenomedullary secretion, and intermediary metabolism are active areas of investigation [237–239].

Although multiple stimuli including hypoxia, hypovolemia, hypoglycemia, pain, and fear cause catecholamine secretion, the exact mechanisms involved in the adrenomedullary control of catecholamine secretion remain poorly understood [242]. Nonhypotensive hemorrhage, which is a potent stimulus for SNS activation, does not increase the adrenomedullary secretion of catecholamines [43]. The latter occurs only when hypotension develops [42]. Increased chemoreceptor drive and decreased high-pressure baroreceptor drive may have minimal effects on adrenomedullary catecholamine secretion when the reflexes are examined in isolation [45, 243]. Conversely, SNS-mediated adrenomedullary catecholamine secretion can occur in the absence of increased cardiac or renal sympathetic nerve activity [244]. SNS activity can be graded and may be distinct from adrenomedullary activation.

The actions of epinephrine and norepinephrine as hormones may be broadly classified as metabolic, hemodynamic, or modulatory. In the liver, epinephrine stimulates glycogenolysis [245], gluconeogenesis [246, 247], lipolysis, and ketogenesis [246]. Among these hepatic actions, epinephrine is the most potent in stimulating glycogenolysis [89]. In adipose tissue, epinephrine increases lipolysis [115], while in skeletal muscle it increases glycogenolysis and inhibits insulin-stimulated glucose uptake [248]. As a result of these actions, epinephrine appears to mediate insulin resistance (stress-induced hyperglycemia) by increasing hepatic glucose production and by decreasing peripheral glucose uptake. Using minimal mathematical models of glucose metabolism, epinephrine has been recently shown to cause impaired acute-phase insulin-induced insulin secretion in humans [239]. Sympathetic blockade by spinal anesthesia blunts the normal insulin response to glucose and arginine and increases the response of glucagon to arginine infusion [237].

The hormonal effects of catecholamines include β-receptor-mediated increases in renin [249] and parathyroid hormone release [250], α-receptor-mediated inhibition of insulin and glucagon secretion, and β-receptor-mediated stimulation of insulin and glucagon secretion [18, 251]. The hormonal effects of catecholamines are dependent on the receptor density and sensitivity of the effector cells. This is observed for the α- and β-islet cells in the pancreas, which secrete glucagon and insulin, respectively, and contain both α- and β-adrenergic receptors. Since the density of α-adrenergic receptors of the β-islet cells is greater than that of the α-islet cells, catecholamine and SNS stimulation of the pancreas results in increased secretion of glucagon and decreased secretion of insulin.

The hemodynamic effects of catecholamines are dose-dependent and include α_1-mediated venous and arterial vasoconstriction; β_2-mediated arterial vasodilatation; and β_1-mediated increases in myocardial rate, contractility, and sinus node recovery period [240]. In low doses, epinephrine acts primarily at β_1- and β_2-receptors, whereas at high doses epinephrine acts primarily at α_1-receptors. In normal physiologic circumstances, norepinephrine is most important in the β_1 and α_2 actions of catecholamines, whereas epinephrine is responsible for β_2 effects [115]. The hemodynamic effects of dopamine are mediated through both dopaminergic and adrenergic receptors. In low circulating concentrations or low doses, dopamine causes renal vasodilatation through dopaminergic receptor action. At greater concentrations, dopamine acts at β- and eventually at α-receptors [252].

Secretion of epinephrine and norepinephrine increases immediately following injury [253]. Increases in each hormone do not always change in parallel; the ratio of epinephrine to norepinephrine varies according to the stimulus. Hemorrhage, a potent stimulus to adrenomedullary secretion, decreases the epinephrine-to-norepinephrine ratio, whereas hypoglycemia maintains it [254]. After elective operation, catecholamine increases are small, and norepinephrine may not increase [237, 253, 255]. Peak plasma catecholamine concentrations are achieved 24–48 h following stimuli, especially in circumstances that involve loss of effective circulating blood volume. Maximal secretion correlates with the Injurity Severity Score [253]. The fact that SNS norepinephrine metabolism does not occur in a single compartment system complicates the interpretation of simple plasma catecholamine levels [236] and underscores the need for further detailed analysis of acute catecholamine kinetics in trauma patients.

Renin and Angiotensin

Renin exists in an inactive form, prorenin, in the myoepithelial cells of the renal afferent arterioles [256]. Proteolytic cleavage of the zymogen and the release of renin are under the control of three intrarenal receptors and the influences of several hormones and ions [19]. The macula densa receptor senses the concentration of chloride in tubular fluid as it passes through the distal nephron. Decreased chloride ion concentration in the tubular fluid stimulates renin release. The neurogenic receptor of the juxtaglomerular apparatus increases renin release by β-adrenergic stimulation. The third renal receptor, the juxtaglomerular cell, acts as a stretch receptor that increases renin release with reduction in stretch (decreased blood pressure). Additional ions and hormones that alter the secretion of renin include potassium, magnesium, calcium, ACTH, AVP, prostaglandins, and glucagon [11].

Renin substrate is converted to angiotensin I in the circulation. The secretion of renin substrate, which is produced by the liver, is increased by ACTH, corticosteroids, and AII [15]. Angiotensin I acts primarily as the precursor for the formation of AII, a process that is mediated in the pulmonary circulation by angiotensin-converting enzyme. Angiotensin-converting enzyme (ACE) also potentiates the release of catecholamines by the adrenal medulla and redistributes blood flow to the renal cortex by decreasing blood flow to the renal medulla [257].

The actions of AII may be broadly classified according to effects on hemodynamics, fluid and electrolyte balance, hormonal regulation, metabolism, and surrounding cells. AII is a potent vasoconstrictor [258] that is vital to the maintenance of normal blood pressure and is implicated in the pathogenesis of hypertension. Additional hemodynamic effects include tachycardia, increased contractility, and increased vascular permeability [15]. The profound effects of AII on fluid and electrolyte homeostasis are mediated by potent stimulation of aldosterone synthesis and secretion, increases in AVP secretion [15], and regulation of thirst

[259]. AII increases CRH release via increased ACTH release [260] and potentiates
the effects of ACTH on the adrenal cortex [261]. AII, like ACE, potentiates the
release of epinephrine by the adrenal medulla [260] and increases sympathetic
neurotransmission [15]. The metabolic actions of AII include the stimulation of
glycogenolysis and gluconeogenesis in the liver through a cAMP-independent, calcium-dependent mechanism [105]. In addition, recent studies have demonstrated a
blood-flow dependent effect of the renin-AII system on insulin action and whole
body glucose utilization [262]. Further evidence for metabolic effects for the renin
system include the fact that insulin and IGF I are secretagogues for AII [263].
Immunologic interactions for the renin system have also been observed: TNF and
IL-1 act as secretagogues for renin release. Interestingly, recent work has observed
mitogen action for AII for human mesangial cells, an action that is partly mediated
by the potent endothelial cell vasoconstrictor, endothelin [264].

Aldosterone

Aldosterone is synthesized and secreted by cells of the adrenal zona glomerulosa in
response to three primary stimuli: AII, ACTH, and potassium ion concentration.
AII is a potent stimulator of aldosterone secretion that acts through a calcium-dependent, cAMP-independent [265, 266] enhancement of the conversion of cholesterol to pregnenolone and of corticosterone to 18-hydroxycorticosterone and aldosterone [267, 268]. Among these steps, the early conversion of cholesterol to
pregnenolone appears to be the most important in the AII-stimulation of aldosterone secretion [267]. ACTH stimulates aldosterone secretion through a calcium-
dependent, cAMP-dependent pathway [265, 266, 268]. ACTH, like angiotensin,
stimulates the early conversion of cholesterol to pregnenolone [267], but does not
appear to stimulate the later steps of aldosterone biosynthesis in humans [267].
Elevation of serum potassium stimulates aldosterone secretion via calcium-
dependent, cAMP-independent increases in the conversion of cholesterol to
pregnenolone [241, 265, 266].

There is also evidence that a pituitary-produced aldosterone-stimulating factor
or hormone (ASF) exists in humans [269]. This glycoprotein has been isolated in
the urine of normal but not of hypophysectomized humans and stimulates aldosterone secretion in vitro [270]. In addition, ASF also causes hypertension and hyper-
aldosteronism in experimental models. Immunofluorescent studies have located it
in the anterior pituitary gland [269], but the exact structure has not been determined.

On a molar basis, ACTH is the most potent stimulator of aldosterone production
[241]. As a result, stress-induced elevations in aldosterone are most likely mediated
through ACTH. However, the stimulatory effects of ACTH on aldosterone production are short-lived; a phenomenon that has been attributed either to down-regula-
tion of ACTH on zona glomerulosa cells or to inhibition of AII synthesis by an increase in the effective circulating volume [241, 271]. This short-lived potency
suggests ACTH has a minor role in the overall control of aldosterone secretion in
chronic states [241]. In chronic conditions, AII is most likely the primary stimulus

for aldosterone secretion. This is supported by the finding that ACTH-deficient persons respond with an appropriate increase in aldosterone release during sodium restriction [271, 272].

The existence of an inhibitory dopaminergic pathway that blocks the later stages of aldosterone synthesis is suggested [241]. This may explain the fact that metaclopropramide, a dopamine antagonist, causes increased secretion of aldosterone, whereas bromocriptine, a dopamine agonist, inhibits the ACTH- or AII-induced secretion of aldosterone but does not alter the basal secretory rate of aldosterone [273]. The dopaminergic pathway may be important in mediating changes in the secretion of aldosterone in response to alterations in the plasma sodium concentration or to the effective circulating volume [274, 275].

The primary actions of aldosterone are increased reabsorption of sodium and of chloride in the early distal convoluted tubule of the kidney epithelia and the gastrointestinal tract. Aldosterone also promotes sodium reabsorption and potassium secretion in the late distal convoluted tubules and the early collecting ducts [86, 271]. On a cellular level, aldosterone acts by binding to surface receptors (rapid response) and by forming activated nuclear-bound complexes similar to those of other steroids (genomic response). The proteins that are induced by aldosterone stimulate an increase in the number of membrane sodium-specific channels and increase the activities of mitochondrial enzymes that generate adenosine triphosphate [63].

Atrial Natriuretic Peptides

Atrial natriuretic peptides (ANP, also termed atrial natriuretic factors) are released by the CNS and by neurosecretory granules in left atrial myocytes in response to changes in atrial wall tension [87]. The biologic half-life of these peptides is approximately 3 min. Centrally, ANP reduces the secretion of AVP from the posterior pituitary [276] and inhibits AVP peripheral action [277]. AVP also stimulates ANP secretion [278]. ANP inhibits aldosterone secretion and blocks perirenal tubular reabsorption of sodium, but the role of ANP in normal control of fluid and electrolyte balance remains controversial [279]. ANP promotes excretion of sodium and water and lowers blood pressure [280]. ANP secretion is also stimulated by angiotensin, AVP, α- and β-agonists, and endothelin. Metabolic effects for ANP are suggested by the finding of ANP-modulation of ACTH, AVP, and AII responses to acute hypoglycemia [281].

Secretion of ANP is unaffected by coronary artery bypass operation [282] but does change during atrial pacing [283] and after surgical reconstructions that involve the atria [284]. ANP may function to balance the effects of the renin-angiotensin-aldosterone system following activation by injury [285]. ANP inhibits the vasopressor effects of norepinephrine and AII and suppresses the release of ACTH and AVP following hemorrhage [286]. Fluid resuscitation does not appear to alter plasma ANP following experimental hemorrhage [287]. Increases in ANP that typically occur following injury are secondary to increased tension of the atrial wall from tachycardia, rather than blood volume contraction (which would decrease ANP secretion) [288]. The most important role for ANP, thought to be the protection of the heart from large acute increases in blood volume [289], may be important in the physiologic response to blunt chest trauma and to acute massive volume resuscitation. The precise physiologic role of ANP in fluid balance and in the metabolic responses to injury remains incompletely understood.

Insulin

Synthesis and secretion of insulin by pancreatic β-islet cells are controlled by the concentration of circulating substrate (glucose, amino acids, and free fatty acids), the activity of the autonomic nervous system, and the direct and indirect effects of several hormones. Increases in the plasma concentration of glucose stimulate the secretion of insulin through central glucoreceptors and through direct pancreatic β-cell activation. Decreases in the concentration of glucose inhibit insulin secretion through similar pathways [251]. The secretion of insulin is also stimulated by increases in amino acids and possibly by increases in free fatty acids and ketone bodies. Under normal physiologic conditions, the plasma concentration of glucose is the most important controller of insulin secretion. However, during injury and stress, the effect of glucose is blunted by neural and humoral mechanisms (termed insulin resistance) [290].

As noted previously, pancreatic β-islet cells have a greater density of α-adrenergic receptors that inhibit insulin secretion than of β-adrenergic receptors that stimulate insulin secretion. As a result, sympathetic stimulation of the pancreas or increases in circulating epinephrine or norepinephrine inhibit insulin secretion. In contrast, the infusion of isoproterenol, a pure β-agonist, results in an increase in the secretion of insulin. Parasympathetic stimulation of the pancreas also increases insulin secretion [18].

Somatostatin is a potent inhibitor of insulin secretion through direct action on the β-islet cells [291]. In contrast, β-endorphin [216], glucagon [292], cortisol [88], estrogen, progesterone, and parathyroid hormone produce hyperinsulinism [30, 88, 216, 293]. Whereas glucagon and β-endorphin increase insulin secretion through a direct action on pancreatic β-cells, cortisol appears to increase insulin secretion by interfering with peripheral insulin activity [293]. Recent work also suggests that insulin release may be mediated by nitric oxide, an endogenous oxygen free radical that causes vasodilatation, and may partially account for the secretagogue properties of arginine [294].

Insulin, by promoting the storage of carbohydrate, protein, and lipid, is the primary anabolic hormone of the body. Although the actions of insulin are primarily on the liver, skeletal muscle, and adipose tissue, it affects most tissues. Notable exceptions include hematopoietic, CNS, and wounded tissues. Insulin promotes the entry of glucose into cells by stimulating glucose membrane transport. The increased intracellular concentrations of glucose are used in glycogenesis and in glycolysis [246]. By stimulating these processes concurrently, the energy necessary for glycogen synthesis is made available by glycolysis. Insulin also inhibits gluconeogenesis in the liver by inhibiting phosphoenolpyruvate carboxylase and by stimulating phosphofructokianse and pyruvate kinase [105, 295].

The major action of insulin in protein metabolism is to promote protein synthesis. This is accomplished by increasing the transport of amino acids into the liver and other peripheral tissues and by inhibiting gluconeogenesis and amino acid oxidation [293]. The actions of insulin on lipid metabolism are directed toward the stimulation of lipid synthesis and the inhibition of lipid degradation. By stimulating lipoprotein lipase, insulin makes triglycerides more available for uptake from the plasma by adipose tissue and by the liver. Glycerol synthesis from glucose and the pentose phosphate shunt are also stimulated by insulin, to provide the elements necessary for lipid synthesis.

Insulin release and activity is suppressed following operation and during the acute phase of injury [237, 255, 296]. This is the result of direct effects on pancreatic islet cell release and catecholamine-related alterations in insulin and glucose activity [239]. Sympathetic blockade by spinal anesthesia blunts the normal insulin response to glucose and arginine and increases the response of glucagon to arginine infusion [237].

Glucagon

Synthesis and secretion of glucagon by the pancreatic α-islet cells are controlled by the concentrations of circulating substrates (glucose, amino acids, and fatty acids), the efferent activity of the central and the autonomic nervous systems, and the action of circulating and paracrine hormones.

As in the case of insulin under normal conditions, the primary stimuli to glucagon release are glucose, amino acids, and exercise [105]. Hyperglycemia stimulates glucagon secretion primarily from a direct action of glucose on the pancreatic α-cell [292]. The potency of different amino acids to stimulate glucagon secretion is variable and unrelated to their ability to stimulate insulin secretion. In general, gluconeogenic amino acids have greater stimulatory effects than nongluconeogenic amino acids [30]. The ability of amino acids to stimulate glucagon secretion is critical for the maintenance of euglycemia when a protein meal is ingested. If this were not the case, the unopposed stimulation of insulin secretion by amino acids after a protein meal would result in hypoglycemia, through a decrease in hepatic glucose production, an increase in protein synthesis, and an increase in glucose uptake in skeletal muscle. However, in the presence of glucagon, the liver increases its production of glucose to oppose the action of insulin and maintain glucose homeostasis [297].

The potency of glucose and amino acids to alter glucagon and insulin secretion depends on the route of administration. Ingestion of a protein meal results in a greater increase in glucagon and insulin secretion than that seen following the intravenous administration of similar concentrations of amino acids [298]. Ingestion of glucose results in greater alterations in insulin and glucagon secretion than that observed following intravenous administration of a similar glucose load [299]. These phenomena may be mediated through the presentation of greater concentrations of substrate to the pancreas by venous drainage from the gastrointestinal tract, through the potentiation by gastrointestinal hormones of substrate-induced pancreatic secretion, or through the effects of neural inputs to the pancreas that are activated by oral ingestion [30]. Pharmacologic administration of cholecystokinin, gastrin, vasoactive intestinal peptide, substance P, neurotensin, and gastric inhibitory peptide (GIP) cause increased secretion of glucagon and insulin [30, 291, 292].

Although the physiologic role of gastrointestinal hormones in the control of pancreatic hormonal secretion is complex, gastrin in physiologic concentrations appears to potentiate amino acid-stimulated release of glucagon and insulin, and GIP appears to potentiate glucose-mediated inhibition of glucagon secretion and stimulation of insulin secretion [292]. Other hormones that increase glucagon secretion include β-endorphin, insulin, and cortisol [216]. Somatostatin is the major hormone that inhibits glucagon secretion [291].

The autonomic nervous system mechanisms controlling glucagon release are opposite to those for insulin: activation of α-adrenergic receptors stimulates glucagon secretion and activation of β-adrenergic receptors or of the parasympathetic efferents to the pancreas inhibits glucagon release [18]. However, unlike the β-islet cell, the α-islet has a much greater density of α-adrenergic receptors than of β-adrenergic receptors. As a consequence, increases in epinephrine or norepinephrine and SNS stimulation of the pancreas cause increases rather than decreases in glucagon secretion.

The physiologic actions of glucagon are limited primarily to the liver and are mediated through an increase in cAMP [105, 246]. Glucagon promotes glycogenolysis and gluconeogenesis [105, 246]. Although glucagon does not increase amino acid transport into the liver *per se,* glucagon does direct amino acids toward gluconeogenesis [300]. The net result is an increase in hepatic glucose production that under basal conditions accounts for 75% of the glucose produced by the liver [292]. In the absence of cortisol, the peak action of glucagon is very brief. In the presence of cortisol, the duration of action for glucagon is prolonged and the initial increase in hepatic glucose is greater [5]. Nevertheless, the effects of glucagon are not long lasting [301]. After 30–60 min, the activity assigned to glucagon decreases, even if the plasma glucagon concentration remains elevated, unless levels again increase (termed "burst effect") [301]. Glucagon also stimulates lipolysis in the liver and in adipose tissue [301], inhibits triglyceride synthesis, and stimulates ketogenesis.

The activity of glucagon is important during the metabolic response to starvation and injury because of effects to increase hepatic glucose production and hepatic ketogenesis. Most studies have observed a delay of approximately 12 h before increases in glucagon occur following injury [253]. In fact, the hyperglycemia that immediately follows injury has been shown to be independent of glucagon secretion [302]. Typically, postoperative glucagon levels fall immediately, then rise to baseline at 6–12 h, increase above baseline level 12 h later, and return to normal after 3 days [303, 304]. Early elevations in serum glucose, reductions in insulin, elevations in catecholamines, and gradually rising glucagon levels are characteristic of the acute response to operation and injury mediated by the SNS.

Somatostatin

Somatostatin, a tetradecapeptide, is a potent inhibitor of both insulin and glucagon secretion (251, 291). In addition to pancreatic δ-cells, somatostatin is found in the hypothalamus, limbic system, brainstem, spinal cord, other neural tissue, salivary glands, parafollicular thyroid cells, and kidney and gastrointestinal tissue [291]. Somatostatin, originally named for its ability to inhibit GH secretion, is now known to inhibit the secretion of TSH, renin, insulin, glucagon, calcitonin, and gastrointestinal hormones such as gastrin, secretin, and cholecystokinin [291]. In addition, somatostatinergic nerve fibers are involved in the projection of impulses from peripheral sensory organs to the neuroaxis [291].

The role of somatostatin in the physiologic regulation of insulin and glucagon secretion is not fully understood. The plasma half-life of somatostatin is approximately 2 min. The α, β, and δ cells have somatostatin receptors that inhibit the secretion of glucagon, insulin, and somatostatin, respectively. Somatostatin acts as a paracrine substance [251, 291]. However, recent evidence suggests that somatostatin reaching the pancreas through the bloodstream may be more important in the control of pancreatic secretion than that produced locally. The effects of somatostatin on α-cells are transient, but the effects on β-cells are long-acting [251]. The difference may account for the relative hyperglycemia that occurs in patients with tumors that produce somatostatin or after long-term somatostatin administration [251]. Complex metabolic changes observed after infusion of somatostatin in burn patients suggests that interesting physiologic roles for this compound will be found with further study [305].

Insulin-Like Growth Factors

The somatomedins are a family of polypeptides that stimulate proteoglycan synthesis in cartilage and DNA synthesis and cell replication in a variety of cell types [306]. Named because of their ability to mediate some of the actions of GH, such as sulfation of cartilage and other aspects of cell growth, the somatomedins possess insulin-like actions. Somatomedin activity includes increased glucose uptake and protein synthesis in skeletal muscle [307, 308], increased glucose uptake and oxidation and increased lipid synthesis in adipose tissue [306], increased protein synthesis and glycogenesis in the liver [309, 310], and decreased glucagon-stimulated hepatic gluconeogenesis [174].

Concurrent with the discovery of the somatomedins, it was learned that human plasma contains large amounts of (noninsulin) insulin-like activity [306]. This nonsuppressible insulin-like activity (NSILA) contains all the known metabolic actions of insulin and is divisible into two chemically and biologically related polypeptides, NSILA-I and NSILA-II. In addition to their insulin-like effects, these two proteins have marked effects on cell growth. As a result, they are now referred to as IGF I and IGF II. At present, it appears that somatomedin C, somatomedin A, and IGF I, are the same molecule [311]. Somatomedin B is the same molecule as epidermal growth factor. A relationship between IGF II and the other somatomedins has not been established.

The somatomedins are found in large quantities in human plasma, primarily as an inactive bound form. Somatomedins have been isolated from liver, muscle, fibroblasts, and kidney and have been shown to have a molecular weight of less than 10,000 [312]. The exact physiologic role of the somatomedins and of IGFs are not yet fully understood, but it is clearly known that the stimulation of protein synthesis by GH is primarily mediated by IGF I.

After injury, IGF I secretion decreases and correlates well with the negative nitrogen balance that is commonly observed in the post-traumatic state [313]. This decrease may in large part be the result of the starvation that accompanies injury because the plasma concentration of IGF is also depressed during fasting [314]. Recent studies of the effects of recombinant IGF I infusion suggest that nitrogen loss [315] and gut atrophy and bacterial translocation [316] may be reduced by administration of this peptide.

Parathyroid Hormone

Parathyroid hormone (PTH), which is synthesized in the parathyroid glands, is not stored in large quantities [317]. As a result, large increases in the secretion of PTH must be accompanied by an increase in PTH synthesis. The major regulator of PTH synthesis and secretion is the serum concentration of ionized calcium [318]. The secretion of PTH varies inversely with the ionized calcium concentration [319]. Within the normal range of serum calcium, small changes in the serum calcium concentration produce small, inverse changes in the secretion of PTH. In contrast, outside the normal range of calcium, small changes in the serum calcium concentration are accompanied by large, inverse changes in the secretion of PTH. Calcium-induced PTH secretion involves cAMP and is affected by magnesium [319]. Although the precise role of the SNS in PTH release is not known, parathyroid cells contain β-adrenergic receptors and PTH release has been observed with infusion of epinephrine and isoproterenol [250, 320]. Unlike glucagon and calcitonin, which stimulate PTH through decrease in the extracellular calcium, epinephrine-induced PTH stimulation appears to be independent of extracellular calcium and may be mediated through intracellular cAMP [317, 319]. The physiologic importance of catecholamine-mediated PTH secretion remains unknown.

The primary target organs for PTH are the kidneys and bone. In the kidneys, PTH increases the distal tubular resorption of calcium, decreases the proximal resorption of phosphorus, and stimulates the renal conversion of 1-hydroxyvitamin D to 1,25-dihydroxyvitamin D (calcitriol) which stimulates the intestinal absorption of calcium and phosphorus. In bone, PTH stimulates calcium mobilization, bone resorption, and bone remodeling. The PTH response to injury has not been fully established.

Summary

The biological response to injury is transmitted through neuroendocrine changes, the release of mediator substances, and alterations in cellular and intermediary metabolism that are tailored to the magnitude and nature of the injury. Primary stimuli to this endocrine response include alterations in effective circulating volume, changes in oxygen, carbon dioxide, or hydrogen ion concentration, the presence of pain, changes in substrate availability, alterations in temperature, and ongoing infection. These stimuli are transduced by specialized receptors to provide afferent signals that are further integrated and modulated by the central and peripheral nervous systems. Efferent output is then engaged through multiple coordinated systems by the hypothalamic-pituitary axis and by the autonomic nervous system. Hormone-induced target cell actions occur through signal transduction mechanisms acting by genomic transcription (e.g., lipid-permeable hormones such as corticosteroids and thyroid hormones) and by ligand binding to cell surface receptors (e.g., catecholamines and insulin). Hormonal signal transduction mechanisms on target cells can involve the activity of enzymes (e.g., kinases), guanine nucleotide-binding proteins (G proteins), and ligand-gated ion channels. Intracellular second messengers include cAMP, cGMP, inositol triphosphate, and calcium ion.

The endocrine response during the acute, catabolic phase of injury is enacted by hormones primarily under the control of hypothalamic-pituitary axis and the autonomic nervous system. Hormones of hypothalamic-pituitary systems include those of the anterior pituitary, CRF–ACTH–cortisol adrenal system, AVP, oxytocin, prolactin, GH, thyroid hormones, gonadotropins, and opioid peptides. Hormones under the primary direction of the autonomic nervous system include the catecholamines, renin and angiotensin, aldosterone, ANP, insulin, glucagon, somatostatin, somatomedins, and, perhaps, PTH. In general, injury and operation cause increased release of all hypothalamic-pituitary axis hormones with the exception of thyroid hormones and the gonadotropins. Hormones primarily controlled by the autonomic nervous system are also increased early following injury, with the exception of insulin and the insulin-like growth factors. Further understanding of the dynamic neuroendocrine response to injury using tools of molecular and cellular physiology, recombinant genetic methods, mathematical models of hormone and substrate kinetics, and controlled clinical trials and observations will launch this exciting field of study into the next century with improved understanding and physiologically directed therapy.

References

1. Cuthbertson DP (1932) Observations on the disturbances of metabolism by injury to the limbs. Q J Med 1:233
2. Cannon WB (1939) The wisdom of the body. Norton, New York
3. Yates FE (1982) Outline of a physical theory of physiological systems. Can J Physiol Pharmacol 60:217–248
4. Waddington CH (1968) The basic ideas of biology. In: Waddington DH (ed) Towards a theoretical biology. Aldine, Chicago
5. Egdahl RH (1959) Pituitary-adrenal response following trauma to the isolated leg. Surgery 46:9–21
6. Hume DM, Egdahl RH (1959) The importance of the brain in the neuroendocrine response to injury. Ann Surg 150:697–712
7. Hume DM, Bell CL, Bartter F (1962) Direct measurement of adrenal secretion during operative trauma and convalescence. Surgery 52:174–187
8. Longnecker DE, McCoy S, Drucker WR (1979) Anesthetic influence on response to hemorrhage in rats. Circ Shock 6:55–60

9. Zimpfer M, Manders WT, Barger AC, Vatner SF (1982) Pentobarbital alters compensatory neural and humoral mechanisms in response to hemorrhage. Am J Physiol 243:H713–21

10. Weissman C, Hollinger I (1988). Modifying systemic responses with anesthetic techniques. Anesthesiol Clin North Am 6:221–236

11. Baertschi AJ, Ward DG, Gann DS (1976) Role of atrial receptors in the control of ACTH. Am J Physiol 231:692–699

12. Gann DS, Ward DG, Baertschi AJ, Carlson DE, Maran JW (1977) Neural control of ACTH release in response to hemorrhage. Ann NY Acad Sci 297:477–497

13. Kircheim HR (1976) Systemic arterial baroreceptor reflexes. Physiol Rev 56:100

14. Korner PI (1971) Integrative neural cardiovascular control. Physiol Rev 51:312–367

15. Peach MJ (1977) Renin-angiotensin system: biochemistry and mechanism of action. Physiol Rev 57:313–370

16. Reid IA, Ganong WF (1977) Control of aldosterone secretion. In: Genest J, Kolw E, Kuchel O (eds) Hypertension. McGraw-Hill, New York

17. Gerich JE, Karam JH, Forsham PH (1973) Stimulation of glucagon secretion by epinephrine in man. J Clin Endocrinol Metab 37:479–481

18. Porte DJ, Smith PH, Ensinck JW (1976) Neurohumoral regulation of the pancreatic islet A and B cells. Metabolism 25:1453–1456

19. Fray JCS, Luch DJ, Valentine AND (1983) Cellular mechanisms of renin secretion. Fed Proc 42:3150–3154

20. Guyton AC (1986) Arterial pressure regulation. I. Rapid pressure control by nervous reflexes and other mechanisms. In: Guyton AC (ed) Textbook, of medical physiology. Saunders, Philadelphia, pp 244–256

21. Guyton AC (1980) Arterial pressure and hypertension. Saunders, Philadelphia

22. Coleridge JCG, Coleridge HM (1979) Chemoreflex regulation of the heart. In: Berne RM (ed) Handbook of physiology, sect. 2: The cardiovascular system. William and Wilkins, Baltimore, pp 653–676

23. West JB (1985) Control of ventilation. In: West JB (ed) Physiological basis of medical practice. Baltimore, pp 605–612

24. Gann DS, Dallman MF, Engeland WC (1981) Reflex control and modulation of ACTH and corticosteroids. In: McCann SM (ed) Endocrine physiology III: international review of physiology. University Park Press, Baltimore, pp 157

25. Cannon WB (1939) The wisdom of the body. Norton, New York

26. Frohman LA (1983) CNS peptides and glucoregulation. Annu Rev Physiol 45:95–107

27. Gerich JE, Chaires MA et al. (1976) Regulation of pancreatic insulin and glucagon secretion. Annu Rev Physiol 38:353–388

28. Metz SA, Halter JB, Robertson RP (1978) Induction of defective insulin secretion and impaired glucose tolerance uptake by clonidine: selective stimulation of metabolic α-adrenergic pathways. Diabetes 27:554–562

29. Miller RE (1981) Pancreatic neuroendocrinology: peripheral neural mechanisms in the regulation of the islets of Langerhans. Endocrinol Rev 4:417–494

30. Porte D, Halter JB (1981) The endocrine pancreas and diabetes mellitus. In: Williams RH (ed) Textbook of endocrinology. Saunders, Philadelphia

31. Bernheim HA, Block LH, Atkins E (1979) Fever: pathogenesis, pathophysiology, and purpose. Ann Intern Med 91:261–270

32. Hensel H (1973) Neural processes in thermoregulation. Physiol Rev 53:948–1017

33. Hume DM, Egdhal RH (1959) Effect of hypothermia and of cold exposure on adrenal cortical and medullary secretion. Ann NY Acad Sci 80:435–444

34. Wood CE, Shinsako J, Keil LC, Ramsay DJ, Dallman MF (1981) Hormonal and hemodynamic responses to 15 ml/kg hemorrhage in conscious dogs: responses correlate to body temperature. Proc Soc Exp Biol Med 167:15–19

35. Egdahl RH, Nelson DH, Hume DM (1955) Adrenal cortical function in hypothermia. Surg Gynecol Obstet 101:715–720

36. Egdahl RH (1959) The differential response of the adrenal cortex and medulla to bacterial endotoxin. J Clin Invest 38:1120–1125

37. Lilly M, Gann DS (1992) The hypothalalmic-pituitary-adrenal-immune axis. Surgery 127:1463–1474

38. Blalock JE (1989) A molecular basis for bidirectional communication between the immune and neuroendocrine systems. Physiol Rev 69:1–32
39. Woloski BM, Smith EM, Meyer WJ III, Fuller GM, Blalock JE (1985) Corticotropin releasing activity of monokines. Science 230:1035–1037
40. Olberg B, White S (1970) Circulatory effects of interruption and stimulation of cardiac vagal afferents. Acta Physiol Scand 80:383–394
41. Pelletier LL, Edis AJ, Shepard JT (1971) Circulatory reflex from vagal afferents in response to hemorrhage in the dog. Circ Res 29:626–634
42. Engeland WC, Demsher DP, Byrnes GJ, Presnell K, Gann DS (1981) The adrenal medullary response to graded hemorrhage in awake dogs. Endocrinology 109:1539–1544
43. Zileli MS, Gedik P, Adalar N, Caglar S (1974) Adrenal medullary response to removal of various amounts of blood. Endocrinology 95:1477–1481
44. Achtel RA, Downing SE (1972) Ventricular responses to hypoxemia following chemoreceptor denervation and adrenalectomy. Am Heart J 84:377–386
45. Fater DC, Sundet WD, Schultz HD, Goetz KL (1983) Arterial baroreceptors have minimal physiological effects on adrenal medullary secretion. Am J Physiol 224:H194–H200
46. Bereiter DA, Zaid AM, Gann DS (1986) Effect of rate of hemorrhage on sympathoadrenal catecholamine release in cats. Am J Physiol 250:E69–E75
47. Bie P (1980) Osmoreceptors, vasopressin, and control of renal water excretion. Physiol Rev 60:961–1048
48. Schrier RW, Berl WT, Anderson RJ (1979) Osmotic and non-osmotic control of vasopressin release. Am J Physiol 236:F321–F332
49. Quest JA, Gebber GL (1972) Modulation of baroreceptor reflexes by somatic afferent nerve stimulation. Am J Physiol 222:1251–1259
50. Sato A, Schmidt RF (1973) Somatosympathetic reflexes: afferent fibers, central pathways, discharge characteristics. Physiol Rev 53:916–947
51. Cowley AW, Quitlen EW, Skelton MM (1983) Role of vasopressin in cardiovascular regulation. Fed Proc 42:3170–3176
52. Goldman WF, Saum WR (1984) A direct excitatory action of catecholamines on rat aortic baroreceptors in vitro. Circ Res 55:18–30
53. Holmes AE, Ledsome JR (1984) Effect of norepinephrine and vasopressin on carotid sinus baroreceptor activity in the anesthetized rabbit. Experientia 40:825–827
54. Engeland WC, Byrnes GJ, Gann DS (1982) The pituitary adrenocortical response to hemorrhage depends on the time of day. Endocrinology 110:1856–1860
55. Overman RR, S.G. W (1947) The contributory role of the afferent nervous factor in experimental shock: sublethal hemorrhage and sciatic nerve stimulation. Am J Physiol 148:289–295
56. Bereiter DA, Plotsky PM, Gann DS (1982) Tooth pulp stimulation potentiates the ACTH response to hemorrhage in cats. Endocrinology 111:1127–1132
57. Gann DS, Cryer GL, Pirkle JC Jr. (1977) Physiological inhibition and facilitation in adrenocortical response to hemorrhage. Am J Physiol 232:R5–R9
58. Lilly MP, Engeland WC, Gann DS (1982) Adrenal response to repeated hemorrhage: implications for studies of trauma. J Trauma 22:809–814
59. Lilly MP, Gann DS (1982) The effect of repeated operation on the response of the adrenal cortex to infused ACTH. Surg Forum 33:10
60. Raff H, Sinsako J, Sallman MF (1983) Surgery potentiates adrenocortical responses to hypoxia in dogs. Proc Soc Exp Biol Med 172:400–406
61. Reichlin S (1993) Neuroendocrine-immune interactions. N Engl J Med 329:1246–1253
62. Kahn CR, Smith RJ, Chin WW (1992) Mechanism of action of hormones that act at the cell surface. In: Wilson JD, Foster DW (eds) Williams textbook of endocrinology. Saunders, Philadelphia, pp 91–135
63. Clark JH, Schrader WT, O'Malley BW (1992) Mechanisms of action of steroid hormones. In: Wilson JD, Foster DW (eds) Williams textbook of endocrinology. Saunders, Philadelphia, pp 35–90
64. Sutherland EW (1972) Studies on the mechanism of hormone action. Science 177:401–408
65. O'Malley BW, Schrader WT (1976) The receptors of steroid hormones. Sci Am 234:32–43
66. Oppenheimer JH (1979) Thyroid hormone action at the cellular level. Science 203:971–979
67. Sterlin K (1979) Thyroid hormone action at the cell level. N Engl J Med 300:117–123

68. Evans RM (1988) The steroid and thyroid hormone receptor superfamily. Science 240:889–895
69. Funder JW (1993) Mineralocorticoids, glucocorticoids, receptors and response elements. Science 259:1132–1133
70. Davis PJ (1991) Cellular actions of thyroid hormone. In: Utiger RD (ed) Werner and Ingbar's the thyroid. Lippincott, Philadelphia, pp 190–203
71. Nelson DH (1980) Corticosteroid-induced changes in phospholipid membranes as mediators of their action. Endocr Rev 1:180–199
72. Segal J (1989) A rapid, extranuclear effect of 3'5,3'-triiodothyronine on sugar uptake by several tissues in the rat in vivo. Endocrinology 124:2755–2764
73. Gilman AG (1984) G proteins and dual control of adenylate cyclase. Cell 36:577–579
74. Gilman AG (1987) G proteins: transducers of receptor-generated signals. Annu Rev Biochem 56:615–649
75. Birnbaumer L, Codina J, Yatani Y (1989) Molecular basis of regulation of ionic channels by G-protein coupled receptors. Recent Prog Horm Res 45:121–206
76. Stryer L, Bourke HR (1986) G proteins: a family of signal transducers. Ann Rev Cell Biol 2:391–419
77. Birnbaumer L (1990) Transduction of receptor signal into modulation of effector activity by G proteins. FASEB J 4:3179–3188
78. Clapham DE, Neer EJ (1993) New roles for G-protein βγ-dimers in transmembrane signalling. Nature 365:403–406
79. Neer EJ, Clapham DE (1988) Roles of G-protein subunits in transmembrane signalling. Nature 333:129–134
80. McCormick F (1993) How receptors turn Ras on. Nature 363:15–16
81. Bers DM (1991) Excitation-contraction coupling and cardiac contractile force. Kluwer, Dordrecht
82. Berridge MJ (1993) Inositol trisphosphate and calcium signalling. Nature 361:315–325
83. Nishizuka Y (1988) The molecular heterogeneity of protein kinase C and its implications for cellular regulation. Nature 334:661–665
84. Takasawa S, Nata K, Yonekura H, Okamoto H (1993) Cyclic-ADP ribose in insulin secretion from pancreatic beta cells. Science 259:370–373
85. Masaki T (1993) Endothelins: homeostatic and compensatory actions in the circulatory and endocrine systems. Endocr Rev 14:253–268
86. Orth DN, Kovacs WJ, DeBold CR (1992) The adrenal cortex. In: Wilson DJ, Foster DW (eds) Williams textbook of endocrinology. Saunders, Philadelphia, pp 489–619
87. Reichlin S (1992) Neuroendocrinology. In: Wilson DJ, Foster DW (eds) Williams textbook of endocrinology. Saunders, Philadelphia, pp 135–219
88. Eigler N, Sacca L, Sherwin RS (1979) Synergistic interactions of physiologic increments of glucagon, epinephrine, and cortisol in the dog. J Clin Invest 63:114–123
89. Felig P, Sherwin RS, Soman V, Warren J, Hendler R, Sacca L, Eigler N, Goldberg D, Walesky M (1979) Hormonal interactions in the regulation of blood glucose. Recent Prog Horm Res 35:501–532
90. Pirkle JCJ, Gann DS (1976) Restitution of blood volume after hemorrhage: role of the adrenal cortex. Am J Physiol 230:1683–1687
91. Lilly MP, Gann DS (1992) The hypothalamic-pituitary-adrenal-immune axis. Arch Sug 127:1463–1474
92. Antoni FA (1993) Vasopressinergic control of pituitary adrenocorticotropin secretion comes of age. Front Neuroendocrinol 14:76–122
93. Makara GB (1992) The relative importance of hypothalamic releasing neurones containing corticotrophin releasing factor or arginine vasopressin in regulation of ACTH secretion. Ciba Found Symp 168:43–51
94. Dohanics J, Linton EA, Lowry PJ, Makara GB (1990) Osmotic stimulation affects neurohypophysial corticotropin releasing factor-41 content: effect of dexamethasone. Peptides 11:51–57
95. Dunn A (1988) Systemic interleukin-1 administration stimulates hypothalamic norepinephrine metabolism paralleling the increased plasma corticosterone. Life Sci 1988:429–435
96. Dinarello CA (1989) Interleukin-1 and its biologically related cytokines. Adv Immunol 44:153–205

97. Brown SL, Smith LR, Blalock JE (1987) Interleukin 1 and interleukin 2 enhance proopiomelanocortin gene expression in pituitary cells. J Immunol 139:3181–3183
98. Besedovsky HØ, Del Rey A (1986) Immunoregulatory feedback between interleukin-1 and glucocorticoid hormones. Science 233:652–654
99. Berman A, Singh A, Kral T, Solomon S (1989) The immune-hypothalamic-pituitary-adrenal axis. Endocrinol Rev 10:92–112
100. Bernhagen J, Calandra T, Mitchell RA, Martin SB, Tracey KJ, Voelter W, Manogue KR, Cerami A, Bucala R (1993) MIF is a pituitary-derived cytokine that potentiates lethal endotoxemia. Nature 365:756–758
101. Frohman L (1981) Diseases of the anterior pituitary. In: Felig P, Barter JD, Broadus AE, Frohman LA (eds) Endocrinology and metabolism. McGraw-Hill, Nes York
102. Haynes RC, Larner J (1975) Adrenocorticotropic hormone: adrenocortical steroids and their synthetic analogs. In: Goodman LS, Gilman A (eds) The pharmacological basis of therapeutics. Macmillan, New York
103. Hems DA, Whitton PD (1980) Control of hepatic glycogenolysis. Physiol Rev 60:1–50
104. Jones HT (1979) Control of adrenocortical hormone secretion. In: James VH (ed) The adrenal gland. Raven, New York
105. Kraus-Friedmann H (1984) Hormonal regulation of hepatic gluconeogenesis. Physiol Rev 64:170–259
106. Yates FE, Marsh DJ, Maran JW (1980) The adrenal cortex. In: Mountcastle VB (ed) Medical physiology. Mosby, St. Louis
107. Engel FL, Federicks J (1957) Contribution to understanding of mechanism of permissive action of corticoids. Proc Soc Exp Biol Med 94:593–596
108. Clark EJ, Rossiter R (1944) Carbohydrate metabolism after burning. J Exp Physiol Cogn Med Sci 32:279–300
109. Chan TM (1984) The permissive effects of glucocorticoids on hepatic gluconeogenesis. J Biol Chem 259:7426–7432
110. Amaral JF, Shearer JD, Caldwell MD Hepatic metabolism following injury and adrenalectomy. (unpublished observation)
111. Caldwell MD, Lacy WW, Exton JH (1978) Effects of adrenalectomy on the amino acid and glucose metabolism of perfused rat hindlimbs. J Biol Chem 253:6837–6844
112. Fisher JE, Hasselgren PO (1991) Cytokines and glucocorticoids in the regulation of the "hepatico-skeletal muscle axis" in sepsis. Am J Surg 162:266–271
113. Fain JN, Kovacev VP, Scow RO (1965) Effect of growth hormone and dexamethasone on lipolysis and metabolism in isolated fat cells of the rat. J Biol Chem 240:3522–3529
114. Fain JN (1979) Inhibition of glucose transport in fat cells and activation of lipolysis by glucocorticoids. In: Baxter JD, Rousseau GG (eds) Glucocorticoid hormone action. Springer, Berlin Heidelberg New York
115. Fain JN, Garcia-Sainz JA (1983) Adrenergic regulation of adipocyte metabolism. J Lipid Res 24:945–966
116. Munck A, Guyre PM, Holbrook NJ (1984) Physiological functions of glucocorticoids in stress and their relation to pharmacological actions. Endocr Rev 5:25–44
117. Parrillo JE, Fauci AS (1979) Mechanisms of glucocorticoid action on immune processes. Annu Rev Pharmacol Toxicol 19:179–201
118. Weissman G, Thomas L (1964) The effects of corticosteroids upon connective tissue and lysosomes. Recent Prog Horm Res 20:215–245
119. Deitch EA (1992) Multiple organ failure: pathophysiology and potential future therapy. Ann Surg 216:117–134
120. Bone RC (1992) Toward an epidemiology and natural history of SRIS (systemic inflammatory response syndrome). JAMA 268:3452–3455
121. Dinarello CA, Gelfand JA, Wolff SM (1993) Anticytokine strategies in the treatment of systemic inflammatory response syndrome. JAMA 269:1829–1835
122. Bereiter DA, DeMaria EJ, Engeland WC, Gann DS (1988) Endocrine responses to multiple sensory input related to injury. Adv Exp Med Biol 245:251–299
123. Udelsman R, Ramp J, Galluci WT, Gorden AA, Norton JA, Loriaux DL, Chrousos GP (1986) Adaptation during surgical stress: a reevaluation of glucocorticoids. J Clin Invest 77:1377–1383

124. Gann DS, Pirkle JC (1975) Role of cortisol in the restitution of blood volume after hemorrhage. Am J Surg 130:565–569
125. Gann DS, Carlson DE, Byrnes GJ (1981) Impaired restitution of blood volume after large hemorrhage. J Trauma 21:598–603
126. McIntosh TK, Lothrop D, Lee A, Jackson B, Nabseth D, Egdahl R (1981) Circadian rhythm of cortisol is altered in post-surgical patients. J Clin Endocrinol Metabol 52:117–223
127. McIntosh TK (1987) Prolonged alteration in plasma cortisol circadian rhythms following trauma in baboons. Am J Physiol 252:R548–563
128. Reeves WB, Andreoli TE (1992) The posterior pituitary and water metabolism. In: Wilson JD, Foster DW (eds) Williams textbook of endocrinology. Saunders, Philadelphia, pp 311–356
129. Haberich FJ (1968) Osmoreception in the portal circulation. Fed Proc 27:1137–1141
130. Sawchenko PE, Friedman MI (1979) Sensory functions of the liver: a review. Am J Physiol 236:R5–R20
131. Baylis PH, Zepre RL, Robertson GL (1981) Arginine vasopressin response to insulin-induced hypoglycemia in man. J Clin Endocrinol Metab 53:935–940
132. Anderson B (1977) Regulation of body fluids. Annu Rev Physiol 39:185–200
133. Spiegel AM, Downs RW Jr. (1981) Guanine nucleotides: key regulators of hormone receptor-adenylate cyclase interaction. Endocrinol Rev 2:275–305
134. Sklar AH, R. W. S. (1983) Central nervous system mediators of vasopressin release. Physiol Rev 63:1243–1280
135. Mouw D, Bonjour J, Malvin RL, Vander A (1971) Central action of angiotensin in stimulating ADH release. Am J Physiol 220:239–242
136. Holaday JW, Black LE, Long JB (1985) Neuropeptides in shock and trauma. In: Gellhoed GW, Chernow B (eds) Endocrine aspects of acute illness. Churchill Livingstone, New York
137. Kendler KS, Weitzman RE, Fisher DA (1978) The effect of pain on plasma arginine vasopressin concentration in man. Clin Endocrinol 8:89–94
138. Star RA, Nonoguchi H, Balaban R et al. (1988) Calcium and cyclic adenosine monophosphate as second messengers for vasopressin in the rat inner medullary collecting tubule. J Clin Invest 81:1879–1888
139. Brown D (1989) Membrane recycling and epithelial cell function. Am J Physiol 256:F1–F6
140. Valenti G, Hugon JS, Bourguet J (1988) To what extent is microtubular network involved in antidiuretic response? Am J Physiol 255:F1098–F1106
141. Kirk CJ, Rodrigues LM, Hems DA (1979) The influence of vasopressin and related peptides on glycogen phosphorylase activity and phosphotidylinositol metabolism in hepatocytes. Biochem J 1978:493–496
142. Williamson DH (1982) Regulation of ketone body metabolism and the effects of injury. Acta Chir Scand [Suppl] 507:22–29
143. Liard JF (1984) Vasopressin in cardiovascular control. Clin Sci 67:473–479
144. Claybaugh JR, Share L (1973) Vasopressin, renin and cardiovascular responses to continuous slow hemorrhage. Am J Physiol 224:519–523
145. Cochrane JPS, Forsling ML, Gow NM, Le Quesne LP (1981) Arginine vasopressin release following surgical operations. Br J Surg 68:209–213
146. Share L (1968) Control of plasma ADH titer in hemorrhage: role of atrial and arterial receptors. Am J Physiol 215:1384–1389
147. Cioffi WGJ, Vaughan GM, Heironimus JD, Jordan BS, Mason ADJ, Pruitt BAJ (1991) Dissociation of blood volume and flow in regulation of salt and water balance in burn patients. Ann Surg 214:218–218
148. Banks RO, Gallavan RF, Zinner MJ, Buckley GB et al. (1985) Vasoactive agents in the control of the mesenteric circulation. Fed Proc 44:2743–2749
149. Errington M, Roch E, Silva M (1972) Vasopressin clearance and secretion during hemorrhage in normal dogs and in dogs with experimental diabetes insipidus. J Physiol 227:395–403
150. Mitchell A, Collin J (1985) Vasopressin effects on the small intestine: a possible factor in paralytic ileus? Br J Surg 72:462–465
151. Herndon DN, Nguyen TT, Gilpin DA (1993) Growth factors. Arch Surg 128:1227–1233
152. Welbourne T, Joshi S, McVie R (1989) Growth hormone effects on hepatic glutamate handling in vivo. Am J Physiol 257:E959–E962

153. Fryburg DA, Gelfand RA, Barrett EJ (1991) Growth hormone acutely stimulates forearm muscle protein synthesis in normal humans. Am J Physiol 260:E499–E504
154. McGrath MH (1990) Peptide growth factors and wound healing. Clin Plast Surg 17:421–432
155. Bazan JF (1990) Haemopoietic receptors and helical cytokines. Immunol Today 11:350–354
156. Newsome HH, Rose JC (1971) The response of adrenocorticotrophic hormone and growth hormone to surgical stress. J Clin Endocrinol Metab 33:481–487
157. Wright PD, Johnston IDA (1975) The effect of surgical operation on growth hormone levels in surgery. Surgery 77:479–486
158. Hawker FH, Stewart PM, Baxter RC, Borkmain M, Tan K, Caterson ID, McWilliam DB (1987) Relationship of somatomedin-C/insulin-like growth factor I levels to conventional nutritional indices in critically ill patients. Crit Care Med 15:732–736
159. Pacitti AJ, Yoshifumi I, Plumley DA, Copeland EM, Souba WW (1992) Growth hormone regulates amino acid transport in human and rat liver. Ann Surg 216:353–361
160. Ziegler TR, Young LS, Manson JM, Wilmore DW (1988) Metabolic effects of recombinant human growth hormone in patients receiving parenteral nutrition. Ann Surg 208:6–14
161. Voerman HJ, S.R.J.M. vS, Groeneveld ABJ, de Boer H, Nauta JP, van der Veen EA, Thijus LG (1992) Effects of recombinant human growth hormone in patients with severe sepsis. Ann Surg 216:648–655
162. Wolf RF, Pearlstone DB, Newman E, Heslin MJ, Gonenne A, Burt ME, Brennan MF (1992) Growth hormone and insulin reverse net whole body and skeletal muscle protein catabolism in cancer patients. Ann Surg 216:280–290
163. Scanlon MF, Lewis M, Weightman DR, Chan V, Hall R (1980) The neuroregulation of human thyrotropin secretion. In: Martini L, Ganong WF (eds) Frontiers in neuroendocrinology. Raven, New York
164. Larsen PR (1982) Thyroid-pituitary interaction. N Engl J Med 306:23–32
165. Otsuki M, Dakoda M, Baba S (1973) Influence of glucocorticoids on TRF-induced TSH response in man. J Clin Endocrinol Metab 36:95–102
166. Vinik AI, Kalk JW, McLaren H, Hendricks S, Pimstone BL (1975) Fasting blunts the TSH response to synthetic TRH. J Clin Endocrinol Metab 40:509–511
167. Edelman IS, Ismail-Beigi F (1974) Thyroid thermogenesis and active sodium transport. Rec Prog Horm Res 30:235–257
168. Ingenbleck Y (1980) Thyroid function in non-thyroid illness. In: DeVisscher M (ed) The thyroid gland. Raven, New York
169. Charters AC, O'Dell MWD, Thompson JC (1969) Anterior pituitary function during surgical stress and convalescence. J Clin Endocrinol Metab 29:63–71
170. Shirani KZ, Vaughan GM, Pruitt BA, Mason AD (1985) Reduced serum T4 and T3 and their altered transport binding after burn injury in rats. J Trauma 25:953–958
171. Aun F, G.A. M-N, Young RN, Birolini D, DeOliveria MR (1983) The effect of major trauma on the pathways of thyroid hormone metabolism. J Trauma 23:1048–1051
172. Ramsden DB, Askew RD, Bradwell RA et al. (1980) Glucocorticoids and peripheral monodeiodination of thyroxine after stress. Proceeddings of VI International Congress of Endocrinology 363
173. Cavalieri RR, Rappoport B (1977) Impaired peripheral conversion of thyroxine to triiodothyronine. Annu Rev Med 28:57
174. Franchimont P (1971) The regulation of follicle stimulating hormone and luteinizing hormone secretion in humans. In: Martini L, Ganong WF (eds) Frontiers in neuroendocrinology. Oxford University Press, New York
175. Carstensen H et al. (1972) Testosterone, luteinizing hormone and growth hormone in blood following surgical trauma. Acta Chir Scand 138:1–5
176. Aono T, Kurachi K, Miyata M, Nakasima A, Koshiyama K, Yozumi T, Matsumoto K (1976) Influence of surgical stress under general anesthesia on serum gonadotropin levels. J Clin Endocrinol Metab 42:144–148
177. Brizio-Molteni L, Molteni A, Warpeha RL, Angelats J, Lewis N, Fors EM (1984) Prolactin, corticotropin and gonadotropin concentrations following thermal injury in adults. J Trauma 24:1–7

178. Woolfe PD, Hammill RW, McDonald JV, Lee LA, Kelly M (1985) Transient hypogonadotropic hypogonadism cause by critical surgical illness. J Clin Endocrinol Metab 66:444–450
179. Xiao E, Luckhaus J, Niemann W, Ferin M (1989) Acute inhibition of gonadotropin secretion by corticotropin-releasing hormone in the primate. Endocrinology 124:1632–1639
180. Novelli GP, Marsili M, Pieraccioli E (1973) Antishock action of steroids other than cortisone. Eur Surg Res 5:169–174
181. Grossman CJ (1984) Regulation of the immune system be sex steroids. Endocr Rev 5:435–448
182. Parker RC, Baxter CR (1885) Divergence in adrenal steroid secretory pattern after thermal injury in adult patients. J Trauma 25:508–510
183. Horrobin DF (1980) Prolactin as a regulator of gluid and electrolyte metabolism in mammals. Fed Proc 39:2567–2570
184. Cerra FB (1991) Nutrient modulation of inflammatory and immune function. Am J Surg 161:230–234
185. Neill JD (1970) Effect of "stress" on serum prolactin and luteinizing hormone levels during the estrous cycle of the rat. Endocrinology 87:1192–1195
186. Klemcke HG, Nienaber JA, Hahn GL (1987) Stressor-associated alterations in porcine plasma prolactin. Proc Soc Exp Biol Med 186:333–343
187. Carlson DE, Klemcke HG, Gann DS (1988) Plasma prolactin parallels response of adrenocorticotropin to moderate hemorrhage in unanesthetized swine. Physiologist 31:A203
188. Noel GL, Suh HK, Stone JG, Frantz AB (1972) Human prolactin and growth hormone release during surgery and other conditions of stress. J Clin Endocrinol Metab 35:840–851
189. Chiolero R, Lemarchand T, Schutz Y, DeTribolet N et al. (1988) Plasma pituitary hormone levels in severe trauma with and without head injury. J Trauma 28:1368–1373
190. Hollt V (1983) Multiple endogenous opioid peptides. Trends Neurosci 6:24–26
191. Udenfriend S, Kilpatrick DG (1983) Biochemistry of the enkephalins and enkephalin-containing peptides. Arch Biochem Biophys 221:309–323
192. DeBold CR, Menefee JK, Nicholson WE, Orth DN (1989) Proopinomelanocorticotropin gene is expressed by many normal human tissues and in tumors not associated with ectopic adrenocorticotropin syndrome. Mol Endocrinol 2:862–870
193. Guillmen R, Vargo T, Rossier J, Minick S, Ling N, Rivier C, Vale W, Bloom R (1977) B-endorphin and adrenocorticotropin are secreted concomitantly by the pituitary gland. Science 197:1367–1369
194. Guyton AC (1986) Somatic sensations: I. pain, visceral pain, headache, and thermal sensations. In: Guyton AC (ed) Textbook of medical physiology. Saunders, Philadelphia
195. Lacoumenta S, Yeo TH, Burrin JM et al. (1987) Fentanyl and the β endorphin, ACTH, and glucoregulatory hormonal response to surgery. Br J Anesth 59:713–719
196. Rossier J, French ED, Rivier C, Ling N, Guillemin R, Bloom FE (1977) Foot-shock induced stress increases B-endorphin levels in blood but not brain. Nature 270:618–620
197. Cox BM, Baizman ER (1982) Physiological functions of the endorphins. In: Malick JB, Bell RMS (eds) Endorphins: chemistry, physiology, pharmacology and clinical relevance. Marcel Dekker, New York
198. Dubois M, Pickar D, Cohen MR, McNamara T, Burrey WE (1981) Surgical stress in humans is accompanied by an increase in plasma β endorphin immunoreactivity. Life Sci 29:1249–1254
199. Levy EM, McIntosh T, Block PH (1986) Elevation of circulatory β-endorphin levels with concomitant depression of immune parameters after traumatic injury. J Trauma 26:246–249
200. Noda M, Furntani Z, Takahashi H, Toyosato M, Hirose T, Inayama S, Nakanishi S, Numa S (1982) Cloning and sequence analysis of cDNA for bovine adrenal preproenkephalin. Nature 295:202–206
201. Chaminade M, Fortz AS, Rossier J (1984) Co-release of enkephalins and precursors with catecholamines from the perfused cat adrenal gland in situ. J Physiol 353:157–169
202. Lang RE, Bruckner UB, Hermann K, Kempff B, Ruscher W, Sturm V (1982) Effect of hemorrhagic shock on the concomitant release of endorphin and enkepphalin like peptides from the pituitary and adrenal gland in the dog. In: Costa E, Trabucchi R (eds) Regulatory peptides: from molecular biology to function. Raven, New York

203. Farrell LD, Harrison TS, Demers LM (1983) Immunoreactive met-enkephalin in the canine adrenal: response to acute hypovolemia. Proc Soc Exp Biol Med 173:515–518
204. Paterson SJ, Robson LE, Kosterlitz HW (1983) Classification of opioid receptors. Br Med Bull 39:31–36
205. Pfeiffer A, Herz A (1984) Endocrine action of opioids. Horm Metab Res 16:386–397
206. Hamilton AJ, Black PM, Carr DB (1985) Contrasting action of naloxone in experimental spinal cord trauma and cerebral ischemia. Neurosurgery 17:845–888
207. Bernton EW, Long J, Holaday JW (1985) Opioids and neuropeptides: mechanisms in circulatory shock. Fed Proc 44:290–299
208. Harbour DV, Galin FS, Hughes TK, Smith EM, Blalock JE (1991) Role of leukocyte-derived proopiomelanocortin peptides in endotoxic shock. Circ Shock 35:181–191
209. Curtis MT, Lefer A (1980) Protective actions of naloxone in hemorrhagic shock. Am J Physiol 239:H416–H421
210. Holaday JW, Faden AI (1980) Naloxone reversal of endotoxin hypotension suggests role of endorphines in shock. Nature 275:450–451
211. Holaday JW, Faden AI (1980) Naloxone acts at central opiate receptors to reverse hypotension, hypothermia and hypoventilation in spinal shock. Brain Res 189:295–300
212. LeMaire R, Tseng R, LeMaire S (1978) Systemic administration of β-endorphin: potent hypotensive effect involving a serotonergic pathway. Proc Natl Acad Sci USA 75:6240–6242
213. Schaz K, Stock G, Simon W, Schlor H, Unger T et al. (1979) Enkephalin effects on blood pressure, heart rate and baroreceptor reflex. Hypertension 2:395–407
214. Eckenhoff JE, Oech SR (1960) The effects of narcotics and antagonists upon respiration and circulation in man. Clin Pharmacol Ther 1:483–524
215. VanLoon GR, Appel NM (1980) β-endorphin-induced increases in plasma dopamine, norepinephrine, and epinephrine. Res Commun Chem Pathol Pharmacol 27:607–610
216. Feldman M, Kiser RS, Unger RH, Li CH (1983) β-endorphin and the endocrine pancreas. N Engl J Med 308:349–353
217. Ippe E, Dobbs R, Unger RH (1978) Morphine and β-endorphin influence the secretion of the endocrine pancreas. Nature 276:190–191
218. Amaral JF, Caldwell MD, Gann DS (1984) Effect of naloxone on glucose metabolism in skeletal muscle. Surg Forum 35:52
219. Amir S, Berstein M (1982) Endogeneous opiates interact in stress-induced hyperglycemia in mice. Physiol Behav 28:575–577
220. Bereiter DA, Plotsky PM, Gann DS (1983) Selective opiate modulation of the physiological responses to hemorrhage in the cat. Endocrinology 113:1439–1446
221. Caldwell MD, Gann DS (1989) Metabolic response to injury. In: Davis JH (ed) Clinical surgery. Mosby, New York
222. Lymangrover JR, Dokas LA, Martin R, Saffran M (1981) Naloxone has a direct effect on the adrenal cortex. Endocrinology 109:1132–1137
223. Morley JE (1983) Neuroendocrine effects of endogenous opioid peptides in human subjects: a review. Psychoneuroendocrinology 8:361–379
224. Grossman A (1983) Brain opiates and neuroendocrine function. Clin Endocrinol Metab 12:725–746
225. McIntosh TK, Faden AI (1986) Opiate antagonists in traumatic shock. Ann Em Med 15:1462–1489
226. Teschemacher H, Koch G, Scheffler H, Hildebrand A, Brantl V (eds) (1990) Opioid peptides: immunological significance? New York Academy of Sciences, New York
227. Shavit Y, Lewis J, Terman G, Gale R, Liebeskind J (1984) Opioid peptides mediate the suppressive effect of stress on natural killer cell cytotoxity. Science 223:188–190
228. Deitch E, Xo D, Bridges R (1988) Opioids modulate neutrophil lymphocyte function: thermal injury alters plasma β-endorphin levels. Surgery 104:41–48
229. Hildebrand A, Preissner KT, Muller-Berghaus G, Teschemacher H (1989) J Biol Chem 264:15429–15434
230. Hildebrand A (1989) Identification of the beta-endorphin-binding subunit of the SCSb-9 complement complex: S protein exhibits, specific beta-endorphin-binding sites upon complex

formation with complement proteins. Mai 15 159(2). Biochem Biophys Res Commun 159:799–806

231. Van Epps DE, Saland L (1984) Beta-endorphin and met-encephalin stimulate human peripheral blood mononuclear cell chemotaxis. 132(6) June 1984. J Immunol 132:3046–3053

232. Parker CJ, Frame MR, Elstad MR (1988) Vitronectin (S protein) augments the functional activity of monocyte receptors for IgG and complement C3b II(I) Jan 1988. Blood 71:86–93

233. Landsberg L, Young JB (1992) Catecholamines and the adrenal medulla. In: Wilson JD, Foster DW (eds) Williams textbook of endocrinology. Saunders, Philadelphia, pp 621–705

234. Cryer PE (1980) Physiology and pathophysiology of the human sympathoadrenal neuroendocrine system. N Engl J Med 303:436–444

235. Esler M, Jennings G, Lamberg G, Meredith I, Horne M, Eisenhofer G (1992) Overflow of catecholamine neurotransmitters to the circulation: source, fate and functions. Physiol Rev 1990:963–985

236. Linares O, Jacquez J, Zech L et al. (1987) Norepinephrine metabolism in humans: kinetic analysis and model. J Clin Invest 80:1332–1341

237. Halter JF, Pflug AE (1980) Effect of sympathetic blockade by spinal anesthesia on pancreatic islet function in man. Am J Physiol 239:E150–E155

238. Marangou AG, Alford FP, Ward G, Liskaser F, Aitken PM, Weber KM, Boston RC, Best JD (1988) Hormonal effects of norepinephrine on acute glucose disposal in humans: a minimal model analysis. Metabolism 37:885–891

239. Morrow LA, Morganroth GS, Herman WH, Bergman RN, Halter JB (1993) Effects of epinephrine on insulin secretion and action in humans. Diabetes 42:307–315

240. Cryer PE (1981) Disease of the adrenal medullae and sympathetic nervous system. In: Felig P, Baxter JD, Broadus AE, Frohman LA (eds) Endocrinology and metabolism. McGraw-Hill, New York

241. Williams GH (1983) Aldosterone. In: Dunn MJ (ed) Renal endocrinology. Williams and Williams, Baltimore

242. Gann DS, Lilly MP (1983) The neuroendocrine response to multiple trauma. World J Surg 7:101–118

243. Achtel RA, Downing SE (1972) Ventricular responses to hypoexemia following chemoreceptorn denervation and adrenalectomy. Am Heart J 84:377–386

244. Gann DS, Amarl JF (1985) The pathophysiological response to injury. In: Zuidema G, Rutherford R, Mallinger WF (eds) The management of trauma. Saunders, Philadelphia

245. Fain JN (1982) Involvement of phosphatidylinositol breakdown in elevation of cytosol Ca^{++} by hormones and relationship to prostaglandin formation. In: Kohn LD (ed) Hormone receptors. Wiley, New York

246. Newsholme EA, Start C (1973) Regulation in metabolism. Wiley, New York

247. Young JB, Landsberg L (1977) Catecholamines and intermediary metabolism. Clin Endocrinol Metab 6:599–631

248. Chaisson JL, Shikama H, Chu DTW, Exton JH (1981) Inhibitory effect of epinephrine on insulin-stimulated glucose uptake by rat skeletal muscle. J Clin Invest 68:706–713

249. Johnson MD, Shier DN, Barger AC (1979) Circulating catecholamines and control of plasma renin activity in conscious dogs. Am J Physiol 236:H463–H470

250. Kukreja SC, Hargis GK, Bowser EN, Henderson WJ, Fisherman EW, Williams GA (1978) Role of adrenergic stimuli in parathyroid secretion in man. J Clin Endocrinol Metab 40:478–481

251. Unger RH, Dobbs RE (1978) Insulin, glucagon and somatostatin secretion in the regulation of metabolism. Annu Rev Physiol 40:307–343

252. Goldberg LI (1974) Dopamine: clinical uses of an endogenous catecholamine. N Engl J Med 291:707–710

253. Barton RN (1987) The neuroendocrinology of physical injury. Bailliere's Clin Endocrinol Metab 1987:355–374

254. Feuerstein GP, Gutman Y (1971) Preferential secretion of adrenaline or noradrenaline by the cat adrenal in vivo in response to different stimuli. Br J Pharmacol 43:764–768

255. Halter J, Pflug A, Porte D (1977) Mechanism of plasma catecholamine increases during surgical stress in man. J Clin Endocrinol Metab 45:936–940

256. Inagami R, Chang JJ, Dykes CW, Takaii T, Kisaragi M, Mosono KS (1983) Renin: structural features of active enzyme and inactive precursor. Fed Proc 42:2729–2734
257. Baer PG, McGiff JC (1980) Hormonal systems and renal hemodynamics. Annu Rev Physiol 42:589–601
258. Averill DB, Scher AM, Feigl EO (1983) Angiotensin causes vasoconstriction during hemorrhage in baroreceptor-denervated dogs. Am J Physiol 245:H667–H673
259. Simpson JB, Routtenberg A (1973) Subfornical organ: site of drinking elicitation by angiotensin II. Science 181:1172–1175
260. Harrison TS, Birbari A, Seaton JF (1973) Reinforcement of reflex epinephrine release by angiotensin II. Am J Physiol 224:31–34
261. Rivier C, Vale W (1983) Effect of angiotensin II on ACTH release in vivo: role of corticotropin-releasing factor. Regul Pep 7:253–258
262. Buchanan TA, Thawani H, Dades W, Modrall JG, Weaver FA, Laurel D, Poppiti R, Xiang A, Hsueh W (1993) Angiotensin II increases glucose utilization during acute hyperinsulinemia via a hemodynamic mechanism. J Clin Invest 92:720–726
263. Antonipillai I, Horton R (1993) Paracrine regulation of the renin-angiotensin system. J Steroid Biochem Mol Biol 45:27–31
264. Bakris GL, Re RN (1993) Endothelin modulates in the angiotensin II-induced mitogenesis of human mesangial cells. Am J Physiol 264:F937–F942
265. Fakunding JL, Chow R, Catt KJ (1979) The role of calcium in the stimulation of aldosterone production by ACTH, angiotensin II, and potassium in isolated glomerulosa cells. Endocrinology 105:327–333
266. Fujita K, Aguilera G, Catt KJ (1979) The role of C-AMP in the aldosterone production by isolated zona glomerulosa cells. J Biol Chem 254:8567–8574
267. Aguilera G, Catt KJ (1980) Loci of action of regulators of aldosterone biosynthesis in isolated glomerulosa cells. Endocrinology 104:1046–1052
268. Kaplan NM (1965) The biosynthesis of adrenal steroids: effects of angiotensin II, adrenocorticotropin and potassium. J Clin Invest 44:2029–2039
269. Sen S, Bravo EL, Bumpus FM (1977) Isolation of a hypertension-producing compound from normal human urine. Circ Res 40 (5 Suppl): I5–I10
270. Bravo EL, Saito F, Zanella T et al. (1980) In vitro steroidogenic properties of a new hypertension-producing compound from normal human urine. J Clin Endocrinol Metab 51:176–178
271. Baxter JD, Tyrell JB, Felig P, Brodus AE, Frohman LA (1981) The adrenal cortex. In: Felig P, Baxter JD, Brodus AE, Frohman LA (eds) Endocrinology and metabolism. McGraw-Hill, New York
272. Kem DL, Gomez-Sanchez C, Kramer WJ (1995) Plasma aldosterone and renin activity response to ACTH infusion in dexamethasone suppressed normal and sodium-depleted man. J Clin Endocrinol Metab 40:116–124
273. McKenna TJ, Island DP, Nicholson WE, Liddle GW (1975) Dopamine inhibits angiotensin-stimulated aldosterone biosynthesis in bovine adrenal cells. J Clin Invest 64:287–291
274. Alexander RW, Gill JRJ, Yambe H (1974) Effects of dietary sodium and of acute saline infusion on the interrelationship between dopamine excretion and adrenergic activity in man. J Clin Invest 54:194–200
275. Carey RM, VanLoon GR, Baines AD et al. (1981) Decreased plasma and urinary dopamine during dietary sodium depletion in man. J Clin Endocrinol Metab 52:903–909
276. Poole CJM, Carter DA, Vallejo M et al. (1987) Atrial natriuretic factor inhibits the stimulated in vivo and in vitro release of vasopressin and oxytocin in the rat. J Endocrinol 112:97–102
277. Dillingham MA, Anderson RJ (1986) Inhibition of vasopressin action by atrial natriuretic factor. Science 231:1572–1573
278. Manning PT, Schwartz D, Katsube NC et al. (1985) Vasopressin-stimulated release of atriopeptin: endocrine antagonists in fluid homeostasis. Science 229:395–397
279. Goetz KL, Wang BC, Greer PG et al. (1986) Atrial stretch increases sodium excretion independently of release of atrial peptides. Am J Physiol 250:R946–R950
280. Standaert DG, Needleman P, Saper CB (1988) Atriopeptin: neuromediator in the central regulation of cardiovascular function. In: Martini L, Ganong WF (eds) Frontiers in neuroendocrinology. Raven, New York

281. Wittert GA, Espiner EA, Richards AM, Donald RA, Livesay JH, Vandle TG (1993) Atrial natriuretic peptide reduces the vasopressin and angiotensin II but not the ACTH response to acute hypoglycemia in normal men. Clin Endocrinol [Oxf] 38:183–189

282. Cross JS, Gruber DP, Gann DS, Singh AK, Moran JM, Burchard KW (1989) Hypertonic saline attenuates the hormonal response to injury. Ann Surg 209:684–692

283. Noll B, Krappe J, Goke B et al. (1990) Influence of pacing mode and rate on peripheral levels of atrial natriuretic peptide. Pacing Clin Electrophysiol 12:1763–1768

284. Stewart JM, Gewitz MH, Clark BJ, Seligman KP, Romano A, Zeballos GA, Chang A, Murdison K, Woolf PK, Norwood WI (1991) The role of vasopressin and atrial natriuretic factor in postoperative fluid retention after the Fontan procedure. J Thorac Cardiovasc Surg 102:821–829

285. Anderson JV, Bloom SR (1986) Atrial natriuretic peptide. J Endocrinol 110:7–47

286. Genest J, Cantin M (1987) Atrial natriuretic factor. Circulation 75:1–11

287. Gala GJ, Lilly MP, Thomas SE, Gann DS, Singh AK, Moran JM, Burchard KW (1989) Interaction of sodium and volume in fluid resuscitation after hemorrhage. J Trauma 31:545–556

288. Shackford SR, Norton CH, Ziegler MG, Wilner KD (1988) The effect of hemorrhage and resuscitation on serum levels of immunoreactive atrial natriuretic factor. Ann Surg 207:195–202

289. Goetz KL (1988) Physiology and pathophysiology of atrial peptides. Am J Physiol 251:1–47

290. Allison SP, Hinton P, Chamberlain MJ (1968) Intravenous glucose tolerance, insulin and free fatty acid levels in burn patients. Lancet 2:1113–1116

291. Reichlin S (1983) Somatostatin. N Engl J Med 309:1495–1501

292. Unger RH, Orci L (1981) Glucagon and the A cell: physiology and pathophysiology. N Engl J Med 304:1575–1580

293. Felig P (1981) The endocrine pancreas: diabetes mellitus. In: Felig P, Baxter JD, Broadus AE, Frohman LA (eds) Endocrinology and metabolism. McGraw-Hill, New York

294. Schmidt HHHW, Warner TD, Ishi K, Sheng H, Murand F (1992) Insulin secretion from pancreatic B cells caused by L-arginine-derived nitrogen oxides. Science 255:721–724

295. Exton JH (1972) Gluconeogenesis. Metabolism 21:945–990

296. Halter JB, Pflug E (1980) Relationship of impaired insulin secretion during surgical stress to anesthesia and catecholamine release. J Clin Endocrinol Metab 51:1093–1098

297. Felig P, Wahren J, Hendler R (1976) Influence of physiologic hyperglucagonemia on basal and insulin inhibited splanchnic glucose output in normal man. J Clin Invest 58:761–765

298. McIntyre J et al. (1965) Intestinal factors in the control of insulin secretion. J Clin Endocrinol 25:1317–1324

299. Raptis S, Dollinger HC, Schroder KE, Schleyer M, Rothen Buchner G, Pfeiffer EF (1973) Differences in insulin, growth hormones and pancreatic enzyme secretion after intravenous and introduodenal administration of mixed amino acids in man. N Engl J Med 288:1199–1202

300. Chiasson JL, Liljenquist JE, Sinclair-Smith B et al. (1975) Gluconeogenesis from alanine in normal postabsorptive man: intrahepatic stimulatory effect of glucagon. Diabetes 24:574–584

301. Fradkin J, Shamoon H, Felig P, Sherwin RS (1980) Evidence of an important role of changes in rather than absolute concentration of glucagon in the regulation of glucose production in humans. J Clin Endocrinol Metab 50:698–703

302. McLeod MK, Carlson DE, Gann DS (1986) Hormonal responses associated with early hyperglycemia after graded hemorrhage in dogs. Am J Physiol 251:E597–E606

303. Meguid MM, Brennan MF, Aoki II et al. (1974) Hormone-substrate interrelationships following trauma. Arch Surg 109:776–783

304. Miyata M, Yamomoto T, Nakao K (1976) Suppression of glucagon secretion during surgery. Hormon Metab Res 8:239–244

305. Wolffe RR, Burk JF (1982) Somatostatin infusion inhibits glucose production in burn patients. Circ Shock 9:521–527

306. Zapf J, Schoenle E, Froesch ER (1978) Insulin-like growth factors I and II: some biological actions and receptor binding characteristics of two purified constituents of nonsuppressible insulin like activity of human serum. Eur J Biochem 87:285–296

307. Monier S, LeCam A, LeMarchand-Brustel W (1982) Insulin and insulin-like growth factor 1. Diabetes 32:392–397

308. Poggi C, e Marchand-Bruste Y, Zapf J, Froesch E, Freychet P (1979) Effects of binding of IGF-I in the isolated soleus muscle of lean and obese mice: comparison with insulin. Endocrinology 105:723–730
309. Baxter RC, Turtle JR (1978) Stimulation of protein synthesis in isolated hepatocytes by somatomedin. Metabolism 27:503–506
310. Widmer U, Schmid C, Zapf J, Froesch ER (1984) Effects of insulin-like growth factors on chick embryo hepatocytes. Acta Endocrinol [Copenh] 108:237–244
311. Enberg G, Carlquist M, Jornvall H, Hall K (1984) The characterization of somatomedin A, isolated by microcomputercontrolled chromatography, reveals an apparent identity to insulin-like growth factor I. Eur J Biochem 143:117–124
312. Perdue JF (1984) Chemistry structure and function of insulin-like growth factors and their receptors: a review. Can J Biochem Cell Biol: 1237–1245
313. Frayn KN, Prete DA, Maycock PF, Carroll SM (1984) Plasma somatomedin activity after injury in man and its relationship to other hormonal and metabolic changes. Clin Endocrinol 20:179–187
314. Merimee TJ, Zapf MJ, Froesch ER (1982) Insulin-like growth factors in the fed and fasted states. J Clin Endocrinol Metab 55:999–1002
315. Thompson WA, Coyle SM, Lazarus D. Fisher E, Van Zee K, Rock C, Moldawer LL, Lowry SF (1991) The metabolic effects of continuous infusion of insulin-like growth factor (IGF-1) in parenterally fed men. Surg Forum 42:23–25
316. Huang KF, Chung DH, Herndon DN (1993) Insulinlike growth factor 1 (IGF-1) reduces gut atrophy and bacterial translocation after severe burn injury. Arch Surg 128:47–54
317. Habener JF, Potts JT Jr (1978) Biosynthesis of parathyroid hormone. N Engl J Med 299:580–585
318. Coop DH (1964) Parathyroids, calcitonin and control of plasma calcium. Recent Prog Horm Res 20:59–88
319. Habener JF, Potts JT Jr (1976) Chemistry, biosynthesis secretion and met abolism of parathyroid hormone. In: Aurbach GD (ed) Handbook of physiology, sect 7, endocrinology, American Physiological Society, Washington DC
320. Fisher JA, Blum JW et al. (1973) Acute parathyroid hormone response to epinephrine in vivo. J Clin Invest 52:2434–2440
321. Widnell CC, Pfenninger KH (1990) Essential cell biology. Williams and Wilkins, Baltimore
322. Kohn CR, Smith RJ, Chin WW (1992) Mechanism of action of hormones that act at the cell surface: In: Wilson JD, Foster DW (eds) Williams textbook of endocrinology, 8th edn. Saunders, Philadelphia

Immunity in the Acute Catabolic State

R. Slejelid and B. Plytycz

Introduction

Acute catabolic states can be caused by surgical trauma, hemorrhage, serious infections, or other large-scale noxious influences. Within minutes or hours, the balance of normal physiology is shifted to pathological processes throughout the body, involving several organ systems.

As far as we know today, specific immunity is not affected in any characteristic way during the first few hours. On the other hand, unspecific immunity – the function of connective tissue, vessels, leukocytes and foremost macrophages (histocytes), – is pivotal in the development of some of the characteristics of acute catabolism. This is so because the macrophages typically react to changes prevailing at sites of trauma, e.g., denatured proteins and other macromolecules, foreign material, bacterial products, complement, and products of coagulation. The molecular mechanisms underlying the reaction of macrophages to these stimuli are not well understood. It is known that macrophages have receptors for lipopolysaccharide (LPS) and complement, but most "foreign surfaces" that are produced in traumatic conditions cannot at present be defined in molecular terms or in terms of known receptors.

However, the reaction patterns of macrophages and other normal connective tissue cells are much better known. On the basis of this knowledge, the effects fall broadly into two main categories: (1) local reaction, i.e., acute inflammation, and (2) systemic effects.

Acute Inflammation

Acute inflammation is basically a process of connective tissue, vessels, and leukocytes of the myeloid lineage and does not typically involve specific immunity.

We owe our present-day understanding of the concept of acute inflammation largely to Metchnikoff [1]. His definition, slightly modified by Podwyssozki, runs as follows:

Inflammation is a local reaction, often beneficial, of the living tissues against the irritant substance. This reaction is chiefly produced by a phagocytic activity of the mesodermic cells. In this reaction, however, may participate not only changes in the vascular system, but also the chemical action of the blood plasma and tissue fluids in liquefying and dissolving the irritant agent.

This 100-year-old definition, first published in 1892, could be used verbatim in a textbook today.

Before Metchnikoff [1], inflammation was considered only to be the detectable signs of destruction, detrimental to the well-being of the organism. Phagocytosis was looked upon by his contemporaries "as a purely accidental phenomenon, which is brought about for the simple reason that mobile cells happen to be present, together with a material capable of being ingested by them."

One of the reasons why Metchnikoff recognized the major elements of inflammation better than the majority of scientists of his day – and also why he understood the essentially beneficial nature of inflammation – was that he regarded the process from a comparative biological perspective. He observed and performed experiments with a large number of different animals – from simple invertebrates to mammals – and thus became aware of the evolution of the process throughout phylogeny. He saw that single cell organisms, protozoa, reacted to attack by other, infective unicellular organisms by phagocytosis. Primitive multicellular organisms reacted to infection or damage by mobilization of special cells of the mesoderm, the phagocytes, which would approach the harmfull agent, try to engulf it or to sequester it, and in many cases to dissolve it. In some higher invertebrates with blood vessels and in all vertebrates, a vascular phenomenon leading to diapedesis of blood-borne phagocytes and effusion of blood plasma could also be observed. Metchnikoff's observations led him to the firm conclusion that the vascular phenomena were secondary to the reaction of the phagocytes, in evolutionary terms and also, probably, in pathogenetic terms.

How do we describe acute inflammation today? As a prototype, let us consider the reaction to a subcutaneous bacterial infection [2].

The earliest change in the host tissues that has been observed with certainty is the occurrence of a novel category of molecules in the plasma membrane of small vessel endothelium. Prototypes of these molecules are intercellular adhesion molecules (ICAM) and endothelial leukocyte adhesion molecules (ELAM), induced by cytokines and functioning as receptors for corresponding ligands on circulating leukocytes, notably granulocytes [3–5].

The first of these molecules to be induced is P-selectin (also called GMP-140 or CD62) [6], which is induced by thrombin, interleukin (IL)-1, or tumor necrosis factor (TNF), and probably subsequently E-selectin (ELAM-1) and ICAM-1 induced by IL-1 and TNF. The expression of the first two of these endothelial membrane molecules makes granulocytes attach loosely to the endothelium and roll along its surface. The molecular basis for this is not well understood at present. The binding between the endothelium and leukocytes is then strengthened by the interaction between the leukocytes' CD11/CD18 integrin heterodimer, induced by IL-8 [7], on the one surface and the ICAM-1 on the other. IL-8 also leads to shedding of other molecules (L-selectins, LAM-1/LECAM-1) that have to be shed before the leukocytes can start to emigrate.

The actual migration of leukocytes through the endothelium may be governed by chemotaxis or by "haptotaxis", i.e., migration along a gradient of surface-bound molecules. This is not entirely clear.

Several strong chemotactic substances are produced in acutely inflamed tissue, e.g., complement factor $C5_a$, leukotriene B_4, platelet-activating factor, and formylated bacterial peptides, to mention a few of the best studied [8].

Granulocytes are avid phagocytes and will immediately start to engulf bacteria and tissue detritus. Numerous granulocytes will die in the process. Dead granulocytes, bacteria, and detritus constitute what we call pus. Very early on in the process, small vessels dilate and permeability increases, although the mechanism is not well understood. The vascular changes appear to be secondary to the influx of leukocytes, since depletion of circulating granulocytes abrogates the increase in permeability [9, 10]. There is also a humoral component. Dilatation and structural changes of the small vessels allow plasma proteins to escape; among other things, this leads to the activation of complement and of coagulation, with the resulting secondary production of kinins and platelet activation.

In the normal, successful case, macrophages, mainly derived from blood monocytes, will finally engulf and dissolve dead bacteria, leukocytes, and tissue detritus. Under the influence of local growth factors, damaged connective tissue cells and extracellular matrix will be replaced, and the whole tissue returns, more or less, to its original composition and morphology.

What starts the process? Or, in the context of today's understanding of inflammation, where does the *first* signal come from, instructing the endothelial cells to expose adhesion molecules, leading to the influx of blood-borne phagocytes and plasma into the extravascular site, with all the secondary effects briefly outlined above?

There are two obvious possibilities:
1. The inflammatory agent may have a direct influence on the blood vessels.
2. The normal connective tissue cells may be triggered by the irritants to produce stimulatory substances.

There is no published evidence in favor of a direct action of microbes or microbial products on capillaries to induce endothelial adhesion molecules of the types referred to. It is known that bacterial products can act as chemoattractants for granulocytes. However, this can have an appreciable effect only after leukocytes have been attached to the endothelium of the inflamed area. Damage to the endothelium by direct chemical or physical (e.g., actinic) action is likely to result in leukocyte adhesion, although this does not appear to be well studied. Furthermore, induction of blood coagulation with the production of thrombin will quickly induce novel adhesion molecules in the plasma membranes of the endothelium [11]. Both these events — initial damage to the endothelium and initial blood coagulation — appear to be relatively uncommon causes of acute inflammation, however.

This leaves us with the second possibility. As far as we know today, the endothelial adhesive molecules of the ICAM and ELAM type are induced by cytokines, mainly IL-1 and TNF. Thus we can reformulate the question: are there cells in normal connective tissue that can react to infection by releasing significant amounts of cytokines? Indeed there are. The likely candidates among the normal connective tissue cells are endothelial cells themselves, fibroblasts, macrophages, and mast cells.

It has been established that endothelium in vitro can produce IL-1 [12] and IL-6 [13], both of which are cytokines implicated in the pathogenesis of acute inflammation. As already pointed out by Metchnikoff, however, it is unlikely that the primary signal stems from the endothelium itself, for the simple reason that inflammation usually occurs as the result of infection or damage in extravascular tissue spaces and can best be elicited experimentally by an extravascular infective agent or irritant. Intravascular application of the same agent does not normally lead to inflammation (but to other pathological processes, as the case may be). Although uncommon, the possibility should not be excluded, therefore, that cytokines produced by the endothelium as an effect of the infectious agent or irritant may sometimes play a role in the initial induction of adhesive molecules in the blood vessel walls. Fibroblasts do not seem to react to relevant stimuli by producing IL-1 or TNF in quantities that can account for the early induction of adhesion molecules in the endothelium [14]. That leaves us with the mast cells and the macrophages. Mast cells contain TNF and other relevant cytokines in their granules [15] and can release these following immunological or nonimmunological stimuli. Histamine, a major product of mast cells, is reported to modify both the production and effect of cytokines [16]. Heparin, a potent inhibitor of esterases, may easily be envisaged to influence the inflammatory reaction, although this seems to be little studied. There is no reported evidence that mast cells can be triggered directly by microbes or microbial products. On the other hand, mechanical stress and other nonspecific, strong stimuli may cause degranulation. Thus, although mast cells are scarce in many tissues, it is very possible that they contribute significantly to the early stages of inflammation.

Macrophages are ubiquitous and, as opposed to other leukocytes, normal constituents of loose connective tissues throughout the body. They are considered to be the prime producers of IL-1 and TNF [17].

Direct evidence for cytokine production by macrophages derives mainly from in vitro studies. The production of cytokines by tissue macrophages in situ has also been investigated, however [18]. On the basis of these studies, it appears likely that an infective agent will immediately trigger connective tissue macrophages to produce and release cytokines such as IL-1 and TNF, thus inducing the early changes in the endothelium that are essential for the margination, arrest, and diapedesis of leukocytes.

The effect of hemorrhage or trauma or the presence of denatured macromolecules on macrophage production of proinflammatory substances has not been much studied. However, it seems pertinent to deduce from the generally nonspecific nature of macrophage reactivity that molecules produced locally under such circumstances may trigger the macrophages. The molecular characteristics of such interactions appear to be a fruitful field of research, especially with respect to general principles of fundamental immunity.

As mentioned above, it has recently been found that thrombin induces P-selectin within minutes [11, 19]. It is also known that macrophages have an effective prothrombinase in their plasma membrane and thus are capable of generating significant amounts of thrombin [20]. These facts also link macrophage products to the induction of endothelial adhesion molecules in the early phase of acute inflammation.

The dilatation and increased permeability of small vessels, a well-known characteristic of inflammation, is conceivably also an effect of tissue macrophage products. It has long been known that E-type prostaglandins are among the most potent vasodilators [8, 9]. Stimulated macrophages produce large amounts of arachidonic acid metabolites [21]. Recently, it has been found that TNF and IL-1 increase vascular permeability by a direct effect on the endothelium [22]. Although other mediators, not of macrophage origin (histamine, serotonin, kinins), are certainly implicated, it is thus likely that the initial encounter between macrophages and microbes or other irritants will lead to the release of highly efficient vasoactive substances at the site of incipient inflammation. It has recently been reported that histamine accentuates IL-1 production by tissue macrophages [23]. This finding appears to link the mechanisms of allergic reaction to the pathogenesis of acute inflammation.

Quantitative studies of inflammation induced by local injections of *Escherichia coli* [2] have confirmed the early influx of neutrophil granulocytes that can be observed by microscopy. It was found that the rate of neutrophil accumulation peaked at 3 h after the induction and was back to zero after 6 h. Thus, the influx of neutrophils is transient. The absolute number of neutrophils that accumulated in the lesions during the first 6 h greatly exceeded the number of monocytes. However, monocytes started to emigrate just as fast as granulocytes and continued to accumulate for much longer. The accumulated monocytes transformed into macrophages, eventually becoming the predominant cell in the later stages of the inflammation. Thus, available data indicate a crucial role for tissue macrophages in the initial events of inflammation and for blood-borne, monocyte-derived macrophages in later stages.

From the days of Metchnikoff it has been acknowledged that phagocytosis and destruction of the infective agent or products of tissue damage is a central phenomenon in acute inflammation. In this process, granulocytes (neutrophils in most cases) are undoubtedly the primary effector cells. On the other hand, the capacity of macrophages to engulf and dissolve particulate matter as well as soluble macromolecules is well documented. The kinetics of leukocyte influx mentioned above also lends support to the contention that macrophages act as the predominant phagocytes during later phases of inflammation. Furthermore, the production of growth factors by stimulated macrophages may be essential for the reconstitution of tissues after an inflammatory event [24].

There is, however, little exact information on the later phases of acute inflammation.

The majority of studies have concentrated on examining the pathogenic mechanisms of initiation and propagation of the acute inflammatory response. However, an equally intriguing aspect is the process whereby the acute phase response is limited and resolution is accomplished.

First of all, many cytokines and RNA species involved in acute inflammation have a short half-life; therefore, the process can simply be turned off by the decay of the initiating events. Second, naturally occurring antagonists of "alarm cytokines" are known, such as IL-1 receptor antagonist (IL-1Ra) and the soluble TNF receptor (sTNFR) [25]. A naturally occurring soluble form of an IL-1 receptor has also been identified in body fluids [26]. Soluble receptors bind specific cytokines and thereby prevent them from binding to their receptors on cells. Naturally occurring IL-1 receptor antagonists bind to cellular IL-1 receptors, but the binding does not initiate a biological response.

The production of IL-1 and IL-1Ra is differentially regulated, even though the same cell may synthesize both cytokines. For example, in a cell stimulated with endotoxin, the expression of the IL-1b gene takes place before IL-1Ra. In addition, triggering of the receptor for immunoglobulin on the monocyte stimulates IL-1Ra, but not IL-1 production. Other cytokines may also contribute to the balance of IL-1 and IL-1Ra production. For example, IL-4, transforming growth factor-β, and IL-10 have the interesting property of increasing the synthesis of IL-1Ra while at the same time decreasing the synthesis of IL-1 [26].

IL-4 causes the downregulation of TNF and IL-1 and the upregulation of IL-1Ra and VCAM, the endothelial adhesion molecule for monocytes; therefore, it mediates the switch to a later phase of acute inflammation in which blood-borne monocytes predominate. On the other hand, IL-4 enhances apoptosis of monocytes, leading to reduced number of these cells in the inflamed tissue. IL-10, produced by Th2 lymphocytes, monocytes, macrophages, and B cells, inhibits monocyte/macrophage synthesis of IL-1, TNF, IL-6, IL-8, and colony-stimulating factor (CSF) and upregulates IL-1Ra.

IL-4 and IL-10 thus appear to be crucial for the termination of the acute inflammatory reaction. The number of Th2 lymphocytes – the main source of the two cytokines – increases due to the action of glucocorticoid hormone, which drives a shift in the Th1/Th2 balance towards Th2. Therefore, it seems that the activity of glucocorticoids and the activity of some cytokines (IL-4 and IL-10) and cytokine receptor antagonists (IL-1Ra) is sufficient to bring about the termination of the acute inflammatory response [25].

Glucocorticoids are produced due to activation of the hypothalamus–pituitary–adrenal (HPA) axis by "alarm" cytokines such as IL-1, IL-6, and TNF and provide a negative feedback loop by the inhibition of cytokine gene expression. This is probably the main and certainly the best-known feedback mechanism leading to the switching off of the inflammatory reaction. There is, however, a growing body of evidence that a lot of backup mechanisms and regulatory loops operate. The alarm cytokines, apart from inducing the "classical" HPA axis response, also alert other nervous and endocrine centers, inducing involvement of the autonomous nervous system (ANS) and the disperse endogenous opioid system (EOPS) in the complex homeostatic reactions. The immune system and the neuroendocrine system share mediators and receptors [27–32] which are used for communication within and between the systems.

Systemic Effects

The local inflammatory response is always accompanied by a spectrum of systemic reactions, as the macrophage-derived alarm cytokines IL-1, IL-6, and TNF released from the site of tissue injury also act on distant organs.

The liver is the principal target of systemic inflammatory mediators released from the site of inflammation, as was first suggested by Koy [33]. The inflammation-induced increase in liver-derived plasma glycoproteins is commonly referred to as the acute phase response [25]. A a result of tissue injury and inflammation, there is a characteristically rapid rise (within 12–24 h) in the plasma concentration of a number of glycoproteins synthesized by the liver, collectively known as acute phase reactants. Their levels undergo changes which appear to be coordinated with the time course of the inflammatory process.

Some acute phase reactants, e.g., C-reactive protein (CRP) and α_2-macroglobulin (α_2M), show dramatic (100- to 1000-fold) increases. Others increase significantly (two- to fivefold), e.g., α_1-acid glycoprotein (α_1AgP), fibrinogen, haptoglobin, α_1-antichymotrypsin (α_1AcH), and α_1-proteinase inhibitor (α_1Pi). Still others (ceruloplasmin and complement component C3) show a modest increase, while some molecules, most notably albumin, demonstrate a significant decrease in plasma concentration. The variations are species dependent and are under unknown control, although the phylogenetic conservation of the acute phase response indicates an important function. The acute phase reactants include transport proteins, proteinase inhibitors, coagulation proteins, and complement proteins. Thus the acute phase response of the hepatocytes has a direct effect on the pathways leading to the inflammatory response — coagulation, complement, kinin function, and fibrinolysis.

The main function of the acute phase response appears in a broad sense to be to restore the homeostatic balance disturbed by tissue injury. Some of the more obvious functions include fibrinogen deposition as a matrix for wound healing and coagulation as well as inhibition of neutrophil proteases by α_1Pi and α_1AcH. Haptoglobin is a transport protein which binds hemoglobin, and the subsequent complex has peroxidase activity. Ceruloplasmin is a copper transport protein, but it also exhibits a dismutase-like activity on superoxide anion and therefore acts as an O_2-scavenger in inflammatory reactions. α_1AgP exhibits some antiheparin activity and may inhibit platelet reaction, whereas α_2M inhibits polymorphonuclear chemotaxis. One of the most abundant acute phase reactants, CRP, interacts with a phosphoryl-choline moiety and can be seen to bind to damaged cells at the site of inflammation. CRP was first described as a molecule which bound to the C-polysaccharide of *Streptococcus pneumoniae*. CRP functions as an opsonin once bound to its ligand by fixing complement, and as such it appears to protect against experimental *Streptococcus pneumoniae* infection. Recently, Badolato and co-workers claimed that serum amyloid A functions as a chemoattractant for leukocytes [34].

One of the clinical signs of the local inflammation is pain. However, immune cells infiltrating the inflamed tissue contribute to local analgesia by the production of opioid peptides acting on opioid receptors present on sensory nerve terminals [35]. Lymphocytes, monocytes, and macrophages infiltrating the inflamed tissue contain not only significant amounts of β-endorphin and enkephalin immunoreactivity, but also the respective mRNA, incidating that these peptides are produced within these cells [35, 28]. In addition, it has been shown that cytokines, e.g., IL-6 and TNF, induce secretion of opioids from leukocytes and lymphocytes [36].

The alarm cytokines released from the inflamed tissue also have other distant targets. They alter the temperature set-point in the hypothalamus and regulate the febrile response through the induction of prostaglandin E_2 (PGE_2) [26]; they also induce adrenal production of glucocorticoid hormone, acting both via the adrenal–pituitary axis [25] and directly on the adrenal cortical cells [37, 38]. Glucocorticosteroids are required for the hepatic acute phase response, but at the same time provide a negative feedback loop, since they inhibit cytokine gene expression [25] and inhibit the recruitment of neutrophils and monocytes/macrophages to the inflammatory site [39].

In most cases, the acute inflammation subsides over 24–28 h and, within a few days, the organism returns to normal, demonstrating the protective and homeostatic nature of this important host response. However, the normal course can be prolonged, perhaps by the persistence of stimulation or disruption of normal control mechanisms, and can become a chronic inflammation. It is at present not known what factors are crucial in this event.

References

1. Metchnikoff E (1968) Comparative pathology of inflammation. Dover, New York
2. Cybulsky MI, Chan MK, Movat HZ (1988) Acute inflammation and microthrombosis induced by endotoxin, interleukin-1, and tumor necrosis factor and their implication in gram-negative infection. Lab Invest 58:365–378
3. Bevilacqua MP, Prober JS, Mendrick DL et al. (1987) Identification of an inducible endothelial-leukocyte adhesion molecule. Proc Natl Acad Sci USA 84:9238–9242
4. Dustin ML, Springer TA (1988) Lymphocyte function-associated antigen-1 (LFA-1) interaction with intercellular adhesion molecule-1 (ICAM-1) is one of at least three mechanisms for lymphocyte adhesion to cultured endothelial cell. J Cell Biol 107:321–331
5. Osborne L (1990) Leucocyte adhesion to endothelium in inflammation. Cell 62:3–6
6. Lawrence MB, Springer TA (1991) Leukocytes roll on a selectin at physiologic flow rates: distinction from and prerequisite for adhesion through integrins. Cell 65:859–873
7. Lo SK, Detmers PA, Levin SM et al. (1989) Transient adhesion of neutrophils to endothelium. J Exp Med 169:1779–1793
8. Williams TJ, Peck MJ (1977) Role of prostaglandin-mediated vasodilatation in inflammation. Nature 270:530–532
9. Kopaniak MM, Hay JB, Movat HZ (1978) The effect of hyperemia on vascular permeability. Microvasc Res 15:77–82
10. Kopaniak MM, Movat HZ (1983) Kinetics of acute inflammation induced by Escherichia coli in rabbits. II. The effect of hyperimmunization, complement depletion, and depletion of leukocytes. Am J Pathol 110:13–29
11. Hattori R, Hamilton KK, Fugate RD et al. (1989) Stimulated secretion of endothelial von Willebrand factor is accompanied by rapid redistribution to the cell surface of the intracellular granule membrane protein GMP-140. J Biol Chem 264:7768–7771
12. Wagner CR, Vetto RM, Burger DR (1984) The mechanism of antigen presentation by endothelial cells. Immunobiology 168:453–469
13. Shalaby MR, Waage A, Espevik T (1989) Cytokine regulation of interleukin 6 production by human endothelial cells. Cell Immunol 121:372–382
14. Iribe H, Koga T, Kotani S et al. (1983) Stimulating effect of MDP and its adjuvant — active analogues on guinea pig fibroblasts for the production of thymocyte-activating factor. J Exp Med 157:2190–2195
15. Gordon JR, Galli SJ (1990) Mast cells as a source of both preformed and immunologically inducible TNF-V8,1α/cachectin. Nature 346:274–276

16. Fabes A, Merety K (1992) Histamine: an early messenger in inflammatory and immune reactions. Immunol Today 13:154–156
17. Oppenheim JJ, Kovacs EJ, Matsushima K et al. (1986) There is more than one interleukin 1. Immunol Today 7:45–48
18. Rasmussen L-T, Fandrem J, Seljelid R (1990) Dynamics of blood components and peritoneal fluid during treatment of murine E. coli sepsis with β-1,3-D-polyglucose derivatives. II. Interleukin 1, tumor necrosis factor, prostaglandin E_2, and leukotriene B_4. Scand J Immunol 32:333–340
19. Lorant DE, Patel KD, McIntyre TM et al. (1991) Coexpression of GMP-140 and PAF by endothelium stimulated by histamine or thrombin: a juxtacrine system for adhesion and activation of neutrophils. J Cell Biol 115:223–234
20. Lindahl U, Pejler G, Bøgwald J et al. (1989) A prothrombinase complex of mouse peritoneal macrophages. Arch Biochem Biophys 273(1):180–188
21. Scott WA, Zrike JM, Hamill AL et al. (1980) Regulation of arachidonic acid metabolites in macrophages. J Exp Med 152:324–335
22. Royall JA, Beckow RL, Beckman JS et al. (1989) Tumor necrosis factor and interleukin 1 alpha increase vascular endothelial permeability. Am J Physiol 257:L399–L410
23. Okamoto H, Nakano K (1990) Regulation of interleukin-1 synthesis by histamine produced by mouse peritoneal macrophages per se. Immunology 69:162–165
24. Ross R, Raines EW, Bowen-Pope DF (1986) The biology of platelet-derived growth factor. Cell 46:155–169
25. Baumann H, Gauldie J (1994) The acute phase response. Immunol Today 15:74–80
26. Dinarello CA, Cannon JG, Mancilla J (1991) Interleukin-6 as an endogenous pyrogen: induction of prostaglandin E_2 in brain but not in peripheral blood mononuclear cells. Brain Res 562:199–206
27. Shavit Y, Terman GW, Martin FC, Lewis JW, Liebenkind JC, Gale RP (1985) Stress, opioid peptides, the immune system, and cancer. J Immunol 135:834s–837s
28. Przewlocki R (1993) Opioid systems and stress. In: Hertz A (ed) Opioids II. Springer, Berlin Heidelberg New York, pp 293–324 (Handbook of experimental pharmacology, vol 104/2)
29. Blalock JE, Smith EM (1985) The immune system: our mobile brain? Immunol Today 6:115–117
30. Felten SY, Felten DL, Bellinger DL et al. (1987) Noradrenergic sympathetic neural interactions with the immune system: structure and function. Immunol Rev 100:225–260
31. Sibinga NE, Goldstein A (1988) Opioid peptides and opioid receptors in cells of the immune system. Annu Rev Immunol 6:219–249
32. Weigent DA, Blalock JE (1987) Interactions between the neuroendocrine and immune systems: common hormones and receptors. Immunol Rev 100:79–108
33. Koy A (1974) Acute phase reactants. In: Allison A (ed) Structure and function of plasma proteins. Plenum, London, pp 73–75
34. Badolato R, Wang JM, Murphy W et al. (1994) Serum amyloid A is a chemoattractant: induction of migration, adhesion, and tissue infiltration of monocytes and polymorphonuclear leukocytes. J Exp Med 180:203–209
35. Stein C, Hassan AHS, Przewlocki R, Gramsch C, Peter K, Herz A (1990) Opioids from immunocytes interact with receptors on sensory nerves to inhibit nociception in inflammation. Proc Natl Acad Sci USA 87:5935–5939
36. Heijnen CJ, Kavelaars A, Ballieux RE (1991) β-Endorphin: cytokine and neuropeptide. Immunol Rev 119:41–59
37. Winter JSD, Gow KW, Perry YS, Greenberg AH (1990) A stimulatory effect of interleukin-1 on the adrenocortical cortisol secretion mediated by prostaglandins. Endocrinology 127:1904–1909
38. Salas MA, Evans SW, Levell MJ, Whicher TJ (1990) Interleukin-6 and ACTH act synergistically to stimulate the release of corticosterone from adrenal gland cells. Clin Exp Immunol 79:470–473
39. Parillo JE, Fauci AS (1979) Mechanisms of glucocorticoid action on immune processes. Annu Rev Pharmacol Toxicol 19:179–201

Skeletal Muscle in the Stress-Induced Catabolic State

J. Wernerman

Although the largest organ in the human body, skeletal muscle is often considered not to have any role of vital importance in the stress-induced catabolic state. This is true in the sence that muscular strength has no relevance in fighting infections or in improving oxygenation during critical illness. Nevertheless, skeletal muscle has two major roles for such patients: (1) to serve as a reservoire for amino acid substrates needed in other tissues during the stress-induced catabolic state and (2) to function as a limiting organ for mobilization during convalescence. This implies that the size of skeletal muscle tissue is a determinant for the size of the store of amino acid substrates available for mobilization during critical illness. This store may be a limiting factor for survival if critical illness is long-standing. Indirect evidence for this hypothesis is the well-documented fact that malnutrition, in general accompanied by muscle wasting, is associated with a poorer outcome after sepsis and surgical trauma. Furthermore, restitution of lean body mass following depletion is a very slow process. In younger individuals, restitution of body composition takes years, and among elderly people it is often not possible to achieve at all. Patients who have to be rehabilitated during the convalescence phase are heavily dependent upon their muscular reserves in this aspect. This means that remains of skeletal muscle tissue and in particular of muscle function are a determining factor for the duration as well as the outcome of convalescense. In addition, susceptibility to late complications is also related to the nutritional state, indirectly depending upon the muscle mass.

To be more precise, maintenance of amino acid substrate export from muscle may become a critical factor during acute illness. This suggests therapeutic efforts to economize with a limiting resource. Thus, nutritional therapy to maintain body composition and to provide necessary nutrients should be instituted. However, conventional nutrition does not prevent wasting of muscle mass. At best muscle depletion is slowed down. Consequently, maintenance of muscle proteins may not be an optimal strategy if it implics an impaired production of amino acids to be exported. The result may be maintenance of muscle tissue at the expense of essential substrates for other tissues. Instead, a nutritional intervention should aim at maintaining the export of amino acids from muscle. In particular, the composition of the amino acid export from muscle may have several advantages, so a nutritional therapy may be most efficient if that composition is imitated.

In the postabsorptive state, amino acids are constantly exported from skeletal muscle to be taken up across the splanchnic area. One third is glutamine, another

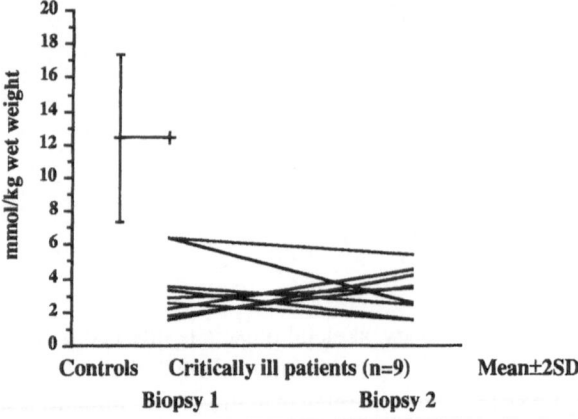

Fig. 1. The free glutamine concentration in skeletal muscle of critically ill patients is distinctly below a 95% confidence interval of muscle glutamine in control subjects. Over time there are few changes in this low glutamine concentration, regardless of whether the patient's condition improves or deteriorates. Consecutive biopsies were taken from intensive care unit (ICU) patients more than 5 days apart [4]

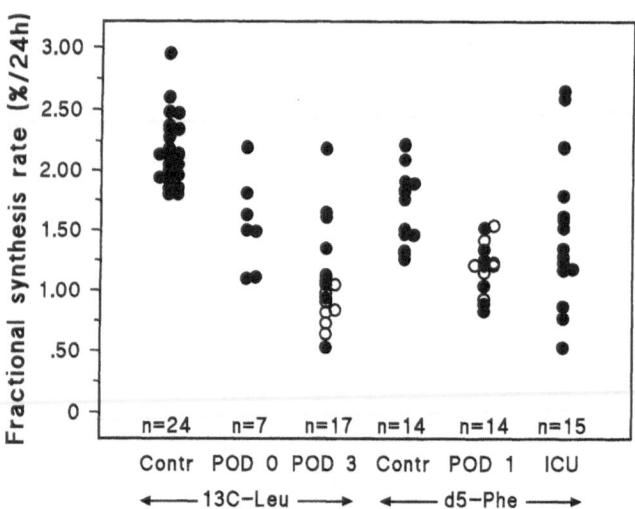

Fig. 2. Protein synthesis rate in skeletal muscle of metabolically healthy patients undergoing open cholecystectomy (*n*=38) and critically ill patients in the intensive care unit (ICU; *n*=15). Biopsies were taken from cholecystectomy patients preoperatively *(Contr),* immediately following the surgical procedure *(POD 0),* and on the first and third postoperative days *(POD 1, 3). Open circles* denote patients receiving postoperative total parenteral nutrition (TPN). Biopsies from the intensive care unit (ICU) patients were taken between the fourth and the 15th day of critical illness, and the patients were fed intravenously. Protein synthesis rate decreased by 30% immediately following surgery and on the first postoperative day, and by 50% on the third postoperative day. In contrast, the ICU patients had a mean value only 15% below controls, although they exhibited a large interindividual scatter. The measurements were performed using ^{13}C-leucine or d5-phenylalanine, the latter giving a 10%–15% lower estimate of protein synthesis rate [5, 6, 25, 26]

third is alanine, and a mixture of all the other amino acids make up the remaining third. Following trauma and during sepsis, the release of free amino acids from the periphery is increased, but the proportion between the individual amino acids remains the same [1]. Concomitantly, a depletion of muscle free glutamine is seen [2, 3]. The intracellular glutamine concentration is diminished to below 25% of normal values (Fig. 1). The decrease in muscle glutamine is not related to the progress or time course of the critical illness [4], and it does not seem to relate to the rate of muscle protein synthesis. Following surgical trauma, there is a dramatic drop in muscle protein synthesis by approximately 50% [5]. Critically ill patients also show a drop of synthesis rate in muscle (Fig. 2), but although statistically significant it is less than 20% [6]. Thus there is no correlation between the low free muscle glutamine concentration and the reduction of muscle protein synthesis. Nevertheless, muscle proteins are lost, suggesting an elevated degradation rate of muscle proteins, as the rate of synthesis is only marginally affected. Following elective surgery, a 10% loss of muscle proteins is reported [7]. This may be explained by the drop in protein synthesis without any concomitant change in protein breakdown. Conventional nutrition may reduce the loss of muscle proteins by a reduced degradation rate following surgical trauma [8]. In the septic state the degradation rate is elevated, as indicated by the efflux of 3-methylhistidine and of aromatic amino acids (Phe+Tyr) from the leg [9]. Simultaneously, low levels of glutathione are seen in muscle [10], suggesting an increased activity of the proteosomes as well as of the cytoplasmatic proteases.

When discussing muscle protein metabolism in the metabolically stressed state, it must be emphasized that a number of methodological difficulties are involved. Protein synthesis may be studied by the use of isotopic techniques [11]. Especially in the fed state, conflicting results are reported in the literature when healthy subjects are studied [12]. The current state of knowledge is that the effects of feeding and fasting upon muscle protein synthesis in man are not established with a satisfying degree of accuracy. Unfortunately, this does not give a solid foundation on which to study the effects of nutritional therapy in different stressed states. The techniques available to estimate muscle protein synthesis should primarily be regarded as qualitative in character. All isotopic techniques depend upon the underlying assumption that the isotopic enrichment in the immediate precursor pool for muscle protein synthesis (the amino acyl–tRNA pool) can be accurately estimated [13]. The major controversies in this field may be traced back to the uncertainty involved in that assumption. Concerning muscle protein degradation, available techniques are even less accurate. The discussion of the methodological difficulties is included here in order to underline the importance of referring to what technique has been used to obtain the different pieces of information that are available in the literature.

In healthy subjects, feeding induces an uptake of amino acids across skeletal muscle [14]. Nevertheless, glutamine and alanine are constantly exported from the periphery, indicating that these two amino acids are manufactured from the other amino acids in muscle. Since amino acids cannot be stored, the net uptake across muscle tissue is only transient following a meal. A large, protein-rich meal affects the intracellular free amino acids only marginally [15]. Muscle protein synthesis is

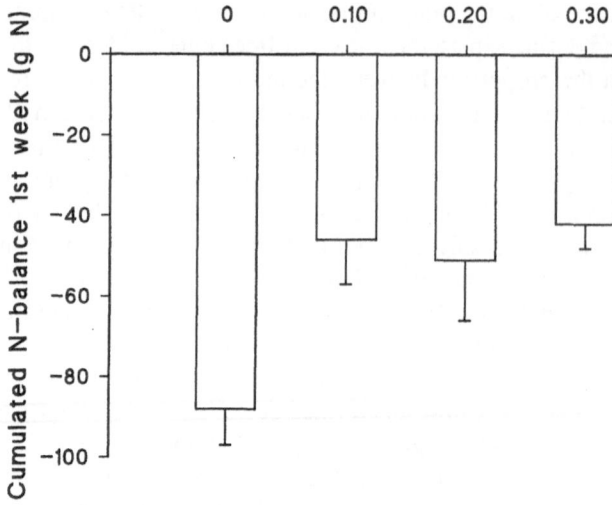

Fig. 3. Accumulated nitrogen balance in critically ill patients during the first week of intensive care. All patients were given intravenous nutrition containing an adequate amount of calories, but they were randomized to receive a different amino acid supply containing 0, 0.10, 0.20, or 0.30 g N/kg body weight per day. The negative nitrogen balance was improved by 50% when an amino acid support corresponding to 0.10 g N/kg body weight per day was given. However, an amino acid support above that level did not improve the nitrogen balance in that group of patients [24]

not influenced by a single meal in any measurable way if studied with regards to the ribosome pattern [16] or by incorporation of ^{13}C-leucine into muscle proteins, when given as a flooding dose [17]. In contrast, a doubling of muscle protein synthesis rate as compared to overnight fasting is seen when the synthesis rate is estimated by the incorporation of ^{13}C-leucine into muscle proteins during a constant infusion [18].

Post-traumatically, muscle protein synthesis decreases regardless of which technique of measurement is used [5, 19]. Conventional nutrition seems to be unable to reverse this decrease (Fig. 2). This contrasts with the situation that occurs when healthy subjects are refed after a short period of starvation. Short-term starvation of healthy volunteers results in a decrease of muscle protein synthesis and in the concentration of muscle free glutamine [20, 21], which are both rapidly normalized upon refeeding [21, 22].

In critically ill patients, conventional nutrition cannot prevent a substantial loss of muscle proteins [23]. Nutrition with a higher caloric content only seems to result in an accumulation of adipose tissue. In addition, a surplus of protein or amino acids does not seem to result in improvement of whole body nitrogen balance when studied carefully. Compared to no nitrogen intake, nutrition including 0.1 g N/kg body weight per day cuts the nitrogen losses by 50%. However, provision of nitrogen above that level does not result in any further nitrogen accretion [24]. These results were obtained when adequate amounts of energy were supplied (Fig. 3).

In summary, the loss of muscle tissue during critical illness may be attenuated to some degree by nutritional treatment. However, the amino acid substrates exported from muscle are vital for the enterocytes and immunocompetent cells in the splanchnic region. Muscle tissue is the substrate provider, which may be a limiting factor for survival when critical illness is long-standing. A reasonable goal for metabolic and nutritional therapy in the stressed state may be to give a treatment similar to the "natural" export from the periphery. Furthermore, such a therapy may save muscle tissue, thus facilitating rehabilitation during the convalescent phase.

References

1. Clowes GHA, Randell HT, Cha C-J (1980) Amino acid and energy metabolism in septic and traumatized patients. JPEN 4:195–203
2. Roth E, Funovics J, Mühlbacher F et al. (1982) Metabolic disorders in severe abdominal sepsis: glutamine deficiency in skeletal muscle. Clin Nutr 1:25–42
3. Vinnars E, Bergström J, Fürst P (1975) Influence of the postoperative state on the intracellular free amino acids in human muscle tissue. Ann Surg 182:665–671
4. Gamrin L, Wernerman J, Vinnars E (1992) The free amino acid pattern in skeletal muscle of critically ill patients does not change over time. Clin Nutr 11 [Suppl]:48 (abstr.)
5. Essén P, McNurlan M, Sonnenfeld T et al. (1993) Muscle protein synthesis after operation: effects of intravenous nutrition. Eur J Surg 159:195–200
6. Essén P, McNurlan M, Tjäder I et al. (1992) Tissue protein synthesis in the critically ill patient. Clin Nutr 11:1–2 (abstr)
7. Wernerman J, Petersson B, Hultman E, Vinnars E (1990) The decline of the protein content in skeletal muscle after uncomplicated surgical trauma is still not resistuted 30 days postoperatively. Clin Nutr 9 [Suppl]:90 (abstr)
8. Rennie MJ, Bennegård K, Edén E, Emery PW, Lundholm K (1984) Urinary excretion and efflux from the leg of 3-metylhistidine before and after major surgical operation. Metabolism 33:250–256
9. Sjölin J, Stjernström H, Friman G, Larsson J, Wahren J (1990) Total and net muscle protein breakdown in infection determined by amino effluxes. Am J Physiol 258:E856–E863
10. Luo J, Hammarqvist F, Andersson K, Wernerman J (1994) Glutathone depletion in human skeletal muscle occurs after surgical trauma. Clin Nutr 131 [Suppl]:24–25 (abstr)
11. Smith K, Rennie M (1990) Protein turnover and amino acid metabolism in human skeletal muscle. Clin Endocr Metab 3:461–498
12. Garlick PJ, Wernerman J, McNurlan MA, Essén P (1990) What is the normal response of protein turnover to nutrient supply? Clin Nutr 9:294–296
13. Garlick PJ, Wernerman J, McNurlan MA, Essén P (1994) Measurement of tissue protein synthesis from the incorporation of labelled amino acids. Am J Physiol 266:E287–E297
14. Elia M, Livesey G (1983) Effects of ingested steak and infused leucine on forelimb metabolism in man, and the fate of the carbon skeletons and amino groups of branched-chain amino acids. Clin Sci 64:517–526
15. Bergström J, Fürst P, Vinnars E (1990) Effect of test meal, without and with protein on muscle and plasma free amino acids. Clin Sci 79:331–337
16. Wernerman J, von der Decken A, Vinnars E (1985) The diurnal pattern of protein synthesis in human skeletal muscle. Clin Nutr 4:203–205
17. McNurlan M, Essén P, Milne E, Vinnars E, Garlick P, Wernerman J (1993) Temporal responses of protein synthesis in human skeletal muscle to feeding. Br J Nutr 69:117–126
18. Rennie M, Edwards R, Halliday D, Matthews D, Wollman S, Millward D (1982) Muscle protein synthesis measured by stable isotope techniques in man: the effects of feeding and fasting. Clin Sci 63:519–523
19. Wernerman J, von der Decken A, Vinnars E (1986) Protein synthesis in skeletal muscle in relation to nitrogen balance after abdominal surgery: the effect of total parenteral nutrition. JPEN 10:578–582
20. Wernerman J, von der Decken A, Vinnars E (1985) Size distribution of ribosomes in biopsy specimens of human skeletal muscle during starvation. Metabolism 34:665–669

21. Andersson K, Luo J, Hammarqvist F, Wernerman J (1994) The effect of fasting on muscle glutathione levels. Clin Nutr 13 [Suppl]:0.12 (abstr)
22. Wernerman J, von der Decken A, Vinnars E (1986) Polyribosome concentration in human skeletal muscle after starvation and parenteral or enteral refeeding. Metabolism 35:447–451
23. Streat Sj, Beddoe AH, Hill GL (1987) Aggressive nutritional support does not prevent protein loss despite fat gain in septic intensive care patients. J Trauma 27:262–266
24. Larsson J, Lennmarken C, Mårtensson J et al. (1990) Nitrogen requirements in severely injured patients. Br J Surg 77:413–416
25 Essén P, McNurlan MA, Wernerman J, Vinnars E, Garlick P (1992) Uncomplicated surgery but not general anesthesia, decreases muscle protein synthesis. Am J Physiol 262:E253–E260
26. Tjäder I, Essén P, McNurlan MA, Garlick PJ, Wernerman J (1992) Protein synthesis rate in human skeletal muscle decrease 24 h after abdominal surgery irrespective of intravenous nutrition. Clin Nutr 11 [Suppl]:49

The Heart and Circulation in the Acute Catabolic State

D. Sørlie, Ø. Irtun, and T. Myrmel

Introduction

The endocrine response to surgical or traumatic stress results in a synergistic interaction between the hypothalamic–pituitary–adrenal axis and the sympathetic nervous system [1]. The heart and vascular systems are effectors in this stress response
and adapt the organism to the stressful situation by a number of compensatory alterations. This adaptation is illustrated by the classic hypovolemic shock with tachycardia, increased stroke work, and elevated systemic vascular resistance normaliz-
ing tissue circulation. In contrast to this adaptory function of a normal cardiovascular system, extreme septic shock is a poorly compensated hyperdynamic state with
reduced systemic vascular resistance, leakage of plasma to the extravascular space,
often a normal or increased cardiac output despite contractile dysfunction, and an elevated central venous oxygen concentration [2]. Although recent emphasis has been
placed on the similarities between such different pathogenic states as surgical stress,
trauma, pancreatitis, and sepsis – commonly called "the systemic inflammatory response" [2] – the different pathogenetic states form a spectrum of dysfunctional en-
vironments for the cardiovascular system. When the responses of the heart and circulation in the acute catabolic state are described, the heterogeneous nature of these
different situations must be kept in mind. The cardiovascular compensation during
surgical stress or bleeding is often sufficient for the organism. On the other hand,
when the systemic inflammatory response is pronounced, as in extreme sepsis, the
heart and vasculature is also affected and the compensatory responses to this distrib-
utive shock might be inadequate for the survival of the organism.

Cardiovascular Dysfunction

During the systemic inflammatory response, as seen in septic shock, the ventricular function is abnormal [2]. Despite an often normal cardiac output, both the right
and left ventricular ejection fractions are reduced and end-diastolic and end-systol-
ic volumes are increased. The reduction in ventricular function usually occurs
24–48 h after the onset of sepsis and subsides 5–10 days after recovery in patients
who survive the septic state. In general, the duration of the hyperdynamic cardiovascular state with reduced ventricular function will determine the outcome for patients in extreme sepsis. Normalization of the hemodynamic parameters within

24 h indicate a favorable prognosis [3]. The exact mechanism for this reduced cardiac function during the systemic inflammatory response is still unkown, but the most likely mediators will be discussed below.

In pure surgical stress, preexisting cardiovascular disease can preclude the normal cardiovascular compensatory adaptation. Every surgeon knows that coronary heart disease makes a major contribution to morbidity and mortality in most surgical patient populations. Tarhan and coworkers reviewed the Mayo Clinic experience with 32 877 general anesthesias from 1967 to 1968 and found that patients operated on within 3 months after an acute myocardial infarction had a 37% reinfarction rate [4]. In the perioperative period, myocardial oxygen requirements may be markedly increased as a result of tachycardia, hypertension, and left ventricular dilatation. Blood oxygen-carrying capacity is often substantially reduced because of anemia and the less optimal characteristics of transfused blood. Marked changes in the neurohormonal milieu may increase vascular tone. Also, other perioperative changes may facilitate coronary thrombosis [5]. There is often an increased coronary shear stress, enhanced platelet aggregation, a generalized hypercoagulable state, and a precipitating coronary vasospasm induced by neurohormonal factors. Thus, in the perioperative period, the presence of coronary disease, but not necessarily preexisting critical stenosis, is the basis for ischemic events.

Cardiac Metabolism

Since the pioneering work by Richard J. Bing, "the father of cardiac metabolism," cardiac substrate metabolism has been viewed as stoichiometrically determined; the heart "eats what it gets" [6]. Thus, the high circulatory level of fatty acids found during catecholamine bursts should increase fatty acid oxidation [7]. This is potentially harmful, as high levels of fatty acids increase oxygen consumption in the myocardium and could increase the occurrence of malignant arrhythmias [8]. However, a number of recent publications point to a more complicated picture of cardiac substrate metabolism in catabolic states.

After uncomplicated cardiac surgery, there seems to be a reduced extraction of fatty acids from the coronary circulation [9, 10]. Whether this indicates a reduced fatty acid oxidation is somewhat controversial [11, 12], but positron emission tomography (PET) scanning after brief episodes of ischemia supports the observation that fatty acid oxidation is reduced [13]. Also, in a model of peritoneal sepsis in rats, a reduced expression of the carnitine palmitoyl transferase gene has been found in liver [14]. The functional consequence of this reduction is a reduced mitochrondrial β-oxidation of fatty acids in septic states. Whether such a reduced gene expression also occurs in the heart has to our knowledge not been investigated. However, the traditional view of cardiac metabolism as a passive consequence of stoichiometric competition between substrates needs to be revised. It is tempting to propose that different stressors could induce a heterogeneous effect on the expression of genes regulating substrate metabolism, possibly through an immediate-early gene response [15, 16]. Thus, substrate preference could theoretically be dependent on the particular pathogenetic state.

An experimental observation from postischemic hearts points to yet another unexplained alteration in cardiac metabolism after metabolic stress. After brief episodes of ischemia, there seems to be a disproportionately high oxygen consumption [17, 18]. The reason for this "oxygen wasting" is still unknown, but could be explained by ventricular dilatation (as seen in septic states), altered substrate metabolism, or an inefficient coupling between excitation and contraction in the myocardium. To what extent this is a general myocardial response to stressful stimuli has not yet been established. To date, this energetically inefficient contractility has also been found in hyperthyroid rabbits [19]. Interestingly, in these rabbits there is an alteration in the expression of myosin-heavy chains from an adult V_3 form to the embryonic V_1 form [20]. Whether this qualitative change of contractile proteins follows other cellular stress responses remains to be clarified.

Morphology

Gotloib et al. [21] found loss of microvascular negative charges accompanied by interstitial edema in septic rat hearts. These authors used a model of multiorgan failure with ruthenium red and polyethylene imine as cationic binding tracers. Twenty-four hours after induction of sepsis, negative charges had decreased in glycocalyx and the basement membrane of myocardial capillary endothelial cells. There was a substantial amount of interstitial edema, but the changes were completely reversed after 13 days. These morphometric data demonstrate the development of protein-rich interstitial edema and defective cell volume regulation observed in cardiac muscle of endotoxin-shocked animals. The authors suggest that this myocardial edema may be the origin of the cardiac dysfunction observed in both experimental and human septic shock.

Mediators

Figure 1 shows an updated number of endogenous mediators shown to be involved in the systemic inflammatory response which hence could play a role in cardiac dysfunction.

During the last 20 years, the myocardial depressant factor has been extensively sought as an explanation for the reduced cardiac function in septic states [2]. Although the nature of such a substance still remains to be unequivocally determined, experimental evidence would indicate that such a substance (or substances) do in fact exist. Parillo and coworkers [22] exposed myocardial cells from newborn rats to serum from septic patients. Compared to myocytes exposed to serum from healthy controls, these myocytes had a reduced extent and velocity of shortening. Also, a high level of this response was associated with a substantially reduced ejection fraction and increased mortality in the patient population [23].

As shown in Fig. 1, it is likely that multiple agents are responsible for causing organ dysfunction in the systemic inflammatory response. To search for the cause

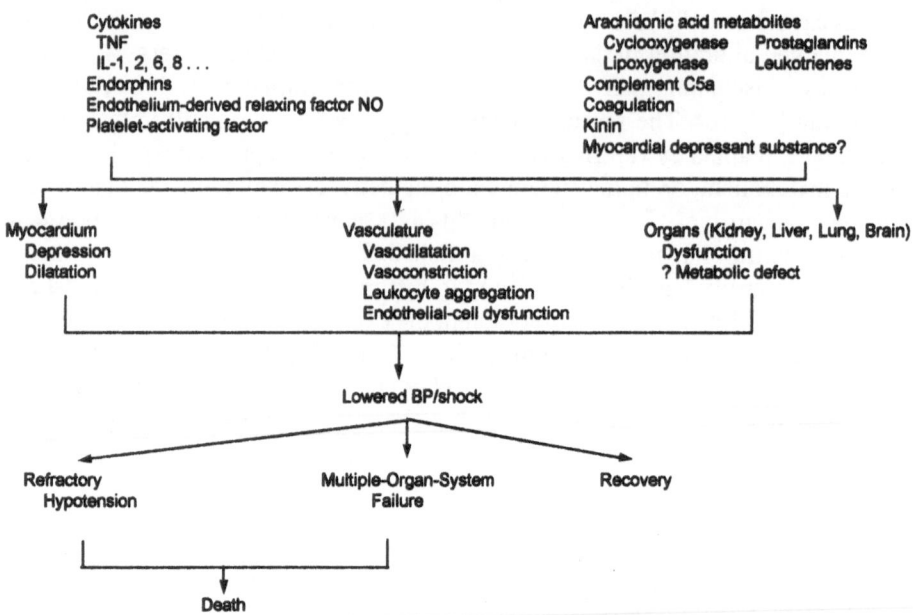

Fig. 1. Endogenous factors influencing cardiovascular performance in the acute catabolic state. *TNF*, tumor necrosis factor; *IL*, interleukin; *BP*, blood pressure. (Modified from [2])

of this response may be a search for something that does not exist as a single entity [24]. However, some of the mediators have been extensively studied. Tumor necrosis factor (TNF) seems to play a particularly central role in the pathogenesis of the systemic inflammatory response. A meta-analysis of 60 articles addressing the role of TNF concluded that this factor may be responsible for initiating many of the observed responses to endotoxin [25]. In an experimental study in dogs, intravenous infusion of recombinant TNF-α was found to decrease systemic vascular resistance, but not intrinsic myocardial performance [26]. The importance of TNF in the septic state has also been demonstrated in adult rhesus monkeys; all animals given monoclonal antibodies to TNF survived a lethal challenge of lipopolysaccharides from salmonella [27]. From a study in guinea pigs, it was concluded that TNF causes in vitro myocardial depression and reduces cardiac responsiveness to norepinephrine [28]. A reduced responsiveness to catecholamines has also been demonstrated in man, suggesting that a β-adrenergic receptor dysfunction might contribute to the reduced myocardial performance [29]. In rats, TNF-α was found to enhance muscle degradation [30].

During the last decade, a vast number of studies has also been published on the possible role of oxygen-derived free radicals as mediators of deleterious effects of the inflammatory response in the myocardium [31]. As these chemical substances are produced in activated polymorphonuclear leukocytes [24], they may be a general cause of organ dysfunction in the body. However, to what extent this response does in fact overshoot during different pathological states and thus contribute to myocardial dysfunction is still somewhat uncertain.

Cellular Stress Response – A Protective Response?

In recent years a family of proteins called the "heat shock proteins" (HSP) has been isolated from a number of cell systems as a response to different stressful stimuli [32]. These proteins are highly conserved throughout evolution and apparently play a basic protective role in the cellular defense system through conservation and transportation of different intracellular proteins. Thus, these proteins have been called intracellular chaperones. In the heart, HSP are induced by a number of stressors such as pressure overload, ischemia, increased temperature, hypoxia, and different metal ions [33]. There is now increasing evidence that HSP induce a general cellular protection independent of the inductory stimulus (the so-called cross-protection) [34]. For example, increasing body temperature in rats prior to myocardial ischemia induces a partial protection towards the ischemic damage. Induction of HSP seems to be a very basic cellular protective response to different stressors.

Interestingly, the combined trauma of laparatomy and bleeding in rats induced a rapid and substantial induction of the HSP70 mRNA in the adrenal medulla and the aortic wall [35]. As shown by the same authors in a subsequent study [36], the induction of HSP70 mRNA in the aortic wall could be completely blocked by α_1-receptor blockers. Thus, this rapid cellular response is induced during the endocrine response to a stressful stimulus. The role of the stress protein induction in this reflex-induced response to catecholamine stress still remains to be explained, but the response seems to be the cellular effector of the hypothalamic–pituitary–adrenal stress reflexes.

Conclusion

The acute catabolic state is a heterogeneous group of events ranging from the modest, hardly recognizable response to moderate trauma to a severe, highly lethal condition, as seen in septic shock. The pathophysiology of the acute catabolic state has been extensively studied in recent years, and we may now start to discern protective and harmful responses. An extensive systemic inflammatory response entails considerable cardiovascular stress and causes morbidity and mortality in susceptible patients. Hopefully our new insights will soon enable us to direct treatment towards hampering deleterious effects and stimulating the protective cellular stress responses.

References

1. Udelsman R, Holbrook NJ (1994) Endocrine and molecular responses to surgical stress. Curr Probl Surg 31:658–720
2. Parrillo JE (1993) Pathogenetic mechanisms of septic shock. N Engl J Med 328:147–177
3. Parker M, Shelhamar JH, Natanson C et al. (1987) Serial cardiovascular variables in survivors and nonsurvivors in human septic shock; heat rate and an early predictor of prognosis. Crit Care Med 15:923–929

4. Tarhan S, Moffit EA, Taylor WF et al. (1972) Myocardial infarction after general anaesthesia. JAMA 220:1451–1454
5. Massie BM, Mangano DT (1993) Risk stratification for noncardiac surgery. Circulation 87:1752–1755
6. Bing RJ (1965) Cardiac metabolism. Physiol Rev 45:171–213
7. Neely JR, Morgan HE (1974) Relationship between carbohydrate and lipid metabolism and the energy balance of heart muscle. Annu Rev Physiol 36:413–419
8. Oliver MT, Kurien VA, Greenwood TW (1968) Relationship between serum-free fatty acids and arrhythmias and death after myocardial infarction. Lancet i:710–715
9. Svennson S, Svedjeholm R, Ekroth R et al. (1990) Trauma metabolism and the heart. J Thorac Cardiovasc Surg 99:1063–1073
10. Teoh KH, Mickle DAG, Weisel RD et al. (1988) Decreased postoperative myocardial fatty acid oxidation. J Surg Res 44:36–44
11. McMillin JB (1990) Myocardial energy metabolism early after cardiac operations. J Thorac Cardiovasc Surg 99:1110–1112
12. Liedtke AJ, Demaison L, Eggleston AI et al. (1988) Changes in substrate metabolism and effects of excess fatty acids in reperfused myocardium. Circ Res 62:535–542
13. Schwaiger M, Schelbert HR, Keen R et al. (1985) Retention and clearance of C-11 palmitic acid in ischemic and reperfused canine myocardium. JACC 6:311–320
14. Barke RA, Brady PS, Roy S et al. (1992) The possible inhibitory role of the leucine-zipper DNA binding protein c-fos in the regulation of hepatic gene expression after sepsis. Surgery 112:412–418
15. Barke RA, Roy S, Chapin RB et al. (1994) Sepsis-induced release of interleukin-6 may activate the immediate-early gene program through a hypothalamic-hypophyseal mechanism. Surgery 116:141–149
16. Izumo S, Nadal-Ginard B, Mahdavi V (1988) Protooncogene induction and reprogramming of cardiac gene expression produced by pressure overload. Proc Natl Acad Sci USA 85:339–343
17. Krukenkamp IB, Silverman NA, Sørlie D et al. (1986) Characterization of postischemic myocardial oxygen utilization. Circulation 74(suppl III):III125–III129
18. Lerch R (1993) Oxidative substrate metabolism during postischemic reperfusion. Basic Res Cardiol 88:525–544
19. Goto Y, Slinker BK, LeWinter MM (1990) Decreased contractile efficiency and increased non-mechanical energy cost in hyperthyroid rabbit heart: relation between oxygen consumption and systolic pressure-volume area or force time integral. Circ Res 66:99–1011
20. Nadal-Ginard B, Mahdavi V (1989) Molecular basis of cardiac performance: plasticity of the myocardium generated through protein isoform switches. J Clin Invest 84:1693–1700
21. Gotloib L, Shostak A, Galdi P, Jaichenko J, Fudin R (1992) Loss of microvascular negative charges accompanied by interstitial edema in septic rat's heart. Circ Shock 36:45–56
22. Parillo JE, Burch C, Shelhamer JH et al. (1985) A circulating myocardial depressant substance in humans with septic shock: septic shock patients with a reduced ejection fraction have a circulating factor that depresses in vitro myocardial cell performance. J Clin Invest 76:1539–1553
23. Reilly JM, Cunnion RE, Burch-Withman C et al. (1989) A circulating myocardial depressant substance is associated with cardiac dysfunction and peripheral hypoperfusion (lactic acidemia) in patients with septic shock. Chest 95:1072–1080
24. Simons RH (1991) Pathogenesis of acute alveolar injury. In: Danzker DR (ed) Cardiopulmonary critical care. Saunders, Philadelphia, pp 3–24
25. Ghosh S, Latimer RD, Gray BM, Harwood RJ, Oduro A (1993) Endotoxin-induced organ injury. Crit Care Med 21: Suppl 2:S19–24
26. Pagani FD, Baker LS, Know MA, Cheng H, Fink MP, Visner MS (1992) Load-insensitive assessment of myocardial performance after tumor necrosis factor-alpha in dogs. Surgery 111:683–693
27. Fiedler VB, Loof I, Sander E, Voehringer V, Galanos C, Fournel MA (1992) Monoclonal antibody of tumor necrosis factor-alpha prevents lethal endotoxin sepsis in adult rhesus monkeys. J Lab Clin Med 120:574–588

28. Heard SO, Perkins MW, Fink MP (1992) Tumor necrosis factor-alpha causes myocardial depression in guinea pigs. Crit Care Med 20:523–527
29. Silverman HJ, Penaranda R, Orens JB, Lee NH (1993) Impaired beta-adrenergic receptor stimulation of cyclic adenosine monophosphate in human septic shock: association with myocardial hyporesponsiveness to catecholamines. Crit Care Med 21:31–39
30. Llovera M, Lopez-Soriano FJ, Argiles JM (1993) Effects of tumor necrosis factor-alpha on muscle-protein turnover in female Wistar rats. J Natl Cancer Inst 85:1334–1339
31. Valen G, Vaage J (1993) Toxic oxygen metabolites and leucocytes in reperfusion injury; a review. Scand J Thorac Cardiovasc Surg 41:19–29
32. Jaattela M, Wissing D (1992) Emerging role of heat shock proteins in biology and medicine. Ann Med 24:249–258
33. Myrmel T, McCully JD, Malikin L et al. (1994) Heat shock protein 70 mRNA is induced by anaerobic metabolism in rat hearts. Circulation 90 [part 2]: II299–II305
34. Yellon DM, Latchmann DS (1992) Stress proteins and myocardial protection. J Mol Cell Cardiol 24:113–124
35. Udelman R, Blake MJ, Holbrook NJ (1991) Molecular response to surgical stress: specific and simultaneous heat shock protein induction in the adrenal cortex, aorta, and vena cava. Surgery 110:1125–1131
36. Udelsman R, Ding-Gang L, Stagg CA et al. (1994) Adrenergic regulation of adrenal and aortic heat shock protein. Surgery 116:177–182

Glutamine, the Gut, and the Acute Catabolic State

B.P. Bode, M. Pan, and W.W. Souba

Introduction

Although the gut was once considered to be an organ of quiescence or inactivity following injury and infection, recent studies have demonstrated that this notion is incorrect. It is now recognized that the bowel plays an important role in nutrition and metabolism in critically ill patients. The relative inaccessibility of the portal vein has made it difficult to study amino acid metabolism by the gut, particularly in human beings. Earlier studies that sampled arterial and hepatic venous blood provided information about the splanchnic bed as a unit, but did not partition the individual contributions of the gut and liver. Changes in arterial–hepatic venous concentration differences in catabolic patients were ascribed primarily to changes in substrate handling by the liver, assuming that the gut played little or no role in amino acid metabolism. This concept has been proven wrong, as a number of more recent studies demonstrate that the gut plays a crucial role in amino acid processing in normal and catabolic states. The amino acid which has received the most attention is glutamine, and a number of studies indicate that glutamine is required for gut metabolism, structure, and function.

Glutamine is a nonessential amino acid and is the most abundant amino acid in the body. The circulating concentration of glutamine is maintained at a farily constant level and is dependent on the relative rates of net glutamine uptake and release by the various organs in the body. As a consequence of changes in these exchange rates, glutamine concentrations in blood and tissues fall markedly following catabolic stresses such as starvation, surgery, trauma, and infection [1, 2]. The decline in glutamine concentrations exceeds that of all other amino acids and persists during recovery from the insult at a time when other amino acid concentrations have normalized.

The small intestine is the principal organ of glutamine uptake and metabolism [3], and a number of factors influence its utilization by the intestinal epithelial cell (Fig. 1). Uptake of glutamine occurs from the gut lumen across the brush border and from the blood stream across the basolateral membrane of the enterocyte. Glutamine oxidation by the gut epithelial cells provides a major energy source for the mucosa and processes nitrogen and carbon from the lumen and from the blood stream into precursors for hepatic ureagenesis and gluconeogenesis. This ability of the gut mucosa to metabolize glutamine may be even more important during catabolic disease states when glutamine depletion may be severe and when oral nutri-

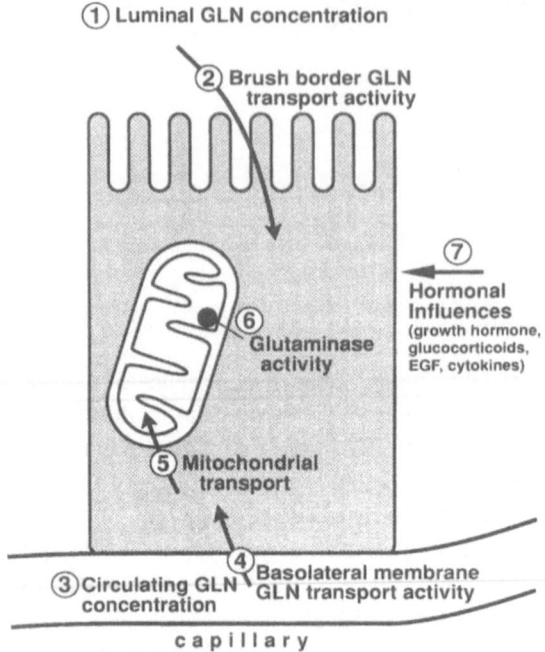

Fig. 1. Factors which can influence glutamine *(GLN)* uptake and metabolism in the small intestinal cell. *EGF,* epithelial growth factor

tion may be interrupted due to the severity of the illness. The dependence of replicating cells on this amino acid may be due to the fact that glutamine is essential for nucleic acid biosynthesis and because high rates of glutamine metabolism ensure adequate amounts of key intermediates for the cell at the time of replication. In the long run, a depleted glutamine state may adversely affect the gut mucosa if its availability in the blood becomes rate limiting or if alterations in metabolic regulation impair intestinal glutamine-utilizing pathways.

In the rat, the entire gastrointestinal tract extracts about 20% of circulating glutamine in the postabsorptive state, which translates into a consumption of 60–80 μmol/h in the adult rat. More than 90% of the glutamine extracted by the small bowel occurs in the mucosal cells. In the autoperfused rat small intestine, approximately 64% of the glutamine carbon is oxidized to carbon dioxide, accounting for a major portion of the total CO_2 produced by the small bowel [4]. Glutamine nitrogen appeared in ammonia (38%), citrulline (28%), and alanine (24%). The gut is well suited to metabolize glutamine, as the ammonia produced when glutamine is hydrolyzed by mitochrondrial glutaminase is released into the portal blood and extracted by the liver before it reaches the systemic circulation. In healthy surgical patients who were studied intraoperatively, glutamine extraction by the portal-drained viscera was approximately 12%–13% [5]. This translates into a net consumption rate of about 1200 nmol/kg body weight per min (approximately 18–20 g glutamine taken up by the portal-drained viscera each day in the average-sized adult). The average amount of glutamine ingested in the diet is in the order of 5–8 g/day. The importance of the small intestine in overall glutamine metabolism is evident from studies which demonstrated that whole body rates of glutamine utilization were diminished by 20% in patients who had undergone massive small-bowel resection [6].

In the postprandial state, uptake of glutamine by the gut also occurs from the lumen, across the brush border. The amount of glutamine reaching the portal blood depends on the luminal concentration. At 6 mM concentrations, only one third of the luminal glutamine was transported intact into the venous blood, while at 45 mM more than two thirds of the luminal glutamine was translocated into the portal circulation [7]. Studies using jejunal brush border membrane vesicles [8] and confluent monolayers of human Caco-2 cells [9] demonstrated that glutamine uptake occurs predominantly via system B, formerly designated the neutral brush border (NBB) transporter. Within the gut epithelial cell, glutamine is metabolized similarly whether it enters the mucosa from the luminal side or from the blood stream.

Intestinal Glutamine Metabolism in Response to Operative Stress

Studies using a catheterized dog model have demonstrated that glutamine uptake by the gastrointestinal tract in vivo nearly doubles following operative stress [10]. Gut glutamine uptake is increased postoperatively despite a fall in the circulating concentration and a reduction in intestinal blood flow, suggesting that an active

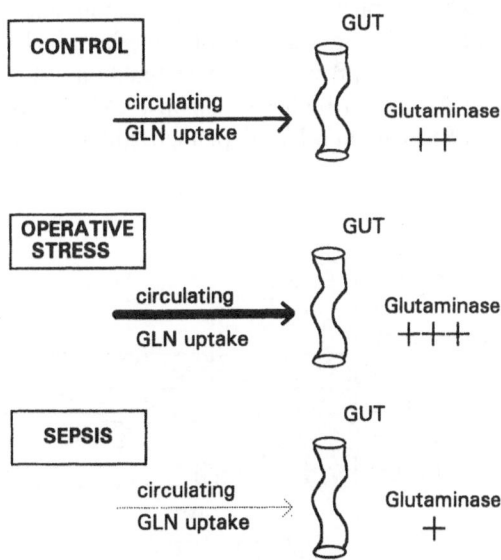

Fig. 2. Differences between intestinal glutamine *(GLN)* uptake and metabolism following operative stress and endotoxemia. Operative stress increases intestinal extraction of circulating glutamine and glutaminase activity, while sepsis results in a decrease in both uptake and metabolism

process for glutamine uptake occurs independent of substrate delivery. This postoperative effect is related to the operative stress itself and not to a decrease in food intake. Further studies showed that gut glutamine uptake more than double following administration of dexamethasone [11]. Glucocorticoids increase the fractional extraction of glutamine from the blood stream [11] and increase the activity of mucosal glutaminase [12]. A single dose of dexamethasone also increases glutaminase mRNA levels in the jejunal mucosa [12], a response which is time dependent. In addition, glucocorticoids increase glutaminase activity and mRNA in mesenteric lymph nodes [13], suggesting an important role for lymphocytes in glutamine metabolism in stress states. During glucocorticoid treatment, the gut switches from an organ of glucose uptake to one of net release, an adaptation that may spare glucose for the wound or for other tissues which are obligate glucose consumers.

The pancreatic hormone glucagon, which is produced in increased amounts after injury, also plays a role in modulating intestinal glutamine consumption. Glucagon administration diminished plasma glutamine concentrations by 25% and caused a threefold enhancement in intestinal glutamine uptake in a canine model [14].

Intestinal Glutamine Metabolism in Response to Severe Infection

A major metabolic difference between sepsis and operative stress is the handling of glutamine by the bowel (Fig. 2). Gut uptake of circulating glutamine is diminished in septic patients and in endotoxemic rats [5], and is associated with a fall in mucosal glutaminase activity and the development of gram-negative bacteremia. Such relationships are only associations and no cause and effect should be inferred, although in other models of bacterial translocation exogenous glutamine has been shown to improve gut barrier function. Glutamine transport across the brush border exhibits a biphasic response to endotoxemia. Early after lipopolysaccharide (LPS) treatment, Na^+-dependent glutamine transport is enhanced [15], a response

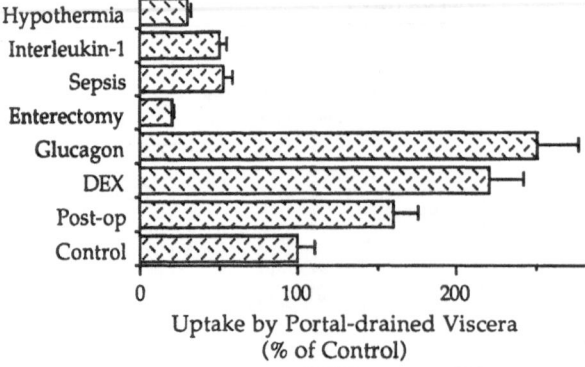

Fig. 3. Effects of different treatments on intestinal uptake of circulating glutamine. *DEX,* dexamethasone

which may support the increased intestinal protein synthesis that is observed in septic animals [16]. At later timepoints (after more than 12 h) during endotoxemia, glutamine transport across the brush border of rats and septic humans is diminished [17]. Likewise, thermally injured rats exhibit a reduced glutamine uptake across the basolateral membrane of the enterocyte [18]. These changes are in contrast to the augmented glutamine uptake that occurs in postoperative and in steroid-treated animals. Interleukin-1 treatment also diminishes intestinal uptake of circulating glutamine [19], while lymphocyte glutaminase activity in mesenteric lymph nodes is increased in septic rats [20]. Studies by Brand et al. [21] have demonstrated that glutamine utilization is tenfold greater in proliferating lymphocytes compared to resting cells. Thus, the reduced gut uptake of glutamine that occurs during sepsis may occur primarily in the mucosal cells as opposed to lymphatic tissues, which may actually consume more glutamine during stress states. A summary of known effectors of glutamine uptake by the gut is presented in Fig. 3.

Despite the reduction in gut glutamine uptake during severe infection, the blood glutamine level remains fairly constant, particularly in view of the magnitude of exchange rates that simultaneously exist. Under these circumstances, the liver becomes the major glutamine consumer in the body [22], exceeding gut glutamine uptake threefold (Fig. 4). Hepatic glutamine uptake increases tenfold following endotoxin treatment secondary to increases in hepatic blood flow and amino acid extraction. Inoue and colleagues [23] have examined the effects of endotoxin on glutamine transport activity in rat hepatic plasma membrane vesicles. Endotoxemia resulted in a time-dependent two- to threefold increase in Na^+-dependent glutamine transport secondary to an increase in the transport V_{max}, consistent with the appearance of increased numbers of corresponding transporter proteins in the hepatocyte plasma membrane.

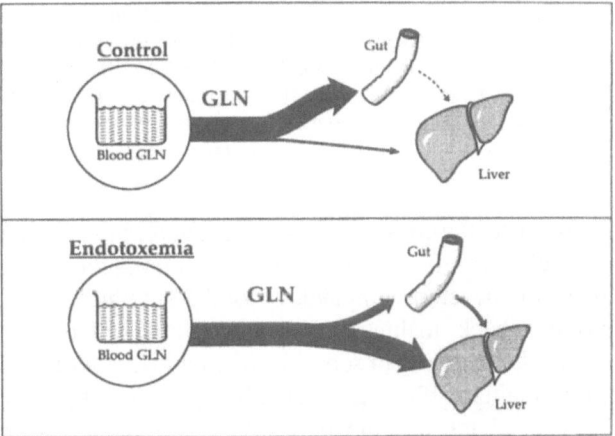

Fig. 4. Redistribution of splanchnic glutamine *(GLN)* flow during endotoxemia. Under normal circumstances, gut glutamine uptake is three to four times greater than uptake by the liver, while following lipopolysaccharide (LPS) administration hepatic uptake exceeds intestinal glutamine consumption threefold

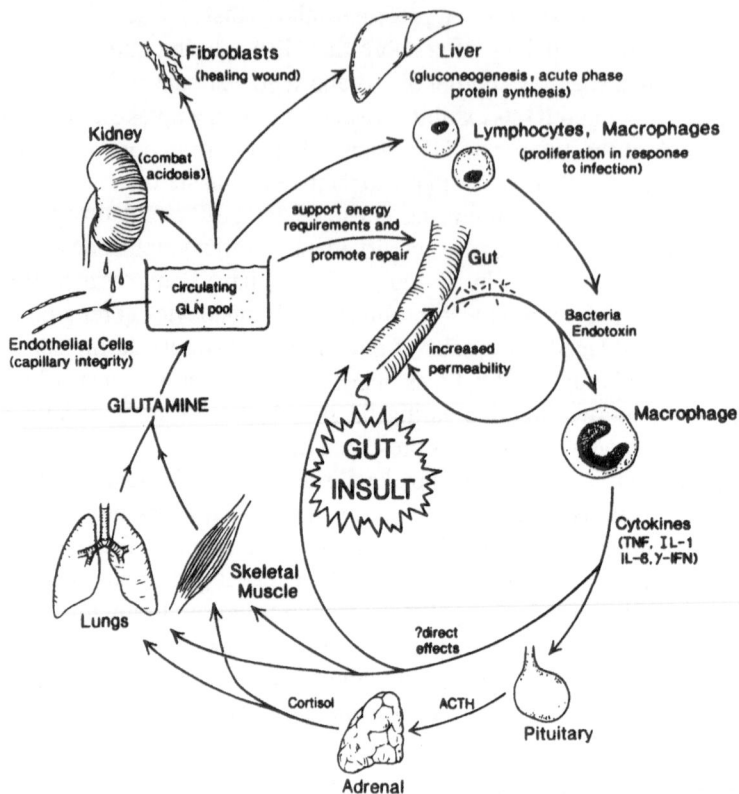

Fig. 5. The interorgan glutamine *(GLN)* cycle can be initiated by any local and/or systemic inflammatory insult and results in the redistribution of circulating glutamine. In the case illustrated here, the patient develops a breakdown in the gut mucosal barrier which causes an increase in bowel permeability and bacterial translocation. Bacteria and endotoxins stimulate macrophages to release cytokines, i.e., tumor necrosis factor *(TNF)*, interleukin *(IL)*-1, IL-6, γ-interferon *(IFN)*, which exert direct and indirect effects on glutamine metabolism in various organs and also stimulate release of glucocorticoids. These mediators work together to mobilize glutamine stores from muscle and to stimulate glutamine production by the lungs. Maintenance of the blood glutamine pool helps provide glutamine to support the increased glutamine requirements in other tissues. It is unclear why organs such as the gut should subserve other tissues, but it is apparent that if the cycle persists, a prolonged catabolic state develops. *ACTH*, adrenocorticotrophic hormone

What are the consequences of this interorgan glutamine cycle in individuals who have chronic sepsis and develop profound glutamine depletion? Consider the patient who develops a breakdown of the gut mucosal barrier from a combination of insults (shock, malnutrition, sepsis, antibiotic therapy, etc.). A central part of the metabolic response to sepsis is the mobilization of glutamine stores in an attempt to maintain the blood glutamine level and thereby "nourish" other tissues (Fig. 5). In skeletal muscle, the intracellular glutamine concentration is a regulator of protein synthesis which may further lead to net catabolism. Under these circumstances, glutamine availability may eventually become rate limiting and result in inadequate amounts of this key substrate for certain cells. Moreover, such critically ill patients often have a gastrointestinal tract which is unusuable and hence they are nourished with total parenteral nutrition (TPN), which currently does not contain glutamine.

Ability of Glutamine to Protect the Gut

Several recent studies indicate that glutamine may be a necessary dietary component for the maintenance of gut mucosal integrity. This may be especially important during critical illness, when the mucosal barrier may be susceptible to breakdown and when additional amounts of glutamine are needed to support the metabolic needs of other tissues. This appears to have important therapeutic implications, since most commercially available parenteral amino acid formulations do not contain glutamine and many enteral diets may contain inadequate amounts of glutamine. It should be pointed out that glutamine-enriched TPN solutions have recently become commercially available in the state of Massachusetts in the USA. Glutamine is readily synthesized in a variety of tissues in the body and because of this

Table 1. Effects of conditionally essential nutrient (glutamine, GLN) absence and repletion

Effect	Evidence/examples
Absence	
Fall in blood and tissue glutamine concentrations	Catabolic states are associated with glutamine depletion
Atrophy or dysfunction of the gut mucosa	Rats on GLN-free TPN develop bacterial translocation, villous atrophy, and a fall in lamina propria lymphocyte populations
	Rats treated with radiation or chemotherapy develop bacteremia and mucosal damage when no GLN is provided
Repletion	
Correction of blood glutamine depletion	Glutamine-enriched diets restore circulating and muscle glutamine concentrations
Enhancement of cellular utilization	GLN-enriched TPN increases gut uptake of circulating glutamine; feeding a GLN diet to rats increases brush border transport
Improvement in tissue morphology and function	GLN-enriched TPN increases villous height and decreases bacterial translocation
	GLN-enriched TPN improves gut morphology and protein synthesis in septic rats
	Glutamine-enriched enteral diets improve recovery and enhance mucosal healing after chemotherapy or radiation therapy
Improvement in protein economy	Glutamine-enriched TPN improves nitrogen balance after bone marrow transplantation
Improvement in outcome	Glutamine nutrition in bone marrow transplant patients decreases infections and shortens hospital stay

TPN, total parenteral nutrition.

fact it has been assumed that glutamine is not required in the diet. The classification of glutamine as a nonessential or nutritionally dispensable amino acid implies that, in its absence from the diet, it can be synthesized in adequate quantities from other amino acids and precursors. For this reason, and because of glutamine's relative instability and short shelf-life compared to other amino acids, it has not been considered necessary to include glutamine in nutritional formulas. Glutamine has been eliminated from TPN solutions and, with few exceptions, glutamine is present in oral and enteral diets only at the relatively low levels characteristic of its concentration in most animal and plant proteins.

Based on our knowledge of the changes in glutamine metabolism that are characteristic of catabolic states, the categorization of glutamine as a nonessential amino acid may be misleading. Under certain circumstances, glutamine may be required in the diet, even though the body has glutamine-synthesizing enzymes in numerous tissues. Several recent studies indicate that glutamine may be a conditionally essential amino acid for the gut during critical illness (Table 1). (A conditionally essential amino acid is one that is usually nonessential but is required in the diet in certain pathophysiologic states because tissue utilization exceeds the capacity for endogenous biosynthesis. This may lead to inadequate amounts of the amino acid to support metabolic needs in some cells, such as the gut mucosal cells.) The studies suggest that during certain pathophysiologic "stress" states, when glutamine depletion in the body is severe or when enteral nutrition is not provided, glutamine is an essential amino acid for the gut mucosa, since its provision in the diet improves intestinal structure and function. These reports also indicate that pharmacologic doses of glutamine are necessary to accomplish this benefit, and thus glutamine may be considered a drug as well as a nutrient.

Impact of Glutamine Nutrition on the Intestinal Mucosa and on Gut Immune Function

Glutamine is found in virtually all foods and in many specialized diets provided to hospitalized patients, but it is present in relatively small amounts. Glutamine comprises 3%–8% of dietary protein [24], and hence enteral feedings may provide as little as 2–6 g glutamine daily, a quantity insufficient to support the requirements of the stressed, depleted individual. In addition, current TPN solutions are glutamine free, which may explain in part the development of villous atrophy in patients receiving long-term TPN. Hwang et al. [25] demonstrated that glutamine enrichment of TPN solutions resulted in an increase in jejunal mucosal weight and DNA content; supplementation also significantly attenuated the villous atrophy associated with standard TPN. Klimberg et al. [26] showed that supplementation of standard TPN solutions with glutamine stimulated gut glutamine utilization. Both enteral [27] and parenteral [28] glutamine accelerate transport of glutamine across the jejunal brush border. Others have demonstrated the ability of glutamine-supplemented intravenous diets to increase villous height and mucosal nitrogen content [29].

Alverdy [30] demonstrated that TPN promotes bacterial translocation from the gut in rats. When rats were allowed to drink a standard TPN solution, bacterial translocation was significantly reduced but, unlike regular chow diet, the rate of bacterial translocation was not abrogated. Subsequent studies by this group [31] showed that glutamine-enriched TPN results in decreased bacterial translocation when compared to standard formulas. This decrease in translocation was associated with a normalization of S-IgA (secretory immunoglobulin A) levels and a decrease in bacterial adherence to enterocytes, suggesting that glutamine-supplemented TPN may enhance gut immune function. Glutamine-supplemented TPN also maintained both B and T cell populations in the lamina propria of the terminal ileum [32]. Other investigators have shown that provision of glutamine-supplemented nutritional support may accelerate the healing of the intestinal injury that occurs secondary to chemotherapy or radiation therapy. Fox et al. [33] showed that the addition of glutamine to an elemental, enteral diet resulted in a significant reduction in the severity of methotrexate-induced enterocolitis, as reflected by improved morphometric parameters in the jejunum and colon. Provision of glutamine reduced endotoxin transmigration from the gut lumen and improved survival. Similar benefits were reported by Jacobs et al. [34], who demonstrated that a glutamine-enriched intravenous diet accelerated healing of the gut mucosa in rats receiving 5-fluorouracil (5-FU). O'Dwyer et al. [35] also showed that, after 5-FU treatment, rats maintained on glutamine-enriched TPN demonstrated greater mean jejunal villous height and an increase in mucosal DNA content. When glutamine-supplemented TPN was given before the administration of 5-FU, there was an even more marked effect on mucosal cellularity and a significantly lower mortality rate than in animals maintained on standard TPN.

Glutamine feeding has been shown to diminish the incidence of bacterial translocation to the mesenteric lymph nodes in an experimental radiation enteritis model [36]. Jejunum from rats receiving the glutamine diet demonstrated increased villous height and number and nearly three times the number of mitoses per crypt [37]. Provision of oral glutamine following abdominal irradiation also supports gut glutamine metabolism and decreases the morbidity and mortality associated with abdominal radiation. Administration of a glutamine-enriched oral diet prior to abdominal radiation was equally effective in exerting a radioprotective effect [38]. Thus, provision of glutamine to patients undergoing abdominal or pelvic irradiation may protect the intestinal mucosa from injury, accelerate healing or irradiated bowel, and possibly attenuate the long-term sequelae of radiation enteritis.

A recent study by Yoshida et al. [39] evaluated the effect of the combination of TPN and sepsis on intestinal mucosal morphology and protein synthesis. Addition of glutamine to the TPN solution attenuated the endotoxin-induced damage to the jejunum and ileum. Sepsis was associated with an increase in mucosal protein synthesis and the increase was greatest when supplemental glutamine was supplied.

Human Clinical Trials

Studies in human volunteers [40] and in hospitalized patients have failed to demonstrate any toxicity associated with glutamine-supplemented parenteral nutrition. Glutamine in solution undergoes hydrolysis in a relatively short period of time, but this process can be slowed considerably by adjusting the pH and temperature of the solution. Breakdown is negligible when the glutamine is added to the TPN mixture at the time the pharmacist prepares the final solution.

One of the best studies to date evaluating the effects of glutamine-enriched TPN is a randomized, double-blind controlled trial [41, 42]. The investigators studied 45 adults receiving allogeneic bone marrow transplants (BMT) for hematologic malignancies. Patients received a standard, glutamine-free TPN solution or an isonitrogenous, isocaloric solution supplemented with L-glutamine (0.57 gm/kg body weight per day). Patients received the diets for approximately 25 days after BMT. Patients receiving glutamine-supplemented TPN after BMT had improved nitrogen balance, a diminished incidence of clinical infections, less fluid accumulation, and a shortened hospital stay. It was not apparent from the study whether supplemental glutamine was beneficial to the gut. However, based on the animal data, which show an improvement in gut histology and barrier function when glutamine-enriched diets are given, and on the reduced incidence of infections that occurred in the glutamine-fed BMT patients, it could be speculated that the patients receiving the glutamine formula had an improvement in mucosal integrity. A recent study strongly supports this concept. Patients receiving glutamine-supplemented TPN for 2 weeks did not develop a defect in intestinal permeability or a fall in villous height as patients receiving standard TPN did [43].

References

1. Vinnars E, Bergstrom J, Furst P (1975) Influence of the postoperative state on the intracellular free amino acids in human muscle tissue. Ann Surg 182:665–671
2. Roth E, Funovics J, Muhlbacher F et al. (1982) Metabolic disorders in severe abdominal sepsis: glutamine deficiency in skeletal muscle. Clin Nutr 1:25–41
3. Windmueller HG (1982) Glutamine utilization by the small intestine. Adv Enzymol 53:202–237
4. Windmueller HG, Spaeth AE (1974) Uptake and metabolism of plasma glutamine by the small intestine. J Biol Chem 249:5070–5079
5. Souba WW, Herskowitz K, Klimberg VS et al. (1990) The effects of sepsis and endotoxemia on gut glutamine metabolism. Ann Surg 211:543–551
6. Darmaun D, Messing B, Just B et al. (1991) Glutamine metabolism after small intestinal resection in humans. Metabolism 40:42–44
7. Windmueller HG, Spaeth AE (1975) Intestinal metabolism of glutamine and glutamate from the lumen as compared to glutamine from blood. Arch Biophys Biochem 171:662–672
8. Said HM, van Voorhis K, Ghishan FK et al. (1989) Transport characteristics of glutamine in human intestinal brush-border membrane vesicles. Am. J. Physiol. 256:G240–G245
9. Souba WW, Pan M, Stevens BR (1992) Kinetics of the sodium-dependent glutamine transporter in human intestinal cell confluent monolayers. Biochem Biophys Res Commun 188:746–753
10. Souba WW, Wilmore DW (1983) Postoperative alterations of arteriovenous exchange of amino acids across the gastrointestinal tract. Surgery 94:342–350
11. Souba WW, Smith RJ, Wilmore DW (1985) Effects of glucocorticoids on glutamine metabolism in visceral organs. Metabolism 34:450–456
12. Sarantos P, Abouhamze A, Souba WW (1992) Glucocorticoids regulate intestinal glutaminase expression. Surgery 112:278–283

13. Dudrick PS, Sarantos P, Ockert K, Chakrabarti R, Copeland EM, Souba WW (1993) Dexamethasone stimulation of glutaminase expression in mesenteric lymph nodes. Am J Surg 165: 34–39
14. Geer RJ, Williams PE, Lairmore T et al. (1987) Glucagon: an important stimulator of gut and hepatic glutamine metabolism. Surg Forum 38:27–29
15. Dudrick PS, Salloum RM, Copeland EM et al. (1992) The early response of the brush border glutamine transporter to endotoxemia. J Surg Res 52:372–377
16. Von Allmen D, Hasselgren PO, Higashiguchi T et al. (1990) Increased intestinal protein synthesis during sepsis. Surg Forum 41:68–70
17. Salloum RM, Copeland EM, Souba WW (1991) Brush border transport of glutamine and other substrates during sepsis and endotoxemia. Ann Surg 213:401–410
18. Peitsch JB, Leonard D, Neblett WW et al. (1989) Burn injury alters intestinal glutamine transport. J Surg Res 46:296–299
19. Austgen TR, Chen MK, Dudrick PS et al. (1991) Cytokine regulation of intestinal glutamine utilization. Am J Surg 163:174–180
20. Sarantos P (1994) Effects of endotoxin on glutaminase expression in mesenteric lymph nodes. Arch Surg (in press)
21. Brand K, Leibold W, Luppa P et al. (1986) Metabolic alterations associated with proliferation of mitogen-activated lymphocytes and of lymphoblastoid cell lines: evaluation of glucose and glutamine metabolism. Immunobiology 173:23–34
22. Austgen TR, Salloum RM, Flynn TC et al. (1991) The effects of endotoxin on splanchnic metabolism of glutamine and related substrates in vivo. J Trauma 31:742–752
23. Inoue Y, Pacitti AJ, Souba WW (1993) Endotoxin increased hepatic glutamine transport activity. J Surg Res 54:393–400
24. Lacey J, Wilmore DW (1990) Is glutamine a conditionally essential amino acid? Nutr Rev 48:297–313
25. Hwang TL, O'Dwyer ST, Smith RJ et al. (1987) Preservation of small bowel mucosa using glutamine-enriched parenteral nutrition. Surg Forum 38:56–58
26. Klimberg VS, Souba WW, Sitren H et al. (1989) Glutamine-enriched total parenteral nutrition supports gut metabolism. Surg Forum 40:175–177
27. Salloum RM, Souba WW, Fernandez A et al. (1990) Dietary modulation of small intestinal glutamine transport in intenstinal brush border membrane vesicles of rats. J Surg Res 48:635–638
28. Salloum RM, Herskowitz K, Souba WW (1990) Intravenous glutamine stimulates brush border gut glutamine transport. Surg Forum 41:195–198
29. Grant J (1988) Use of L-glutamine in total parenteral nutrition. J Surg 44:506–513
30. Alverdy JC (1990) Effects of glutamine-supplemented diets on immunology of the gut. JPEN J Parenter Enteral Nutr Suppl 14(4):109S–113S
31. Burke D, Alverdy JC, Aoys E et al. (1989) Glutamine supplemented TPN improves gut immune function. Arch Surg 124:1396–1399
32. Alverdy JC, Aoys E, Weiss-Carrington P et al. (1992) The effect of glutamine-enriched TPN on gut immune cellularity. J Surg Res 52:34–38
33. Fox AD, Kripke SA, DePaula J et al. (1988) Effect of a glutamine supplemented enteral diet on methotrexate-induced enterocolitis. JPEN J Parenter Enteral Nutr 12:325–331
34. Jacobs DO, Evans DA, O'Dwyer ST, Smith RJ, Wilmore DW (1987) Disparate effects of 5-fluorouracil on the ileum and colon of enterally fed rats with protection by dietary glutamine. Surg Forum 38:45–47
35. O'Dwyer ST, Scott T, Smith JR, Wilmore DW (1987) 5-Fluorouracil toxicity on small intestinal mucosa but not white blood cells is decreased by glutamine (Abstr). Clin Res 35:369a
36. Souba WW, Klimberg VS, Hautamaki RD et al. (1990) Oral glutamine reduces bacterial translocation following abdominal radiation. J Surg Res 48:1–5
37. Klimberg VS, Salloum RM, Kasper M et al. (1990) Oral glutamine accelerates healing of the small intestine and improves outcome following whole abdominal radiation. Arch Surg 125:1040–1045
38. Klimberg VS, Souba WW, Dolson DJ et al. (1990) Prophylactic glutamine protects the intestinal mucosa from radiation injury. Cancer 66:62–68

39. Yoshida S, Leskiw MJ, Schulter MD et al. (1992) Effect of total parenteral nutrition, systemic sepsis, and glutamine on gut mucosa in rats. Am J Physiol 26:E368–E373
40. Ziegler TR, Benfell K, Smith RJ et al. (1990) Safety and metabolic effects of L-glutamine administration in humans. JPEN J Parenter Enteral Nutr Suppl 14(4):137S–146S
41. Ziegler TR, Young LS, Benfell K et al. (1992) Glutamine-supplemented parenteral nutrition improves nitrogen retention and reduces hospital mortality versus standard parenteral nutrition following bone marrow transplantation: a randomized, double-blind trial. Ann Intern Med 116:821–828
42. Scheltinga MR, Young LS, Benfell K et al. (1991) Glutamine-enriched intravenous feedings attenuate extracellular fluid expansion after standard stress. Ann Surg 214:385–395
43. Van der Hulst RR, van Kreel BK, von Meyerfeldt MF et al. (1993) Glutamine and the preservation of gut integrity. Lancet 341:1363–1367

Renal Failure in the Acute Catabolic State

T. G. Jenssen

Introduction

Renal failure is a common problem in patients suffering from trauma, burn injury, sepsis, or shock of any other cause. Impaired renal function may supervene on these conditions in a way that causes the patient's condition to further deteriorate. In the acute state of renal failure, defined as a potentially reversible failure in originally normal unobstructed kidneys, the mortality rate improved from 90% to some 50% after the introduction of hemodialysis 40–50 years ago [1]. In the subsequent years, mortality has not improved further. One cause for this may be that the population of patients being treated today is a group at higher risk with more complicated conditions than 40 years ago. In multiorgan failure, mortality increases in proportion to the number of organs that are involved. The mortality rate is 8% when only the kidneys are failing [1] and increases up to 100% when three or more organs are involved [2].

A review of the literature shows us that acute renal failure is better prevented than treated and that much can be achieved by avoiding situations that may leave the patient with this condition. This is also underscored in previous reviews [1, 3, 4].

In experimental models, renal ischemia may be well tolerated in situ for some 30–60 min before permanent functional and structural changes take place. The scope of this paper is to outline mechanisms that are operative within this time frame to impair kidney function and to relate these mechanisms to treatment.

Regulation of Renal Blood Flow

Renal blood flow is regulated at an optimum level despite variations in the systemic blood pressure ranging from 80 to 180 mmHg [5, 6]. The major mechanisms involved in this instant regulation are related to the pre- and postglomerular arteriolar tone. Both direct myogenic responses in the arterioles and tubuloglomerular feedback mechanisms have been discussed. The current belief is that the main regulation of blood flow is operated by a myogenic response in the afferent arterioles. This myogenic response is measurable within seconds when renal perfusion pressure is decreased [7].

Several mediators generated within or outside the kidney itself may contribute to the homeostasis of renal blood flow, e.g., angiotensin II, prostaglandins, kinins, vasopressin, atrial natriuretic peptide (ANP), endothelin, and adenosine (for reviews, see [5–7]). It has been shown that up to 20% of the amount of angiotensin I that passes through the kidneys is converted to angiotensin II [7].

Prostaglandins do not seem to be of importance in the minute to minute regulation of basal renal blood flow, but they become important once blood flow is impaired [7]. The overall effect of prostaglandins is to reduce renal vascular resistance and to maintain renal blood flow [7–10].

Mechanisms of Acute Renal Failure in Experimental Models

Although much is known about renal autoregulation in healthy subjects, the pathophysiology involved in acute renal failure is very complex. A common denominator seems to be renal ischemia with or without the presence of nephrotoxins. Several mechanisms may be operative in this setting, e.g., altered intracellular handling of calcium, renal release of vasoconstrictive agents, microthrombi, impaired prostaglandin synthesis, and reperfusion oxidant injury.

Clinical studies cannot outline in detail the early changes that take place in the hypoperfused kidney. We have to rely on experimental models, although they may be hampered by species differences, the influence of anesthesia [11], and the fact that they are most often performed on healthy animals. Furthermore, the outcome of renal ischemia partly depends on the particular kind of trauma that is initiated. A common model used to study the acute ischemic kidney is renal artery occlusion or intrarenal infusion of epinephrine. In rats, renal artery occlusion leads to more profound metabolic changes than, for instance, different kinds of systemic shocks [12, 13]. This must be due to differences in ischemic injury when renal perfusion is totally shut off during renal artery occlusion. Furthermore, in shock models the kidneys also have an intact external innervation and are exposed to circulating hormones and metabolites as well. The kidneys are less susceptible to cardiogenic shock than to other kinds of shock, probably due to less activation of the sympathetic tone [14, 15] and less suppressed release of ANP.

Oxygen and Energy Status

Renal oxygen levels are crucial for the kidneys to maintain their normal function. Although glomerular filtration is a totally passive process not requiring energy, oxygen deprivation may affect the renal function severely. Ninety-nine percent of all sodium filtered through the glomeruli is reabsorbed in the tubules. There is an almost linear relationship between the sodium reabsorption rate and the oxygen consumption in the kidneys [16].

However, the oxygen need is not evenly distributed in kidneys, being highest in the cortex [4]; even within the cortex there may be a wide scatter in oxygen tension ranging from zero to arterial values [17]. In this way hypoperfusion of the kidney may have a different impact in different parenchymal zones. Earlier studies on patients suffering from acute renal failure showed that kidney dysfunction was primarily related to the cortical area, indicating that impaired renal blood flow and oxygen delivery may have been important in inducing renal failure [18]. In later experimental studies, it was evident that an ischemic insult primarily disturbs the postglomerular perfusion, leading to tubular damage especially in the medulla [19]. The medulla is also the area with the lowest oxygen tension [17], thereby leaving it susceptible to ischemic injury. However, it must be remembered that the renal need for oxygen supply is dramatically reduced when the renal perfusion is lowered and glomerular filtration goes down. This sparing mechanism probably reflects the fact that sodium reabsorption and other energy-requiring processes in the tubules are lowered when glomerular filtration is reduced.

Studies in intact rats show that the renal energy status – as judged by the adenosine triphosphate to diphosphate (ATP/ADP) ratio as well as the total content of renal adenylates – is rather resistant to profound drops in kidney perfusion, as long as this is of limited duration. It has been shown that a sustained drop in blood pressure down to 30–40 mmHg during a 30-min hemorrhagic shock is required to alter the adenylate energy status in rats [12]. This occurs simultaneously with histological changes showing blebbing of the S3 tubular brush border, and these changes are reversible after reperfusion. Free radical scavengers and allopurinol, a xanthine oxidase inhibitor, protect against reperfusion injury after long-standing renal ischemia [20–22], but this is not a consistent finding in the early reperfusion phase [12]. In septic shock, the ATP/ADP balance is apparently preserved, despite a 30%–50% drop in blood pressure for up to 60 min [12, 23].

Nephrotoxins

Both man-made and endogenous nephrotoxic substances may place an extra burden on kidneys exposed to hypoperfusion. In man, the picture of nephrotoxin-induced renal failure does not differ much from what is seen in shock-induced renal failure, neither in terms of renal hemodynamics nor in terms of angiographic findings [18, 24]. However, it is quite clear that the ability of the kidneys to resist ischemia is greatly reduced when renal hypoperfusion and nephrotoxins occur simultaneously.

Although the adenylate status of the kidney is not greatly hampered in the early minutes of ischemia [12], the situation is quite different when a nephrotoxin as for instance gentamicin is added. The renal ATP/ADP ratio is greatly reduced, and this occurs simultaneously with morphologic tubular changes that are not reversed upon reperfusion [25]. The effect of gentamicin seems preferentially to be a post-ischemic one, since changes are the same regardless of whether gentamicin is administered before or after ischemia [26, 27]. This indicates that gentamicin impairs the renal energetics in the reperfusion phase. This effect, however, does not seem to be mediated through hydroxyl radical formation [27].

A major problem in crush injury patients is the generation of acid, myoglobin, and urate from the muscle [3]. Experimentally, myoglobin is able to reduce renal ATP stores by some 25% without the presence of shock. This reduction in renal ATP stores is magnified three- to fourfold when myoglobinuria is superimposed on a hemorrhagic state [28]. Early histologic changes in the proximal tubules are far more pronounced in the presence of myoglobinuria. The mechanism by which myoglobin further causes the ischemic kidney to deteriorate is not clear, but since some of its effects can be reproduced experimentally by other low molecular weight proteins, a mechanism related to tubular protein overload has been suggested [28]. In the myoglobinuric patient, bicarbonate infusion has been advocated to avoid pigment nephropathy and may also reduce acid-induced swelling and intratubular cast formation [3]. Bicarbonate infusion may also have the advantage of reducing the dangerous hyperkalemia that is frequently seen in rhabdomyolysis [3, 29]. However, once oliguria is present, salt volume should be restricted, and renal replacement therapy may be needed.

Calcium

Calcium-mediated cell injury is probably an important mechanism in acute renal failure. Both cellular and mitochondrial accumulation of calcium develop upon postischemic reperfusion (for a review, see [30]). The line of evidence showing that this may be pathogenic for acute renal failure stems from several studies in which verapamil and dihydropyridines seem to protect the ischemic kidney when administered before or after occlusive renal ischemia [31–33]. However, published studies are conflicting as to whether calcium channel blockers can be given before or after the insult to obtain this effect. Furthermore, one study found an effect of verapamil after intrarenal epinephrine infusion, but not after renal artery occlusion [32]. Burke et al. [33] observed that the beneficial effect of verapamil on kidney ischemia was associated with the reversal of mitochondrial calcium accumulation together with normalized mitochondrial respiration. This suggests that verapamil has a direct cytoprotective effect during renal ischemia.

In experimental models with hemorrhagic shock, verapamil protects renal function in rats [13], and felodipine (a dihydropyridine) partly restores renal function in dogs regardless of whether it is given before or after the injury [34]. On the other hand, diltiazem does not protect renal function during hemorrhagic shock in pigs [35]. Whether this can be ascribed to differences in species, calcium channel blockers, or some other factor is not known.

There are several effects of calcium channel blockers that may be of benefit for the ischemic kidney [30]. First, calcium channel blockers may improve cellular respiration by attenuating mitochondrial calcium accumulation. Second, they may protect the cytoskeleton by reducing phospholipase activation and thereby cell membrane degradation. Third, they may induce vascular myogenic relaxation and improve renal blood flow. However, this mechanism may not be very important, since other vasodilators such as acetylcholine or α-receptor blockers do not protect renal function after an ischemic insult [36, 37].

In clinical trials, the application of calcium channel blockers have been tried only in the setting of ischemia after renal graft transplantation. The agents tend to reduce the rate of delayed graft function, but they fail to improve 1-year graft survival (for a review, see [38]). In critically ill patients, concern has been raised about using agents with negative inotropic and chronotropic effects [3]. This is a relevant concern. So far, general use of calcium channel blockers cannot be advocated in these patients. However, newly developed agents such as the latest generation of dihydropyridines (e.g., felodipine, amlodipine, isradipine) do not have profound negative inotropic effects on myocardial function. We still need clinical trials to establish whether these agents can be beneficial for the patient with incipient or established acute renal failure.

Mediators of Inflammation

Renal function during the early phase of septic or endotoxin shock has been extensively studied. However, most models have studied the high-resistance, low-flow state and not the low-resistance, hyperdynamic state that is frequently seen in early sepsis in humans. Experimentally, this condition can be obtained with infusion of live bacteria combined with a rapid infusion of saline [39, 40]. Recently, low-resistance, hyperdynamic sepsis was obtained by inducing peritonitis in sheep [41].

In experiments performed on monkeys with hyperdynamic sepsis, a biphasic response in renal vascular resistance is observed [40]. Renal vascular resistance increases over the first hour, before it drops and then rises again. The drop in renal resistance correlates to increased renal excretion of prostaglandin E_2, which points to an intrarenal compensatory prostaglandin production trying to restore renal blood flow [40]. Cyclooxygenase inhibitors do not have adverse effects on renal blood flow in normal, salt-repleted humans [7, 8], but once salt depletion, endotoxinemia, or hypovolemia occurs, the agents may be deleterious on renal function [8–10]. During a 1-h suprarenal aortic clamping, intact prostaglandin synthesis is crucial to preserve the renal function [42].

The lipopolysaccharide (LPS) fraction of endotoxin produces a well-known fall in glomerular filtration rate [43]. Badr et al. [44] showed that this fall in glomerular filtration may be mediated by vasoconstrictive metabolites of the eicosanoid pathway. Blocking the production of thromboxane A_2 or leukotrienes during endotoxin shock partly restored renal blood flow and glomerular filtration rate in rats. In the perfused, isolated rat kidney, polymorphonuclear white cells release oxygen metabolites and proteinases such as elastase when exposed to LPS and formyl-methionyl-leucyl-phenylalanine (FMLP). FMLP is a chemotactic peptide derived from the bacterial cell wall [45]. The consequent fall in glomerular filtration rate is prevented by scavenging oxygen metabolites and inhibiting elastase action [45].

Other factors proposed to be involved in LPS-induced renal failure are tumor necrosis factor, interleukin-I, and platelet-activating factor. Furthermore, it has recently been shown that mediators generated during inflammation such as leukotriene D4 and interleukin-2 may act on the branching and arcuate arteries to reduce renal blood perfusion as well [6].

Nitric oxide (NO) can be a secondary mediator in endotoxinemia. LPS stimulates NO production in macrophages and vascular cells [46] as well as in glomerular mesangial cells [47]. Besides being a local vasodilator, NO may also prevent platelet aggregation and adhesion to damaged endothelium [48]. Recently it was

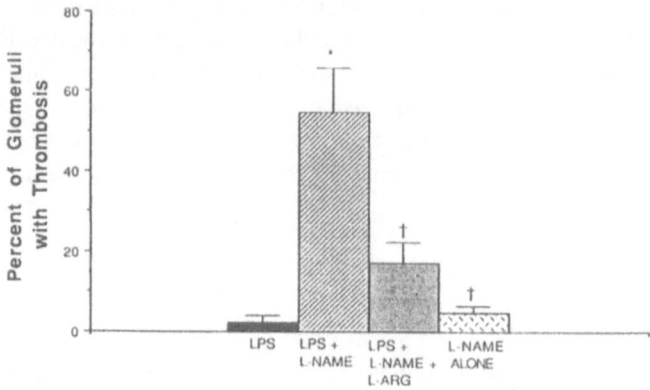

Fig. 1. Percentage of glomeruli with thrombosis in kidneys from rats exposed to *Escherichia coli* lipopolysaccharide *(LPS)* alone, LPS and nitric oxide synthesis inhibitor *(L-NAME)*, LPS, L-NAME, and nitric oxide precursor (L-arginine, *L-ARG*), and L-NAME alone. *$p<0.001$ compared to LPS; '<0.01 compared to LPS+L-NAME. (From [49]).
Reproduced by copyright permission of The Society for Clinical Investigation.

shown [49] that blocking of NO synthesis during *Escherichia coli* endotoxin administration in rats led to profound glomerular thrombosis in rat kidneys. This was partly reversed when NO production was restored by L-arginine (Fig. 1). Integrity of the renal NO production may therefore be of importance to prevent endotoxin-induced renal failure. However, the effect of NO may vary in different settings, since blocking of NO synthesis seems to protect tubular cells from ischemia in vitro [50].

Glomerular thrombosis in endotoxinemia may also be provoked by glomerular generation of type 1 plasminogen activator inhibitor (PAI-1) [51]. PAI-1 is a potent antifibrinolytic agent and probably the most important inhibitor of both tissue-type and urokinase-type plasminogen activators [52].

Endothelin

The polypeptide endothelin is recognized to be the most potent vasoconstrictor in the body, and in the kidneys a dose–response effect has been demonstrated in interlobular as well as arteriolar vessels [53]. Endothelin exists as three isoforms, ET-1, ET-2, and ET-3, with different affinities for the two known endothelin receptors, ET_A and ET_B. The ET_A receptor preferentially binds ET-1, and it is considered to transmit the potent vasoconstrictive effect of ET-1 through increases in intracellular calcium [54].

Both renal ischemia and endotoxinemia induce an immediate and profound increase in systemic endothelin [42, 55, 56]. ET-1 mRNA increases in the rat kidney within 2 h after clamping of the renal pedicle [57]. The ET_A receptor blocker BQ-123 attenuates renal vasoconstriction after aortic cross-clamping, but it does not change the fall in glomerular filtration rate [56]. It has been speculated that either the decline in glomerular filtration rate is mediated by some other factor (e.g., an-

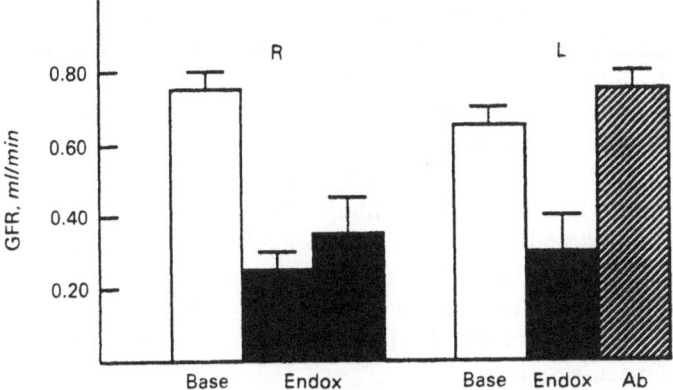

Fig. 2. Glomerular filtration rate *(GFR)* in the right *(R)* and left *(L)* kidney from rats during baseline *(open bars)*, systemic administration of endotoxin *(black bars)*, and during infusion of antiendothelin serum into the artery of the left kidney *(stippled bar)*. (From [55])

giotensin) or the ET_B receptor may also be involved. The fact that ET antibodies, preventing endothelin interaction with any receptor subtype, are able to cancel the fall in glomerular filtration during endotoxinemia [55] suggests that the latter is the case (Fig. 2).

Established Treatment in Kidney Support

Hyperalimentation regimens (caloric and amino acid supply exceeding daily expenditure) with essential amino acids were reported to improve both renal function and survival some 20 years ago [58, 59]. Later studies have not confirmed the beneficial effects of essential amino acids [60]. The number of patients involved in most studies is small, and the patients studied are not necessarily comparable in terms of underlying diseases. Today hyperalimentation in acute renal failure is not considered to improve patient morbidity or mortality, but adequate nutrition is advocated as supportive therapy while the patient is in a critical condition. Volume replacement is important to avoid aggravation of renal hypoperfusion. On the other hand, volume loads may be a problem in the oliguric patient unless renal replacement therapy is performed.

A series of studies involving a relatively small number of patients showed encouraging effects of furosemide or mannitol together with low-dose dopamine in reversing the oliguric phase of acute renal failure [61, 62]. Mannitol may act in the kidney by inducing capillary dilation, improving tubular flow, and scavenging free oxygen radicals. The use of mannitol may be especially beneficial in the management of the crush syndrome, since it also tends to reduce muscle cell edema and lead to decompression of muscle tamponade [3].

Uncontrolled studies suggested that dopamine could be useful even when not combined with diuretics. However, a recent randomized, controlled trial showed that low-dose dopamine as monotherapy is of no use to protect renal function after surgery on the abdominal aorta [63]. On the contrary, dopamine may be associated with serious side effects [64] and in most cases should probably be avoided unless its administration is mandatory to maintain systemic blood pressure.

Sepsis is the most common cause of death in patients with acute renal failure [1, 60, 65] and should be thoroughly treated and monitored. However, nephrotoxic antibiotics must be avoided, and the dosage of drugs cleared by the kidneys should be prescribed according to the renal function. Patients undergoing surgery for obstructive jaundice are especially prone to suffer from acute renal failure [66]. An explanation for this may be that absence of the bile-related detergent effect on the bacterial wall promotes endotoxinemia. The incidence of endotoxinemia is reduced when this category of patients is given bile salts orally before surgery [66].

Any patient with renal insufficiency given radiocontrast media intravenously should be treated with volume expansion (saline) with or without furosemide/mannitol both before and after the procedure [67]. Any other nephrotoxic drug should be avoided and, if the drug is mandatory, plasma levels should be carefully monitored. Special attention must be paid to the common use of nonsteroid anti-inflammatory agents. These drugs must be abandoned during hypovolemia, salt depletion, renal insufficiency, or any intervention/surgery that might produce renal ischemia [8]. The presence of myoglobinuria should be treated with urine alkalinization and removal of the devitalized tissue that is responsible for the problem [3].

Potential Treatments in the Future

Several interventions other than those mentioned above have been tried in experimental acute renal failure. Beneficial effects have been reported on administration of ATP magnesium chloride, potassium, glycine, glutathione, sodium azide, and other substances. Common to all experiments is that the agent has been introduced *before* the ischemic insult to the kidney, which limits its possible clinical application. The most promising findings to date have been reported on ANP and growth factors, especially insulin-like growth factor I (IGF I).

Atrial Natriuretic Peptide

Several years ago, ANP was shown to improve renal function when applied *after* ischemia in rats [68, 69]. However, till now we have been reluctant to apply ANP in the clinical situation because of its possible hypotensive side effects.

Recently Rahman et al. reported the first controlled trial on ANP in patients with acute renal failure, primarily of ischemic origin [70]. ANP, either given intra-arterially in both kidneys for 8 h or intravenously for 24 h, reversed acute renal failure significantly. No serious side effects were observed with the doses employed (0.16–0.24 μg ANP/kg body weight per min intravenously). Compared to the control group, creatinine clearance significantly improved over 24 h (Fig. 3), and the number of patients that had to be dialyzed was reduced by some 50% [70].

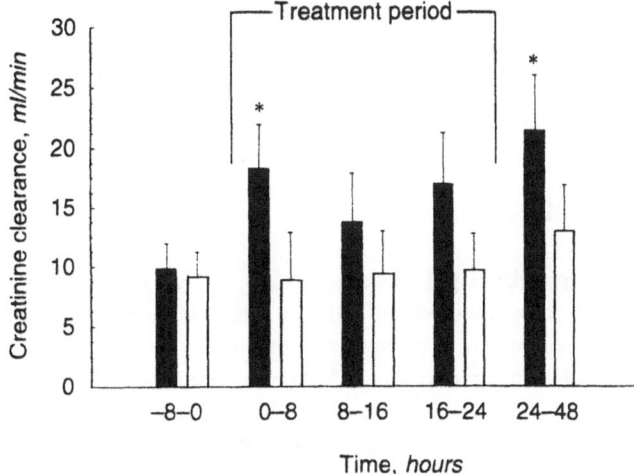

Fig. 3. Changes in glomerular filtration rate in patients with acute renal failure given atrial natriuretic peptide *(solid bars)* compared to controls *(open bars)*. *$p<0.05$ compared to controls. (From [70]).
Reprinted by permission of Blackwell Scientific Publications, Inc.

ANP may modulate several mechanisms involved in acute renal failure. First, it may increase the capillary hydraulic pressure in the glomeruli by changing pre- and postglomerular vascular tone [71]. Second, it has a direct diuretic and natriuretic effect on the distal nephron [72]. Third, ANP prevents an increase in circulating endothelin [42]. Regardless of the mechanism, ANP is a promising agent in the treatment of acute renal failure, but further trials should be conducted to confirm its effect and settle the question of dosage and safety profile.

Insulin-Like Growth Factor I

Treatment with recombinant growth hormone seems to induce a positive nitrogen balance in patients on maintenance hemodialysis [73]. However, most of the effects of growth hormone are mediated through IGF I. Since catabolic conditions such as sepsis and renal failure may cause failure of growth hormone to increase IGF I, direct treatment with IGF I seems more tempting [74]. IGF I stimulates protein synthesis and other anabolic processes [75]. IGF I receptors have been identified in the glomeruli and proximal tubules [76], and IGF I acutely increases renal plasma flow and the glomerular filtration rate in normal man [77]. A recent report on experimental acute renal failure in rats showed that IGF I given *after* renal ischemia may have two beneficial effects [78]:

1. It improves postischemic renal function and enhances formation of new tubular cells.
2. It reduces whole body catabolism by increasing protein synthesis and decreasing protein degradation.

The relevance of these findings for patients with acute renal failure is awaited with interest. On the other hand, growth factors including IGF I may not have the same beneficial effect on kidney function and survival in chronic renal failure (for a review, see [79]).

Conclusions

Impaired renal perfusion and oxygenation may lead to acute renal failure. The situation is aggravated when nephrotoxins or endotoxins are present. Several mechanisms are involved, e.g., intracellular and intramitochondrial accumulation of calcium, generation of free oxygen radicals, leukocyte-related cytokines, vasoconstrictive eicosanoid products, fibrinolytic inhibitors as well as increased endothelin release. The prognosis of acute renal failure has not improved dramatically since renal replacement therapy was introduced. However, volume replacement, mannitol treatment, and avoidance of myoglobinuria and nephrotoxins may improve the course of the disease. Preliminary reports suggest that treatment with ANP and IGF-I may be beneficial.

Acknowledgement. The present work was supported by the Research Council of Norway.

References

1. Cameron JS (1986) Acute renal failure in the intensive care unit today. Intensive Care Med 12:64–70
2. Fry DE, Garrison RN, Heitsch RC, Calhoun K, Polk HC Jr (1980) Determinants of death in patients with intra-abdominal abscess. Surgery 88:517–523
3. Better OS, Rubinstein I, Winaver J (1992) Recent insights into the pathogenesis and early management of the crush syndrome. Semin Nephrol 12:217–222
4. Sandin R (1993) Kidney function in shock. Acta Anaesthesiol Scand 37 Suppl 98:14–19
5. Ofstad J, Aukland K (1985) Renal circulation. In: Seldin DW, Giebisch G (eds) The kidney: physiology and pathophysiology. Raven, New York, pp 471–496
6. Steinhausen M, Endlich K, Wiegman DL (1990) Glomerular blood flow. Kidney Int 38:769–784
7. Stein JH (1990) Regulation of the renal circulation. Kidney Int 38:571–576
8. Clive DM, Stoff JS (1984) Renal syndromes associated with nonsteroidal antiinflammatory drugs. N Engl J Med 310:563–572
9. Oliver JA, Sciacca RR, Pinto J, Cannon PJ (1981) Participation of the prostaglandins in the control of renal blood flow during acute reduction of cardiac output in the dog. J Clin Invest 67:229–237
10. Fink MP, MacVittie TJ, Casey LC (1984) Effects of nonsteroidal anti-inflammatory drugs on renal function in septic dogs. J Surg Res 36:516–525
11. Conger JD, Burke TJ (1976) Effects of anesthetic agents on autoregulation of renal hemodynamics in the rat and dog. Am J Physiol 230:652–657
12. Zager RA (1991) Adenine nucleotide changes in kidney, liver, and small intestine during different forms of ischemic injury. Circ Res 68:185–196
13. Yu L, Seguro AC, Rocha AS (1992) Acute renal failure following hemorrhagic shock: protective and aggravating factors. Renal Failure 14:49–55
14. Weaver LC (1977) Cardiopulmonary sympathetic afferent influences on renal nerve activity. Am J Physiol 233:H592–H599

15. Thames MD, Abboud FM (1979) Reflex inhibition of renal sympathetic nerve activity during myocardial ischemia mediated by left ventricular receptors with vagal afferents in dogs. J Clin Invest 63:395–402
16. Parekh N, Veith U (1981) Renal hemodynamics and oxygen consumption during postischemic acute renal failure in the rat. Kidney Int 19:306–316
17. Baumgärtl H, Leichtweiss HP, Lübbers DW, Weiss C, Huland H (1972) The oxygen supply of the dog kidney: measurements of intrarenal pO_2. Microvasc Res 4:247–257
18. Hollenberg NK, Epstein M, Rosen SM, Basch RI, Oken DE, Merrill JP (1968) Acute oliguric renal failure in man: evidence for preferential renal cortical ischemia. Medicine (Baltimore) 47:455–474
19. Vetterlein F, Pethö A, Schmidt G (1986) Distribution of capillary blood flow in rat kidney during postischemic renal failure. Am J Physiol 251:H510–H519
20. Paller MS, Hoidal JR, Ferris TF (1984) Oxygen free radicals in ischemic acute renal failure in the rat. J Clin Invest 74:1156–1164
21. Bayati A, Frödin L, Källskog Ö, Hellberg O, Wolgast M (1985) Prevention of acute renal failure by long term treatment with alopurinol. Acta Physiol Scand 124 Suppl 542:383
22. Hansson R, Johanson S, Jonsson O, Petterson S, Schersten T, Waldenstrom J (1986) Kidney protection by pretreatment with free radical scavengers and allopurinol: renal function at recirculation after warm ischemia in rabbits. Clin Sci 71:245–251
23. Van Lambalgen AA, van Kraats AA, van den Bos GC et al. (1993) Development of renal failure in endotoxemic rats: can it be explained by early changes in renal energy metabolism? Nephron 65:88–94
24. Hollenberg NK, Adams DF, Oken DE, Abrams HL, Merrill JP (1970) Acute renal failure due to nephrotoxins. Renal hemodynamic and angiographic studies in man. N Engl J Med 282:1329–1334
25. Zager RA (1988) Gentamicin nephrotoxicity in the setting of acute renal hypoperfusion. Am J Physiol 254:F574–F581
26. Spiegel DM, Shanley PF, Molitoris BA (1990) Mild ischemia predisposes the S_3 segment to gentamicin toxicity. Kidney Int 38:459–464
27. Zager RA (1992) Gentamicin effects on renal ischemia/reperfusion injury. Circ Res 70:20–28
28. Zager RA (1991) Myoglobin depletes renal adenine nucleotide pools in the presence and absence of shock. Kidney Int 39:111–119
29. Fraley DS, Adler S (1977) Correction of hyperkalemia by bicarbonate despite constant blood pH. Kidney Int 12:354–360
30. Humes DH (1986) Role of calcium in pathogenesis of acute renal failure. Am J Physiol 250:F579–F589
31. Goldfarb D, Iaina A, Serban I, Gavendo S, Kapuler S, Eliahou HE (1983) Beneficial effects of verapamil in ischemic acute renal failure in the rat. Proc Soc Exp Biol Med 172:389–392
32. Malis CD, Cheung JY, Leaf A, Bonventre JV (1983) Effects of verapamil in models of ischemic acute renal failure in the rat. Am J Physiol 245:F735–F742
33. Burke TJ, Arnold PE, Gordon JA, Bulger RE, Dobyan DC, Schrier RW (1984) Protective effect of intrarenal calcium membrane blockers before or after renal ischemia. J Clin Invest 74:1830–1841
34. Chintala MS, Jandhyala BS (1990) Renal failure in haemorrhagic shock in dogs: salutary effects of the calcium entry blocker felodipine. Naunyn Schmiedebergs Arch Pharmacol 341:357–363
35. Sandin R, Feuk U, Wahlberg J, Modig J (1991) Effects of diltiazem on postischemic renal cortical microcirculation in the pig. Acta Anaesthesiol Scand 35:424–429
36. Conger JD, Robinette JB, Guggenheim SJ (1981) Effect of acetylcholine on the early phase of reversible norepinephrine-induced acute renal failure. Kidney Int 19:399–409
37. Eliahou HE, Brodman RR, Friedman EA (1973) Adrenergic blockers in ischemic acute renal failure in the rat. In: Friedman EA, Eliahou HE (eds) Proceedings of the conference on acute renal failure. National Institute of Health, New York, pp 265–280 (DHEW publication no (NIH) 74-608)
38. Russell JD, Churchill DN (1989) Calcium antagonists and acute renal failure. Am J Med 87:306–315

39. Caroll GC, Snyder JV (1982) Hyperdynamic severe intravascular sepsis depends on fluid administration in cynomolgus monkey. Am J Physiol 243:R131–R141
40. Schaer GL, Fink MP, Chernow B, Ahmed S, Parrillo JE (1990) Renal hemodynamics and prostaglandin E_2 excretion in a nonhuman primate model of septic shock. Crit Care Med 18:52–59
41. Cumming AD, Kline R, Linton AL (1988) Association between renal and sympathetic responses to nonhypotensive systemic sepsis. Crit Care Med 16:1132–1137
42. Sandok EK, Lerman A, Stingo AJ, Perrella MA, Gloviczki P, Burnett JC Jr (1992) Endothelin in a model of acute ischemic renal dysfunction: modulating action of atrial natriuretic factor. J Am Soc Nephrol 3:196–202
43. Henrich WL, Hamasaki Y, Said SI, Campbell WB, Cronin RE (1982) Dissociation of systemic and renal effects in endotoxinemia. Prostaglandin inhibition uncovers an important role of renal nerves. J Clin Invest 69:691–699
44. Badr KF, Kelley VE, Rennke HG, Brenner BM (1986) Roles for thromboxane A_2 and leukotrienes in endotoxin-induced acute renal failure. Kidney Int 30:474–480
45. Linas SL, Whittenburg D, Repine JE (1991) Role of neutrophil derived oxidants and elastase in lipopolysaccharide-mediated renal injury. Kidney Int 39:618–623
46. Marletta MA, Yoon PS, Iyengar R, Leaf CD, Wishnok JS (1988) Macrophage oxidation of L-arginine to nitrite and nitrate: nitric oxide is an intermediate. Biochemistry 27:8706–8711
47. Shultz PJ, Tayeh MA, Marletta MA, Raij L (1991) Synthesis and action of nitric oxide in rat glomerular mesangial cells. Am J Physiol 261:F600–F606
48. Radomski MW, Palmer RMJ, Moncada S (1987) The role of nitric oxide and cGMP in platelet adhesion to vascular endothelium. Biochem Biophys Res Commun 148:1482–1489
49. Shultz PJ, Raij L (1992) Endogenously synthesized nitric oxide prevents endotoxin-induced glomerular thrombosis. J Clin Invest 90:1718–1725
50. Schrier RW, Burke TJ (1994) New aspects in pathogenesis of acute renal failure. Nephrol Dial Transplant 9 Suppl 4:9–14
51. Keeton M, Eguchi Y, Sawdey M, Ahn C, Loskutoff DJ (1993) Cellular localization of type 1 plasminogen activator inhibitor messenger RNA and protein in murine renal tissue. Am J Pathol 142:59–70
52. Hekman CM, Loskutoff DJ (1988) Kinetic analysis of the interactions between plasminogen activator inhibitor 1 and both urokinase and tissue plasminogen activator. Arch Biochem Biophys 262:199–210
53. Bloom ITM, Bentley FR, Wilson MA, Garrison RN (1993) In vivo effects of endothelin on the renal microcirculation. J Surg Res 54:274–280
54. Masaki T, Kimura S, Yanagisawa M, Goto K (1991) Molecular and cellular mechanism of endothelin regulation. Implications for vascular function. Circulation 84:1457–1468
55. Kon V, Badr KF (1991) Biological actions and pathophysiologic significance of endothelin in the kidney. Kidney Int 40:1–12
56. Stingo AJ, Clavell AL, Aarhus LL, Burnett JC Jr (1993) Biological role for the endothelin-A receptor in aortic cross-clamping. Hypertension 22:62–66
57. Firth JD, Ratcliffe PJ (1992) Organ distribution of the three rat endothelin messenger RNAs and the effects of ischemia on renal gene expression. J Clin Invest 90:1023–1031
58. Wilmore DW, Dudrick SJ (1969) Treatment of acute renal failure with intravenous essential L-amino acids. Arch Surg 99:669–673
59. Abel RM, Beck Ch Jr, Abbott WM, Ryan JA Jr, Barnett GO, Fischer JE (1973) Improved survival from acute renal failure after treatment with intravenous essential L-amino acids and glucose. N Engl J Med 288:695–699
60. Feinstein EI, Blumenkrantz MJ, Healy M et al. (1981) Clinical and metabolic responses to parenteral nutrition in acute renal failure. Medicine (Baltimore) 60:124–137
61. Graziani G, Casati S, Cantaluppi A (1982) Dopamine-furosemide therapy in acute renal failure. Proc Eur Dial Transplant Assoc 19:319–325
62. Lumlertgul D, Keoplung M, Sitprija V, Moollaor P, Suwangool P (1989) Furosemide and dopamine in malarial acute renal failure. Nephron 52:40–44
63. Baldwin L, Henderson A, Hickman P (1994) Effect of postoperative low-dose dopamine on renal function after elective major vascular surgery. Ann Intern Med 120:744–747
64. Thompson BT, Cockrill BA (1994) Renal-dose dopamine: a siren song? Lancet 344:7–8

65. Kleinknecht D, Jungers P, Chanard J, Barbanel C, Ganeval D (1972) Uremic and non-uremic complications in acute renal failure: evaluation of early and frequent dialysis on prognosis. Kidney Int 1:190–196
66. Cahill CJ (1983) Prevention of postoperative renal failure in patients with obstructive jaundice — the role of bile salts. Br J Surg 70:590–595
67. Brezis M, Epstein FH (1989) A closer look at radiocontrast-induced nephropathy. N Engl J Med 320:179–181
68. Schafferhans K, Heidbreder E, Grimm D, Heidland A (1986) Norepinephrine-induced acute renal failure: beneficial effects of atrial natriuretic factor. Nephron 44:240–244
69. Shaw SG, Weidmann P, Hodler J, Zimmermann A, Paternostro A (1987) Atrial natriuretic peptide protects against acute ischemic renal failure in the rat. J Clin Invest 80:1232–1237
70. Rahman SN, Kim GE, Mathew AS et al. (1994) Effects of atrial natriuretic peptide in clinical acute renal failure. Kidney Int 45:1731–1738
71. Conger JD, Falk SA, Yuan BH, Schrier RW (1989) Atrial natriuretic peptide and dopamine in a rat model of ischemic acute renal failure. Kidney Int 35:1126–1132
72. Roy DR (1986) Effect of synthetic ANP on renal and loop of Henle functions in the young rat. Am J Physiol 251:F220–F225
73. Ziegler TR, Lazarus JM, Young LS, Hakim R, Wilmore DW (1991) Effects of recombinant human growth hormone in adults receiving maintenance hemodialysis. J Am Soc Nephrol 2:1130–1135
74. Mehls O, Tönshoff B, Blum WF, Heinrich U, Seidel C (1990) Growth hormone and insulin-like growth factor 1 in chronic renal failure — pathophysiology and rationale for growth hormone treatment. Acta Pædiatr Scand Suppl 370:28–34
75. Thomas FM, Knowles SE, Owens PC et al. (1991) Effects of full-length and truncated insulin-like growth factor-I on nitrogen balance and muscle protein metabolism in nitrogen-restricted rats. J Endocrinol 128:97–105
76. Pillion DJ, Haskell JF, Meezan E (1988) Distinct receptors for insulin-like growth factor I in rat renal glomeruli and tubules. Am J Physiol 255:E504–E512
77. Hirschberg R, Brunori G, Kopple JD, Guler HP (1993) Effects of insulin-like growth factor I on renal function in normal men. Kidney Int 43:387–397
78. Ding HU, Kopple JD, Cohen A, Hirschberg R (1993) Recombinant human insulin-like growth factor-I accelerates recovery and reduces catabolism in rats with ischemic acute renal failure. J Clin Invest 91:2281–2287
79. O'Shea MH, Layish DT (1992) Growth hormone and the kidney: a case presentation and review of the literature. J Am Soc Nephrol 3:157–161

The Liver in the Induction and Regulation of the Acute Stress Response

C. Meijer, M. G. Statius Muller, and P. A. M. van Leeuwen

Introduction

The liver is an important organ that plays a key regulatory role in the metabolism of the human body. It performs many functions, but is especially important in the normal host defense. This host response is characterized by a coordinated series of metabolic reactions, which is due to a complex interaction between the Kupffer cell (KC) and the hepatocyte. KC, the fixed macrophages of the liver, are situated at an interface with the blood stream in a location that allows constant exposure to antigens, endotoxins, and other potentially immunostimulatory materials. In this position, the KC can become activated by bacterial products from both the portal vein and the systemic circulation. After scavenging the bacterial products, the KC become activated and produce a myriad of biological mediators and other reactants that can have an impact on adjacent hepatocytes as well as on distant organs. An excessive and uncontrolled production of these inflammatory mediators can lead to the development of a systemic inflammatory response. In addition, profound changes in the plasma concentrations of liver-derived plasma proteins occur, while the synthesis of acute phase proteins in the liver is dramatically increased. Other responses include increased gluconeogenesis and glycogenolysis and a negative nitrogen balance. In the following manuscript we will focus on the immunologic and metabolic response of the liver in the acute state with special reference to the function of the reticuloendothelial system (RES), its substrates during stress, and its interaction with the hepatocytes.

Reticuloendothelial System in the Acute Metabolic State

The RES, also called the mononuclear phagocyte system (MPS), consists of tissue-bound macrophages and blood-borne monocytes. Reticular cells of the spleen, central nervous system, lymph nodes, and bone marrow as well as specialized endothelial cells (capillary lining or sinusoidal cells) in the liver (KC), spleen, lymph nodes, bone marrow, adrenal glands, hypophyseal system, and lungs belong to the fixed phagocytes of the RES. Blood monocytes, tissue macrophages, and connective tissue histiocytes are known as blood-borne monocytes [1–4]. The major sites of RES intravascular activity are located in the liver and spleen, which comprise about 85% and 10% of total body activity, respectively [5]. The Kupffer cells and the endothelial cells of the liver are capable of scavenging antigens, immune complexes, and endotoxins from the portal vein and the systemic circulation. However, KC are generally regarded as the major site of endotoxin detoxification, especially in the acute state. KC reside in the liver for a few weeks and are then replaced by circulating monocytes that subsequently differentiate into new KC. In response to injury or liver resection, Kupffer cells can divide and proliferate locally to restore the hepatic phagocytic function. In addition, liver size will be restored by extrahepatic recruitment of macrophages and monocytes [6, 7], which subsequently stimulates liver regeneration by the production of growth factors. It is well established that phagocytosis by the reticuloendothelial (RE) cells depends upon recognition of appropriate material at the cell surface. In the circulation, recognition is mediated by circulating recognition factors, the opsonins; at the cellular level it is mediated by cell surface receptors. The opsonins can be divided into two groups: those that are nonimmunospecific, e.g., fibronectin, and those that are immunospecific, in particular immunoglobulin (Ig)G and IgM antibodies, which recognize specific antigenic material. Concerning the cell surface-mediated phagocytosis, antigen binding to either complement (C3) receptors or Fc receptors alone produces modest phagocytosis, whereas attachment to both receptor types synergistically induces rapid phagocytosis [6]. RES phagocytic function is of major importance in defending the host against systemic stress and is found to be profoundly depressed in a number of pathological states, such as bacterial infection, neoplasia, and diseases of altered immunity [8, 9]. After major surgery, burn injury, multiple trauma, disseminated intravascular coagulation, and bacterial sepsis it is also disturbed [10–14]. This temporary RES depression lasts for 12–18 h and is followed by a rapid recovery. The transient RES depression is most likely mediated by a decreased activity of C3 receptors, possibly due to endotoxin overload, and results in endotoxin spillover in the systemic circulation. A long-lasting depression of the RES, as seen after liver resection, hepatitis, bile duct obstruction, and cirrhosis, will also give rise to a systemic endotoxemia. The KC and circulating monocytes are thought to be primed by systemic circulating endotoxin and can rapidly produce large amounts of inflammatory mediators when stimulated again by endotoxin.

Integrity of the Gut in Relation to the Reticuloendothelial System

Translocation of bacteria or endotoxin, which takes place in patients subjected to host-compromising effects such as hospitalization, surgery, blood loss, or liver resection, is of clinical importance [15]. Integrity of the intestinal structures, which preserves the mucosal barrier function, determines whether translocation of bacteria or endotoxin takes place. The integrity of the gut wall is determined by a variety of mechanisms, which include an intact mucosa, sufficient mucus protection, an ecological balance of normal gut-related intestinal microflora, immunologic defense mechanisms including IgA from the bile, intestinal peristalsis, and intraluminal secretion of saliva, gastric, and bile acids. The maintenance of a normal cellular structure of the gut wall prevents transepithelial migration of particles from the intestinal lumen, and preservation of the tight junction between the epithelial cells prevents movement through the paracellular channels. A thick mucus layer sustains this epithelial barrier function. The mucosal epithelium is a dynamic, rapidly dividing tissue and is, therefore, highly dependent on adequate nutritional supply. Changes in composition, amount, and even the route of administration of nutrition can easily effect the integrity of the mucosa. Furthermore, disturbance of the normal gut flora, especially the gut wall-associated anaerobic layer, can initiate translocation. Attachment of potential pathogenic aerobic bacteria to the mucosal surface is regarded as the initial event and a prerequisite in the pathogenesis of a systemic infection. Immunologic defense mechanisms include intraepithelial and lamina propria lymphocytes, lymphoid follicles, Peyer's patches, macrophages of the lamina propria, and mesenteric lymph nodes. Peyer's patches are especially important because of their antigen-sampling function through specialized M cells. These antigens are presented to lymphocytes which leave the intestinal tract, migrate through the mesenteric lymph nodes and the thoracic duct, and reach the systemic circulation. After transforming into plasma cells capable of IgA production, these cells home back to the intestinal tract, where IgA is secreted intraluminally and in bile. IgA can bind to endotoxin and bacteria, and this complex is excreted in the feces. This process provides an immune tolerance, thereby preventing unnecessary immune responses which could otherwise trigger an inflammatory response resulting in mucosal damage and subsequent translocation of bacteria and/or endotoxin. In addition, bile acids are capable of binding endotoxin and are thus important in the prevention of endotoxin translocation. Translocation of minute amounts of endogenous endotoxin occurs under physiological conditions and might be important in stimulating the RES and maintaining normal phagocytic capacity [16, 17]. However, during periods of severe stress, such as portal venous thrombosis, mesenteric artery occlusion, bowel ischemia, hypovolemic shock, and other pathological conditions that affect RES function or harm the gut mucosa, translocation of large amounts of endotoxin takes place. These high concentrations of portal venous endotoxin can enhance an already ongoing inflammatory reponse in the liver. For instance, it is highly conceivable that liver failure after liver resection is the consequence of an inflammatory response in the remnant liver necessary to regenerate the liver, but that this response is dramatically augmented by gut-derived endotoxins [18]. Severe liver failure in combination with systemic endotoxemia might then result in an overwhelming sepsis-like inflammatory respons. Gut-derived endotoxins may also enhance inflammation in the liver during liver failure due to bile duct obstruction, liver cirrhosis, hepatitis, and liver transplantation, among others. This idea is sustained by the fact that postoperative complications in patients with cirrhosis or obstructive jaundice is related to a significant increase in blood endotoxin. In conclusion, a delicate balance between RES phagocytic function and the integrity of the gut wall is important in preventing systemic endotoxemia and a systemic inflammatory response.

Kupffer Cells in the Acute State

Recent studies have revealed that binding of lipopolysaccharide (LPS, endotoxin) to monocytes and macrophages involves specific receptors called CD14 [19]. CD14 recognizes complexes of LPS and LPS-binding protein (LBP). In addition, LBP–LPS complexes have an increased capacity, compared to LPS alone, to stimulate monocytes and macrophages. Binding of these complexes to CD14 on the cell surface induces the production of inflammatory mediators. Activated KC and blood mononuclear cells release potent endogenous inflammatory substances, which can mediate deleterious pathophysiological reactions, previously attributed to endotoxin alone [20, 21]. These mediators include tumor necrosis factor (TNF), interleukin-1 (IL-1), interleukin-6 (IL-6), interleukin-8 (IL-8), arachidonic acid metabolites, interferon (IFN), reactive oxygen species, nitric oxide (NO), and platelet-activating factor (PAF), among others. TNF and IL-1 are the first cytokines appearing in the circulation during acute inflammation and induce the production of IL-6 and IL-8. IL-6 is the main regulator of the acute phase protein synthesis by hepatocytes, which is known to protect the body against the potentially harmful effects of inflammatory mediators. IL-8 is a small peptide with important neutrophil-activating properties. Both IL-6 and IL-8 are known to induce the activation of the complement, coagulation, and fibrinolytic systems. IL-1 as well as IL-6 act on the central nervous system, resulting in fever and production of adrenocorticotropic hormone (ACTH) [22, 23]. The eventual release of cortisol may be an effective negative feedback loop, since cortisol is a potent inhibitor of IL-1 and IL-6 synthesis [24]. Many other systemic effects of these two cytokines augment host defense, such as the margination and chemotaxis of neutrophils and monocytes [24, 25]. The inflammatory mediators among themselves are capable of influencing each other. For example, the arachidonic acid metabolites, primarily prostaglandin E_2 (PGE_2), seem to act as endogenous regulators of cytokine production such as IL-6 and TNF. The early increase of in vitro IL-6 and TNF production by LPS-activated KC was limited by a concurrent production of PGE_2 [26, 27]. Since the production of these cytokines is excessively increased in systemic inflammation, PGE_2 may be a major regulator of the production of inflammatory cytokines by KC. Altered monocyte behavior with respect to the production of mediators is observed after massive tissue injury and during severe sepsis. A suppressed IL-1 and IL-8 production by isolated monocytes to LPS was found which correlated to the severity of the injury, whereas the production of TNF and IL-6 was upregulated in these patients [28]. These observations illustrate the complexity of changes in mediator release after activation of monocytes by various amounts of endotoxin. The mechanisms involved in changes in KC activation and clearance function are still unclear. Possibly, initial impaired phagocytic function is followed by a hyperreactive state with release of inflammatory mediators, leading to a generalized inflammatory response. Alternatively, impaired hepatic phagocytosis and increased induction of mediator production by KC may exist at the same time, involving different receptor mechanisms. Clearly, KC are much more than scavenging phagocytes and their functions have both local and systemic consequences for the host. The acute physiological stress response, in which the KC play a pivotal role, normally provides a well-functioning immune system and protects the human body against invading antigens, bacteria, or endotoxin.

Role of Mediators in Tissue Injury

The inflammatory mediators are known to have a stimulatory function in the host defense to immune balance-affecting events. On the other hand, some of the inflammatory mediators exert direct or indirect toxic effects on surrounding tissue, leading to tissue damage. An uncontrolled release of inflammatory mediators will lead to damage of organ microcirculation. TNF and IL-1 induce the expression of the adhesion molecules endothelial leukocyte adhesion molecule (ELAM)-1 and intercellular adhesion molecule (ICAM)-1 on endothelial cells, which in turn induces a procoagulant state of the endothelium. Neutrophils then become activated, either directly by endotoxin or indirectly by complement cascade products or cytokines. Adhesion of these activated neutrophils, through their adhesion proteins, leads to the release of cytotoxic oxygen radicals and proteolytic enzymes and will result in endothelial damage. Subsequent expression of tissue factor and adhesion of platelets, complement products, and fibrin to the injured wall induces formation of microthrombi. Microvascular injury with microthrombosis leads to a disturbance of oxygen availability at cellular level, followed by tissue necrosis. Development of extracellular edema due to increased vascular permeability further compromises organ function. In addition to mediating tissue damage by their release of cytotoxic mediators, the activated "stiff" neutrophils will get jammed in the narrow blood capillaries, thereby reducing blood flow through the liver, which might contribute to the development of liver failure. Release of reactive oxygen-derived free radicals by activated KC and or neutrophils has been found to contribute to hepatic injury [29, 30]. These active toxic metabolites, including superoxide, hydrogen peroxide, and the hydroxyl radical, may damage the cellular membrane as well as the envelope of organelles through the peroxidation of the polyunsaturated fatty acids within the phospholipid structure of the membrane. PAF might be an important inflammatory mediator that enhances the release of toxic oxygen-derived radicals, which may contribute to organ failure during endotoxemia or sepsis. It was shown that PAF stimulates KC and neutrophils to release superoxide anion [31]. Moreover, a specific inorganic signal molecule, NO, is synthesized and excreted by in vitro LPS-activated KC [32] and by hepatocytes when exposed to conditioned medium from activated KC [33]. NO is produced from the guanidino nitrogen of L-arginine by an enzyme, NO synthase (NOS), that forms the free radical NO, with citrulline as the byproduct. NO is rapidly oxidized to the stable, inactive end products nitrite and nitrate. NO produced by the KC has important antimicrobial [34] and antitumor [35] functions. Hepatocyte NO production by in vitro activation results in the suppression of hepatocyte total protein synthesis [32] and in the inhibition of hepatocyte mitochondrial respiration [36]. Although these latter two findings s uggest a stimulatory effect of NO in the development of LPS-induced liver damage, it was found that inhibition of NO synthesis by N^G-monomethyl-L-arginine administration 6 h after injection of LPS in mice promotes hepatic damage, as was determined by plasma levels of hepatocellular enzymes [37]. Histological examination of the liver revealed microvascular thrombosis and multiple infarctions associated with increased liver enzymes in the animals that had NO synthesis inhibited [38]. This protective role for NO in the liver is probably due to the vasodilative effect and the inhibition of platelet and neutrophil aggregation caused by NO in a slow-flow sinusoidal vascular bed, thereby preventing vessel thrombosis and organ infarction. Of interest is the fact that superoxide anion is postulated to be a potent endogenous inhibitor of NO [39]. Other cell types, such as endothelial cells, tumor cells, fibroblasts, and cerebellar neurons also produce NO in response to LPS stimulation. An excessive production of NO by LPS- and cytokine-stimulated vascular smooth muscle cells in sepsis may result in massive dilatation of blood vessels and sustained hypotension commonly encountered in septic shock [40, 41]. Thus, although NO seems to have important physiological functions, it can also contribute to pathophysiological conditions. The above-mentioned complex interactions between inflammatory mediators might all contribute to the development of a systemic inflammatory response and (multi-)organ failure.

Acute Phase Protein Synthesis

Cytokines stimulate the liver to enhance the synthesis and secretion of a broad spectrum of plasma proteins called the acute phase proteins or the acute phase reactants (APR). Concomitantly, the synthesis of some so-called negative acute phase proteins is reduced (e.g., albumin). The majority of APR are synthesized in hepatocytes. The major contributions of APR involve neutralizing the harmful consequences of tissue injury such as inhibiting proteases, clearing superoxide anions, removing freed hemoglobin, and opsonizing particulate matter. Moreover, APR contribute to blood clotting, modulate the activity of the immune system, and provide substrates for tissue repair. Many transport proteins of minerals and trace elements are APR. Changes in their synthesis lead to considerable changes in the plasma levels of iron, copper, and zinc. It should be noted that serum levels of C-reactive protein and serum amyloid A can increase by several 100-fold. Many of the APR that increase by approximately two to five times are protease inhibitors with the obvious role of modifying the untoward tissue-damaging effects of the inflammatory response. Several other plasma APR with well-defined functions, such as fibronectin, fibrinogen, and the complement components, increase in concentration by only 50%. The most active cytokine for induction at transcriptional level of several, but not all, APR is IL-6 [42–44]. IL-6 fulfills its critical role in the induction and regulation of APR in collaboration with other inflammatory cytokines, including IL-1 [45], TNF-α [46], and IFN-γ [47]. Interestingly, IL-1 and TNF appear to act synergistically with IL-6 on the synthesis of some APR, while downregulating the synthesis of albumin [46, 48]. In vitro it has been demonstrated that glucocorticoids can also directly induce hepatocyte APR synthesis [49]. It became clear, however, that APR synthesis can be modulated by glucocorticoids, but its presence is not an absolute requirement for the action of IL-6 [50, 51]. Clearly, activated KC are uniquely equiped to regulate the acute phase response: they can directly induce the acute phase response of neighboring hepatocytes by producing IL-6, the main regulator of the acute phase response [52].

Metabolic Response of the Liver During Stress

During the acute phase response, an increase of protein catabolism in the muscle and a simultaneous rise of amino acid uptake by hepatocytes lead to an amino acid shift from the muscles to the liver. Concomitantly, APR synthesis and gluconeogenesis in the liver are enhanced [53]. The liver is the main glucose-producing organ in the body. In times of stress the glycogen content of the liver is very rapidly depleted and the hepatocytes start the production of glucose from the amino acid precursors, mainly alanine. Therefore, in these catabolic states the release of alanine from skeletal muscle tissue is increased in order to provide the necessary substrate for gluconeogenesis [54, 55]. Clearly, increased gluconeogenesis is important in maintaining normoglycemia in sepsis [56, 57]. In addition, glutamine is released from skeletal muscle to be consumed by enterocytes. In the intestinal conversion of glutamine, alanine is one of the end products. In this way glutamine indirectly stimulates gluconeogenesis [58]. In the response to stress the liver shifts to the production of APR, while the synthesis of albumin is decreased. The precise mechanism leading to this change in the type of protein that is synthesized by the liver remains to be elucidated. As mentioned before, the initiating factors, however, have been recognized as the inflammatory cytokines IL-6, TNF, and IL-1. Although a number of studies suggest an important role of KC in the above-mentioned metabolic responses, their precise role remains to be established. The function of KC is dependent on an adequate supply of oxidative fuels, such as glucose and glutamine. The increased uptake of glutamine by the liver as reported in animals following endotoxin administration [59] might be the result of an increased consumption of glutamine by the KC. Since activated KC produce large amounts of inflammatory cytokines and a number of cytokines have been related to the metabolic changes as observed during stress situations [60–62], KC might play a regulatory role in amino acid and carbohydrate metabolism during the acute phase response of the liver.

Future Therapeutic Interventions

In the current manuscript, evidence was provided for the pivotal role of the KC and its biological mediators in the regulation of the acute metabolic response of the liver to stress situations. A depressed phagocytic capacity of the KC and/or disturbance of gut barrier function might lead to spillover of endotoxins in the systemic circulation. This is the first step in the development of a systemic inflammatory response, which is enhanced by the release of inflammatory mediators by the activated KC and blood mononuclear cells. The toxic effects of some of the inflammatory mediators might result in tissue damage and organ failure. Concomitantly, a complex interaction between the KC and hepatocytes results in an increased APR synthesis, while gluconeogenesis and glycogenolysis is strongly enhanced and a shift of amino acids takes place from the muscles to the liver. Although the liver is known to play a very important role in the induction and regulation of the host response to stress, the precise mechanisms leading to a generalized inflammatory response, tissue injury, and a catabolic state of the human body need to be further clarified. Based on results of recent experiments, however, we will discuss some therapeutic strategies that might be beneficial in the prevention of systemic endotoxemia, endotoxin-induced tissue injury, and the catabolic response of the human body in the acute state of host defense against stress.

In clinical situations in which we can anticipate a reduced clearance function of the liver, prophylactic use of endotoxin-binding therapeutics could be beneficial. Patients undergoing major liver resection, for example, become at risk for liver failure and subsequent impaired clearance function. In these patients, high operative blood loss increases the risk of a temporary low-flow state of the gut with increased endotoxin translocation, and resection of a substantial part of the RES decreases the hepatic phagocytic capacity. In conclusion, after major liver resection, spillover of gut-derived endotoxin is most likely to occur, resulting in systemic endotoxemia. The concept of endotoxemia originating from the gut lumen within the first few hours after liver surgery was confirmed by our experiments with rats undergoing a two thirds liver resection. Pretreatment with enteral cholestyramine, an endotoxin-binding agent, during 7 days prior to surgery almost completely prevented postoperative endotoxemia and liver failure as determined by plasma levels of hepatic enzymes. Furthermore, no deaths occurred in the cholestyramine-treated animals, in contrast to a high mortality rate in the control group [63].

Another potential therapeutic agent to prevent (postoperative) systemic endotoxemia is recombinant bactericidal/permeability-increasing protein (rBPI), because of its bactericidal and endotoxin-binding capacities. We have shown that perioperative treatment with rBPI in rats undergoing partial hepatectomy largely prevented the development of liver failure, a systemic inflammatory response, and hemodynamic derangements such as hypotension and a decreased cardiac output in the early postoperative period [18].

As mentioned earlier, IL-1 is one of the primary inflammatory mediators that are released from (endotoxin-)activated KC and monocytes. It is well known that IL-1 induces the activation of other cytokines and mediator systems, such as the complement, coagulation and fibrinolytic system, which might result in a generalized inflammatory response. Therefore, we also investigated the effect of perioperative treatment with the natural inhibitor of IL-1, IL-1 receptor antagonist (IL-1ra), in the same rat model. Both, perioperative treatment with rBPI and IL-1ra, reduced hepatic inflammation and partially prevented liver failure [7]. Moreover, lipid accumulation after partial hepatectomy, resulting in a "fatty" liver, was significantly reduced in the rBPI and IL-1ra treatment groups, as compared to the control groups [64].

Scavengers of oxygen-derived free radicals should also be mentioned as potential therapeutic agents in the prevention of tissue injury. Oxidative mechanisms have clearly been shown to play an important role in tissue injury in ischemia–reperfusion, radiation, chemotherapy, and inflammation. These oxidative mechanisms, mediated by the xanthine oxidase system and activated neutrophils, might also be important in endotoxin-induced tissue injury. Individual studies have demonstrated varying levels of protection by any single antioxidant. However, administration of antioxidant, such as superoxide dismutase (SOD), catalase, allopurinol, glutathione, and alpha tocopherol, to endotoxin-injured animals clearly was shown to have protective effects. Among other things, an increased survival rate, decreased lipid peroxidation, maintenance of hepatic adenosine triphosphate (ATP) levels and mild attenuation of hemodynamic parameters of shock were reported as beneficial effects of antioxidant administration in endotoxin-challenged animals [65–68].

In nutritional support, glutamine-enriched diets might have beneficial effects in acute metabolic states. Glutamine is the most abundant amino acid in the body and plays a key role in oxidative metabolism of enterocytes and lymphocytes [69]. In catabolic states, glutamine muscle stores become rapidly depleted and plasma levels drop. Dietary supplementation with glutamine, however, restores glutamine availability and has potentially beneficial effects on the liver [69]. Glutamine is the precursor for glutathione synthesis in the liver, and glutamine-enriched nutrition has been shown to sustain glutathione levels after hepatic injury [70]. Since glutathione is an important antioxidant, glutamine indirectly protects the liver and the human body against tissue damage due to oxidative stress. Furthermore, it has recently been shown that a glutamine-enriched enteral diet increases total hepatic blood flow [71]. Thus, glutamine may contribute to liver perfusion and maintenance of RES activity. Finally, as mentioned before, glutamine might be an important oxidative fuel for KC [59].

References

1. Aschoff L (1924) Das reticulo-endotheliale System. Ergeb Inn Med Kinderheilkd 26:1–118
2. Metchnikoff E (1905) Immunity in infective disease. Cambridge University Press, Cambridge
3. Stuart AE (1970) The reticulo-endothelial system. Livingstone, Edinburgh
4. Vernon-Roberts B (1972) The macrophage. Cambridge University Press, Cambridge
5. Biozzi G, Stiffel C (1965) The physiopathology of the reticuloendothelial cells of the liver and spleen. Prog Liver Dis 2:166–191
6. Lanser ME (1990) Reticuloendothelial system failure. In: Deitch EA (ed) Multiple organ failure. Pathology and basic concepts of therapy. Thieme, New York, pp 72–86
7. Boermeester M, Straatsburg IH, Houdijk APJ et al. (1995) Endotoxin and interleukin-1 related hepatic inflammatory response promotes liver failure following partial hepatectomy (submitted for publication) Hepatology 22:1499–1506
8. Saba TM (1970) Physiology and pathophysiology of the reticulo-endothelial system. Arch Intern Med 126:1031
9. Beermeester MA, Houdijk APJ, van Leeuwen PAM (1993) The importance of endotoxin in the development of MOF
   In: Vincent J-L (ed) Yearbook of intensive care and emergency medi-cine. Springer-Verlag, Berlin Heidelberg, pp 64–74
10. Saba TM, Blumenstock FA, Scovill WA, Bernard H (1978) Cryoprecipitate reversal of opsonic α2 surface binding glycoprotein deficiency in septic surgical and trauma patients. Science 201:622
11. Saba TM, Blumenstock FA, Weber P, Kaplan JE (1978) Physiologic role for cold-insoluble globulin in systemic host defense. Implications of its characterization as the opsonic α2SB glycoprotein. Ann NY Acad Sci 312:43
12. Scovill WA, Saba TM, Kaplan JE, Bernard H, Powers S (1976) Deficits in reticuloendothelial humoral control mechanisms in patients after trauma. J Trauma 16:898

13. Schildt B, Gertz I, Wide L (1974) Differentiated reticuloendothelial system (RES) function in some critical surgical conditions. Acta Chir Scand 140:611
14. Scovill WA, Saba TM, Kaplan JE, Bernard HR, Powers SR (1977) Disturbances in circulating opsonic activity in man after operative and blunt trauma. J Surg Res 22:709
15. Van Leeuwen PAM, Boermeester MA, Houdijk APJ et al. (1994) Clinical significance of translocation. Gut 1994:35 (Suppl 1); S28–S34
16. Gonnella PA, Helton WS, Robinson M, Wilmore DW (1992) O-Side chain of Escherichia coli endotoxin 0111:B4 is transported across the intestinal epithelium in the rat: evidence for increased transport during total parenteral nutrition. Eur J Cell Biol 59:224–227
17. Steffan AM, Hirn A (1986) C3 mediated phagocytosis induced in murine Kupffer cells by in vitro activation with endotoxin. Gastro Clin Biol 10:117–121
18. Boermeester MA, Houdijk APJ, Meijer S et al. (1995) Liver failure due to partial hepatectomy in rats induces a systemic inflammatory response. Prevention by recombinant N-terminal bactericidal/permeability-increasing protein. Am J Pathol 147:1428–1440
19. Ulevitch RJ, Mathison JC, Schumann RR, Tobias PS (1990) A new model of macrophage stimulation by bacterial lipopolysaccharide. J Trauma 30:189–192
20. Rogoff TM, Lipsky PE (1981) Role of the Kupffer cells in local and systemic immune responses. Gastroenterology 80:854
21. Border JR (1988) Hypothesis: sepsis, multiple system organ failure, and the macrophage. Arch Surg 123:285–286
22. Ballou S, Kushner I (1992) C-reactive protein and the acute phase response. Adv Intern Med 37:313–336
23. Le J, Vilcek J (1989) Interleukin-6: a multifunctional cytokine regulating immune reactions and the acute phase response. Lab Invest 61:558–602
24. Balkwill FR, Burke F (1989) The cytokine network. Immunol Today 10:299–303
25. Wong GC, Clark SC (1988) Multiple actions of IL-6 within a cytokine network. Immunol Today 9:137
26. Decker T, Lohmann-Matthes ML, Karck U, Peters T, Decker K (1989) Comparative study of cytotoxicity, tumor necrosis factor, and prostaglandin release after stimulation of rat Kupffer cells, murine Kupffer cells, and murine inflammatory macrophages. J Leukoc Biol 45:139–146
27. Callery MP, Mangino MJ, Kamei T, Flye MW (1990) Interleukin-6 production by endotoxin-stimulated Kupffer cells is regulated by prostaglandin-E$_2$. J Surg Res 48:523–527
28. Faist E, Storck M, Hultner L et al. (1992) Functional analysis of monocyte activity through synthesis patterns of proinflammatory cytokines and neopterin in patients in surgical intensive care. Surgery 112:562–572
29. Arthur MJP, Bentley IS, Tanner AR, Kowalski Saunders P, Millward-Sadler GH, Wright R (1985) Oxygen-derived free radicals promote hepatic injury in the rat. Gastroenterology 89:1114–1122
30. Bautista AP, Meszaros K, Bojta J, Spitzer JJ (1990) Superoxide anion generation in the liver during the early stage of endotoxemia in rats. J Leukoc Biol 48:123–128
31. Bautista AP, Spitzer JJ (1992) Platelet activating factor stimulates and primes the liver, Kupffer cells and neutrophils to release superoxide anion. Free Rad Res Comm 17:195–209
32. Billiar TR, Curran RD, Stuehr DJ, West MA, Bentz BG, Simmons RL (1989) An L-arginine-dependant mechanism mediates Kupffer cell inhibition of hepatocyte protein synthesis in vitro. J Exp Med 169:1467–1472
33. Curran RD, Billiar TR, Stuehr DJ, Hofmann K, Simmons RL (1989) Hepatocytes produce nitrogen oxides from L-arginine in response to inflammatory products from Kupffer cells. J Exp Med 170:1769–1774
34. Granger DL, Hibbs JB, Perfect JR, Durack DT (1990) Metabolic fate of L-arginine in relation to microbiostatic capability of murine macrophages. J Clin Invest 85:264–273
35. Hibbs JB Jr, Taintor RR, Vavrin Z (1987) L-Arginine is required for expression in the activated macrophage effector mechanism causing selective metabolic inhibition in target cells. Science 235:473–476
36. Stadler J, Curran RD, Ochoa JB et al. (1991) Effect of endogenous nitric oxide on mitochondrial respiration of rat hepatocytes in vitro and in vivo. Arch Surg 126:186–191

37. Harbrecht BG, Billiar TR, Stadler J et al. (1992) Nitric oxide synthesis serves to reduce hepatic damage during acute murine endotoxemia. Crit Care Med 20:1568–1574
38. Harbrecht BG, Billiar TR, Stadler J et al. (1992) Inhibition of nitric oxide synthesis during endotoxemia promotes intrahepatic thrombosis and an oxygen radical-mediated hepatic injury. J Leukoc Biol 52:39–44
39. Gryglewski RJ, Palmer RMJ, Moncada S (1986) Superoxide anion is involved in the breakdown of endothelium-derived vascular relaxing factor. Nature 320:454–456
40. Kilbourn RG, Jubran A, Gross SS et al. (1991) Endotoxin-mediated shock by N^G-methyl-L-arginine, an inhibitor of nitric oxide synthesis. Biochem Biophys Res Commun 172:1132–1138
41. Petros A, Bennett D, Vallance P (1991) Effect of nitric oxide synthase inhibitor on hypotension in patients with septic shock. Lancet 338:1557–1558
42. Ganter U, Arcone R, Toniatti C, Morrone G, Ciliberto G (1989) Dual control of C-reactive protein gene expression by IL-1 and IL-6. EMBO J 8:3773–3779
43. Li S, Liu T, Goldman N (1990) Cis-acting elements responsible for IL-6 inducible C-reactive protein gene expression. J Biol Chem 265:4136–4142
44. Steel D, Whitehead A (1991) Heterogenous modulation of acute-phase-reactant mRNA levels by interleukin-1β and interleukin-6 in the human hepatoma cell line PLC/PRF/5. Biochem J 277:477–482
45. Prowse KR, Baumann H (1989) Interleukin-1 and interleukin-6 stimulate acute phase protein production in primary mouse hepatocytes. J Leukoc Biol 45:66–71
46. Perlmutter DH, Dinarello CA, Punsal PI, Colten HR (1986) Cachectin/tumor necrosis factor regulates hepatic acute-phase expression. J Clin Invest 78:1349–1354
47. Koj A (1989) The role of interleukin-6 as the hepatocyte stimulating factor in the network of inflammatory cytokines. Ann NY Acad Sci 557:1–8
48. Mortensen RF, Shapiro J, Lin BF et al. (1988) Interaction of recombinant Il-1 and recombinant tumor necrosis factor in the induction of mouse acute phase proteins. J Immunol 140:2260–2266
49. Vannice JL, Ringold GM, McLean JW et al. (1983) Induction of the acute-phase reactant, α1-acid glycoprotein, by glucocorticoids in rat hepatoma cells. DNA 2:205–212
50. Baumann H, Richards C, Gauldie J (1987) Interaction among hepatocyte-stimulating factors, interleukin-1 and glucocorticoids for regulation of acute phase protein in human hepatoma (Hep G2) cells. J Immunol 139:4122–4128
51. Castell JV, Andus T, Kunz D, Heinrich PC (1989) Interleukin-6: the major regulator of acute phase protein synthesis in man and rat. Ann NY Acad Sci 557:87–101
52. Callery MP, Kamei T, Flye MW (1992) Endotoxin stimulates interleukin-6 production by human Kupffer cells. Circ Shock 37:185–188
53. Bibby DC, Grimble RF (1989) Temperature and metabolic changes in rats after various doses of tumour necrosis factor α. J Physiol (Lond) 410:367–380
54. Romanosky AJ, Bagby GJ, Bockman EL et al. (1980) Increased muscle glucose uptake and lactate release after endotoxin administration. Am J Physiol 239:E311–E316
55. Aikawa T, Matsutaka H, Yamamoto H et al. (1973) Gluconeogenesis and amino acid metabolism. II. Interorganal relations and roles of glutamine and alanine in the amino acid metabolism of fasted rats. J Biochem 74:1003–1017
56. Curnow RT, Rayfield EJ, George DT et al. (1976) Altered hepatic glycogen and glucoregulatory hormones during sepsis. Am J Physiol 230:1296–1301
57. Filkins JP, Cornell RP (1974) Depression of hepatic gluconeogenesis and the hypoglycemia of shock. Am J Physiol 227:778–781
58. Souba WW, Smith RJ, Wilmore DW (1985) Glutamine metabolism by the intestinal tract. JPEN 9:608–616
59. Austgen TR, Chen MK, Flynn TC, Souba WW (1991) The effects of endotoxin on the splanchnic metabolism of glutamine and related substrates. J Trauma 31:742–752
60. Argilés JM, Lopez-Soriano FJ, Wiggins D, Williamson DH (1989) Comparative effects of tumour necrosis factor-α (cachectin), interleukin-1-beta and tumour growth on amino acid metabolism in the rat in vivo: absorption and tissue uptake of α-amino[1-14C]isobutyrate. Biochem J 261:357–362

61. Roh MS, Moldawer LL, Ekman LG et al. (1986) Stimulatory effect of interleukin-1 upon hepatic metabolism. Metabolism 35:419–424
62. Bereta J, Kurdowska A, Koj A et al. (1989) Different preparations of natural and recombinant human interleukin-6 (IFN-β2, BSF-2) similarly stimulate acute phase protein synthesis and uptake of α-aminoisobutyric acid by cultured rat hepatocytes. Int J Biochem 21:361–366
63. Van Leeuwen PAM, Hong RW, Rounds JD, Rodrick ML, Wilmore DW (1991) Hepatic failure and coma after liver resection is reversed by manipulation of gut contents: the role of endotoxin. Surgery 110:169–175
64. Straatsburg IH, Boermeester MA, Houdijk APJ et al. Endotoxin- and cytokine-mediated effects on liver cell proliferation and lipid metabolism after partial hepatectomy. A study with recombinant N-terminal bactericidal/permeability-increasing protein and interleukin-1 receptor antagonist. Accepted in: J Pathol on 12 sept. '95
65. McKechnie K, Furman BL, Parratt JR (1986) Modification by oxygen free radical scavengers of the metabolic and cardiovascular effects of endotoxin infusion in conscious rate. Circ Shock 19:429–439
66. Sumida S, Yagi H (1981) Experimental study on the inhibition of kinin release in endotoxin shock by GSH, proteinase inhibitors, hydrocortisone, and hyperbaric oxygen. Jpn Circ J 45:1364–1368
67. Broner CW, Shenep JL, Stidham GL, Stokes DC, Hildner WK (1988) Effect of scavengers of oxygen derived free radicals on mortality in endotoxin challenged mice. Crit Care Med 16:848–851
68. Sugino K, Kiyohiko D, Yamada K, Kawasaki T (1989) Changes in the levels of endogenous antioxidants in the liver of mice with experimental endotoxemia and the protective effects of the antioxidants. Surgery 105:200–206
69. Souba WW, Herskowitz K, Austgen TR, Chen MK, Salloum RM (1990) Glutamine nutrition: theoretical considerations and therapeutic impact. JPEN 14:S237–S243
70. Hong RW, Rounds JD, Helton WS, Robinson MK, Wilmore DW (1992) Glutamine preserves liver glutathione after lethal hepatic injury. Ann Surg 215:114–119
71. Houdijk APJ, Van Leeuwen PAM, Boermeester MA et al. (1994) Glutamine-enriched enteral diet increases splanchnic blood flow in the rat. Am J Physiol 1994:267; G1035–1040

The Role of the Pancreas in the Induction of the Acute Catabolic State

B. Vonen

The pancreas is a supplier of enzymes and hormones that are essential for the utilization of nutrients.

Endocrine Pancreas

Insulin is the most important pancreatic hormone. Its actions have an anabolic end point and in clinical terms it is the most essential anabolic hormone. During acute stress, the sympathetic alpha receptor-mediated inhibition of insulin secretion [1], together with the influence of circulating catecholamines and the general circulatory instability, might be responsible for an initial reduction of plasma insulin in the hyperacute ebb phase that has occasionally been reported [2]. This early low plasma insulin is only demonstrated in the most dramatic clinical settings with an immediate need for resuscitation with fluids, oxygen, and other stabilizing therapy. However, a stable insulin level has also been reported in several low-flow states including cardiodepressive, hemorrhagic, and endotoxin-induced shock [3–5]. Thus most surgical procedures and other physical trauma leading to acute catabolic states are not associated with an initial lowering of plasma insulin levels [6]. Later in the hypermetabolic flow phase, plasma insulin levels rise [6], in part as a response both to an increased glucose and insulin resistance in peripheral tissues.

Somatostatin generally inhibits biological processes. The precise role of pancreatic somatostatin is unclear. Circulating somatostatin originates from several sources, and the pancreas represents only a minor source, even after strong selective stimulation of the delta cells [7]. It seems that the physiological effects of pancreatic somatostatin are mainly within the gland, where it might participate in modulating the secretion of insulin and glucagon. The delta cells are located downstream from the beta and alpha cells [8]; thus somatostatin cannot exert an effect on insulin or glucagon secretion through a vascular route. A paracrine somatostatin effect is, however, feasible, but current evidence for such an effect is only indirect [6, 9–11]. The final role for pancreatic somatostatin remains to be elucidated, but it is most likely not an important peripheral effector substance in the responses following acute critical illness.

Plasma levels of pancreatic polypeptide (PP) are reported to rise five- to tenfold during initial phases of shock [3–5]. The role of PP in this situation has not yet been elucidated. PP is not reported to have profound effects on the metabolism of fuels and most likely it does not play a significant role in the initiation or maintenance of the acute catabolic state.

The major source of "true" glucagon in adult humans is the pancreatic islet alpha cell. Physiological glucagon effects usually oppose those of insulin, and glucagon has classically been considered as a catabolic hormone [12]. The molar ratio of insulin to glucagon has classically been used to determine whether a metabolic setting is mainly anabolic or catabolic. Glucagon effects include degrading glycogen deposits, mobilizing ketones, and directing essential fuels to vital organs. Elevated glucagon levels are observed during the ebb phase, and physiological glucagon effects are considered to contribute to the development of the acute catabolic state [13]. The catabolic effects of increased plasma levels of glucagon alone are minor, and it has been demonstrated that a synergism exists between several counterregulatory stress hormones (hydrocortisone, glucagon, and epinephrine). This synergism seems in part to be responsible for the more profound metabolic responses to acute injury [14]. Infusion of such triple-hormone combinations have, however, failed to produce a considerable net degradation of skeletal muscle, which is one hallmark of a profound catabolic state [14]. Such breakdown of skeletal muscle is seen only when the triple therapy is supplemented with octreotide infusion to radically lower plasma insulin levels [15]. This experimental model was designed to mimic the actual ebb phase in unstable patients in whom the initial insulin values had been reported to be lower than those normally reported [2]. However, most patients do not pass through a period of low plasma insulin before entering the more prolonged hypermetabolic flow phase, and this experimental model might be relevant only for a select group of patients entering an acute catabolic state.

The combination of cortisone and epinephrine [14] has been proposed as the main effector of the increased metabolic rate, whereas cortisol alone is claimed to be responsible for the hormone-mediated nitrogen loss [16]. These hormones do not only induce catabolic effects; epinephrine facilitates muscular amino acid uptake [17]. The complete role of glucagon in this context has not been finally determined. The effects on fuel mobilization have been well documented, and Vilstrup and coworkers have suggested that increased glucagon levels enhance hepatic efficacy for urea production by facilitating the hepatic amino acid turnover [18]. On the other hand, glucagon has a dose-dependent stimulatory effect on insulin secretion [19, 20] even at an infusion concentration close to basal systemic levels of glucagon [21]. This effect obviously counteracts the inhibitory effects from the sympathetic nervous system and the circulating inhibitory hormones. The net glucagon effect might thus be not only to facilitate circulating fuels from body deposits, but also to facilitate insulin secretion in clinical situations with an increased demand for this hormone. This corresponds well with the result of Pipeleers et al., who demonstrated that a functional cooperation between islet cells is a prerequisite for adequate insulin secretion. They suggest that glucagon, in addition to mobilizing fuel from internal stores, has an important role in facilitating glucose-induced insulin secretion, thereby stimulating an anabolic process [22]. The reduction of plasma glucagon eventually seen in the hypermetabolic flow phase corresponds well with the concomitant increase in plasma insulin seen in this phase. It has been well documented that insulin both suppresses basal pancreatic glucagon secretion [23, 24] and inhibits arginine-induced glucagon secretion [11].

Exocrine Pancreas

Impaired exocrine secretion or leakage of activated exocrine enzymes from the ductal system might be possible initiators of an acute catabolic situation. Long-standing malnutrition leads to atrophy of acinar tissue, regional vacuolization, loss of exocrine tissue architecture, and a reduction in protein output [25]. This natural-ly leads to a catabolic state, but without the dramatic ebb phase and a hardly man-ifest hypermetabolic phase. Stress effects on exocrine pancreatic secretion have not been well characterized. An experimental in vivo model using acoustic and physi-cal restraint stress in dogs has revealed that pancreatic exocrine secretion diminish-es during stress [26]. The clinical effect is moderate, and this reduction in exocrine pancreatic secretions can parallel a fasting situation.

The dramatic metabolic and circulatory effects of fulminate acute pancreatitis are initiated following leakage of activated digestive enzymes from the exocrine ductal system into the circulation and the interstitium of the pancreas and later also into the abdominal cavity. The activated digestive enzymes trigger all lines of body defense mechanisms and can as such initiate the ebb phase in a most dra-matic manner. These enzymes are, however, not catabolic in their biological ef-fects, and they are only relevant in terms of initiating a dramatic clinical situation. Low-flow states such as septic, circulatory, and cardiogenic shock are reported to initiate acute pancreatitis [27]. Morphological changes following shock include indentation of the perinuclear membrane, marked intracellular edema, dilatation of the endoplasmic reticulum, and breaks in the plasma membrane [28]. In a study of peritonitis-induced shock, membrane-bound vacuoles were observed [29]. These vacuoles contained digested intracellular material and were thus auto-phagic, indicating that autodigestion can be initiated by shock. When the pancr-eatitis becomes manifest, the process will of course contribute to the ebb phase characteristics.

References

1. Woods SC, Porte D Jr (1974) Neural control of the endocrine pancreas. Physiol Rev 54:596 619
2. Allison SP, Hinton P, Chamberlain MJ (1968) Intravenous glucose-tolerance, insulin, and free fatty acid levels in burned patients. Lancet 2:1113–1116
3. Revhaug A, Lygren I, Lundgren TI et al. (1985) Release of gastrointestinal hormones in cardiodepressive shock. Acta Anaesthesiol Scand 29:371–374
4. Revhaug A, Jenssen TG, Røkke O, Jorde R, Burhol PG, Giercksky KE (1985) Gastrointestinal peptide responses to severe upper gastrointestinal haemorrhage. Gastrointestinal peptides in low flow states. PhD Thesis, University of Tromsø, Tromsø
5. Revhaug A, Jenssen TG, Røkke O, Jorde R, Burhol PG, Giercksky KE (1985) Changes in plas-ma levels of gastrointestinal regulatory peptides during haemorrhage shock in pigs. Gastroin-testinal peptides in low flow states. PhD Thesis, University of Tromsø, Tromsø

6. Black PR, Brooks DC, Bessey PQ et al. (1982) Mechanisms of insulin resistance following injury. Ann Surg 196:420
7. Taborsky GJ Jr (1983) Evidence of a paracrine role for pancreatic somatostatin in vivo. Am J Physiol 245:E595–E603
8. Samols E, Stagner JI, Ewart RBL, Marks V (1988) The order of islet microvascular cellular perfusion is B-A-D in perfused rat pancreas. J Clin Invest 82:350–353
9. Itoh M, Mandarino L, Gerich JE (1980) Antisomatostatin gamma globulin augments secretion of both insulin and glucagon in vitro. Evidence for a physiologic role for endogenous somatostatin in the regulation of pancreatic A- and B-cell function. Diabetes 29:693–696
10. Taniguchi H, Utsumi M, Hasegawa M (1977) Physiologic role of somatostatin. Insulin release from rat islets treated by somatostatin antiserum. Diabetes 26:700–702
11. Vonen B, Florholmen J, Malm D, Torjesen PA, Burhol PG (1991) Glucagon mediates arginine induced somatostatin secretion from isolated rat pancreatic islets. Scand J Clin Lab Invest 52:107–112
12. Unger RH, Orci L (1976) Physiology and pathophysiology of glucagon. Phys Rev 56:778–826
13. Wilmore DW, Moylan JA, Pruitt BA, Lindsey CA, Faloona GR, Unger RH (1974) Hyperglucagonæmia after burns. Lancet 19:73–75
14. Bessey PQ, Watters JM, Aoki TT, Wilmore DW (1984) Combined hormonal infusion stimulates the metabolic response to injury. Ann Surg 200:264–280
15. Bessey PQ, Lowe KA (1993) Early hormonal changes affect the catabolic response to trauma. Ann Surg 218:476–491
16. Gelfand RA, Matthews DW, Bier DM, Sherwin RS (1983) Is the catabolic response to major stress mediated by counter-regulatory hormones? Clin Res 31:241A
17. Shamoon HM, Hendler R, Sherwin RS (1981) Synergistic interactions among anti-insulin hormones in the pathogenesis of stress hyperglycemia in humans. J Clin Endocrinol Metab 52:1235–1241
18. Vilstrup H, Hansen BA, Aldal T (1988) Glucagon enhances hepatic efficacy for urea production. Clin Nutr 7 (suppl):35
19. Weir GC, Samols E, Ramseur R, Day JA, Patel YC (1977) Influence of glucose and glucagon upon somatostatin secretion from the isolated perfused canine pancreas. Clin Res 25:403A
20. Weir GC, Samols E, Day JA, Patel YC (1978) Glucose and glucagon stimulate the secretion of somatostatin from the perfused canine pancreas. Metabolism 27 [Suppl 1]:1223–1226
21. Kawai K, Rouiller D (1981) Evidence that the islet interstitium contains functionally separate "arterial" and "venous" compartments. Diabetes 30 (Suppl 1):14A
22. Pipeleers D, int'Veld PI, Maes E, Van de Winkel M (1982) Glucose-induced insulin release depends on functional co-operation between islet cells. Proc Natl Acad Sci USA 79:7322–7325
23. Samos E, Tyler J, Marks V, Mialhe P (1969) The physiologic role of glucagon in different species. In: Gual C, Ebling FJG (eds) Progress in endocrinology. Excerpta Medica, Amsterdam, pp 206–219
24. Maruyama H, Hisatomi L, Orci L, Grodsky GM, Unger RH (1984) Insulin within islets is a physiologic glucagon release inhibitor. J Clin Invest 74:2296–2299
25. Geldof AA, Becking JL, de Vries CD, van der Veen EA (1992) Histopathological changes in rat pancreas after fasting and cassava feeding. In Vivo 6:545–551
26. Lenz HJ, Messmer B, Zimmerman FG (1992) Noradrenergic inhibition of canine gallbladder concentration and murine pancreatic secretion during stress by corticotropin-releasing factor. J Clin Invest 89:437–443
27. Florholmen J (1985) A study on human and porcine cationic trypsin-like immunoreactivity. Thesis, University of Tromsø, Tromsø
28. Florholmen J, Lindal S, Røkke O, Olsen R, Burhol PG, Revhaug A (1988) Effects of endotoxin on the pancreatic ultrastructure. APMIS 96:991–996
29. Florholmen J, Riepl R, Almdahl SM et al. (1987) Impact of experimental endogenous gram-negative peritonitis on the pancreas of the rat as evaluated by cationic trypsin-like immunoreactivity in peritoneal fluid and serum and by electron microscopy of pancreatic tissue. Scand J Gastroenterol 22:313–320

The Lungs and the Catabolic State

J. Kjæve

Introduction

Infection, trauma, and surgery induce a catabolic state characterized by hypermetabolism. This catabolic state usually resolves spontaneously after minor insults to the organism such as elective surgery. However, in sepsis, multiple trauma, and major surgery hypermetabolism may persist and organ failure develop. The sequential failure of lungs, liver, and kidneys has been recognized for many years as a potential sequela of ruptured aneurysm, acute pancreatitis, septic shock, and surgical complications, as well as burns and other trauma. Acute lung injury is the earliest and most frequent organ complication in prolonged catabolic states. Injurious agents such as endotoxin and fibrin split products have been suggested as mediators of acute lung injury. In experimental studies it has been found that a large number of agents may cause lung injury. The bulk of these studies have focused on damage to the pulmonary vascular endothelium. Less attention has been paid to the metabolic function of the lungs with respect to energy utilization as well as specific metabolic functions. This review is concerned with: (1) metabolic changes in the lungs with respect to injurious agents released in sepsis, and following multiple trauma and major surgery; (2) interorgan metabolism in catabolic states with respect to the lungs.

The Catabolic State

The response to major injury, operations, and sepsis is characterized by increased metabolic activity. There is a shift to fatty acid oxidation for energy requirements. Gluconeogenesis increases in the liver. Amino acids from breakdown of proteins in skeletal muscle are main substrates for gluconeogenesis in the catabolic state. Whereas alanine is the main gluconeogenetic amino acid, glutamine serves as substrate for energy utilization in replicating tissue such as intestinal tract and the lymphoid tissue.

Hormones such as insulin, corticosteroids, catecholamines, and glucagon play important roles in the metabolic responses to stress. There is increasing evidence that cytokines such as tumor necrosis factor (TNF) and interleukins, and arachidonic acid metabolites may modify the metabolic response to stress as well.

The Lungs and the Catabolic State

When considered in the context of the whole human organism, the lungs have one function, the transfer of oxygen from the environment to the blood and carbon dioxide from the blood to the environment. Following laparotomy, reduced functional residual capacity (FRC) and stagnant secretions may lead to atelectasis and infections in the lungs with arterial hypoxemia [1]. These changes in lung function usually resolve spontaneously in uncomplicated elective surgery. However, sepsis, major injuries, and major operations may lead to acute lung injury characterized by: (1) severe arterial hypoxemia, (2) increased intrapulmonary shunting, (3) decreased lung compliance, and (4) decreased lung volumes. The major pathophysiologic finding in acute lung injury is damage to the pulmonary vascular endothelium, which causes permeability edema and loss of vasomotor control. The alterations in pulmonary vascular smooth muscle control favor exaggerated pulmonary vasoconstriction [2]. Additionally, hypoxic pulmonary vasoconstriction (HPV) and other mechanisms aiming at diverting blood away from poorly ventilated areas of the lungs are modified, leading to increased ventilation/perfusion mismatching [2].

Metabolic Properties of the Lungs

Nonrespiratory functions of the lungs include handling of vasoactive substances and possibly the net uptake/release of substrates such as amino acids. Taking into account that the lungs receive the entire cardiac output, any altered metabolic function of the lungs in acute lung injury may have systemic effects on vascular resistance and interorgan metabolism. With respect to gas exchange, lung metabolism, including energy utilization, is of importance for the function of the pulmonary vascular endothelium, the alveolar lining cells, and regulation of vascular tone.

In order to achieve gas exchange, the blood is spread out in a very thin film over the pulmonary capillary surface and is separated from the air by a structure consisting of a thin alveolar epithelium, some basement membrane, and another thin, vascular endothelium. The pulmonary vascular endothelium is continuous and offers a total surface area of about 70 m^2. Thus the structure maximizing gas exchange between blood and air also maximizes contact between the blood and the largest endothelial cell surface in the body. The cells covering the alveolar space and the vessel walls are the most prominent cells in the lungs with respect to function and quantity. The pulmonary endothelial cells and the alveolar type II cells are 45% and 16%, respectively, of the cellular population in the lungs [3].

Energy Utilization

The oxygen uptake in the lungs is low and comparable to that of the intestine and resting skeletal muscle [4]. The main substrate for energy utilization is fatty acids, and the rates of uptake and oxidation of fatty acids by the lungs are high compared with those in other tissues [5]. The lungs do not have a significant capacity to store glucose as glycogen or lipid, unlike the liver and adipose tissue [6]. The lungs most resemble skeletal muscle in that lactate is a major product of glucose metabolism. However, in contrast to muscle, which relies on glycolysis as an important energy source during contraction or during hypoxia, the lungs derive little energy from this pathway under aerobic or anaerobic conditions [6]. This suggests that glycolysis in the lungs is not regulated by energy need and that perhaps glycolysis serves other biochemical functions. This does not exclude the possibility that some lung cells such as alveolar type I cells with only a small number of mitochondria, are dependent upon glycolysis for energy production. Animals studies suggest that the lungs lack enzymes necessary for using keton bodies as fuel [7]. Glutamine may be an important fuel for endothelial cells and alveolar type II cells [7].

Glucose Metabolism

The role of glucose metabolism in the lungs is controversial. Glucose is of minor importance for energy utilization, and isolated lungs may be perfused for 2 h without glucose before edema develops. On the other hand, addition of glucose to the preservation fluid during lung transplantation has been reported to be beneficial [8].

Glucose enters lung cells via active cotransport with sodium or facilitated diffusion [9]: this is the rate-limiting step for glucose utilization in the lungs. Insulin is probably of minor importance in the regulation of glucose uptake in the lungs, but insulin has been reported to enhance glucose uptake in hypoglycemia [10]. Probably, the relationship between concentrations of glucose and fatty acids in the blood is the major determinant of glucose uptake in the lungs. This suggests that the fluctuations in glucose and fatty acids plasma levels seen with catabolic states influence glucose metabolism in the lungs.

The major fate of utilized glucose in the lungs is glycolytic conversion to lactate, which probably accounts for 75% of the glucose consumed [6]. Conversion of glucose into amino acids accounts for 10% of the utilized glucose [6]. Incorporation into lipids occurs to a lesser degree and represents mostly α-glycerophosphate in phospholipids [6]. However, taking into account that phospholipids are the main component of alveolar surfactant and that glucose is the main source of α-glycerophosphate in the lungs, this may be an important function of glucose. The activity of the pentose cycle in the lungs is reportedly high and accounts for 5%–10% of the glucose consumed [10].

The glycolytic pathway to lactate is of interest since the lungs are one of the most aerobic organs in the body. Since this pathway is of minor importance for energy production in the lungs, it must serve other important functions. Being located in the cytoplasma, it has been suggested that glycolysis provides adenosine triphosphate (ATP) for membrane functions such as the ATP-denpendent K+ channels [10]. This implicates a role for glucose in the regulation of vascular tone. Experimentally, hyperglycemia has been shown to hamper HPV [11]. There is evidence that altered cytoplasmatic ATP concentrations induced by changes in glycolytic activity may mediate these effects by activating or inactivating K+ channels. The clinical implication of this hypothesis is that altered levels of glucose and fatty acids in catabolic states may modify pulmonary vascular tone.

Toxic oxygen metabolites derived from activated leukocytes in sepsis and major trauma may cause injury to the microvascular endothelium in lungs. The key enzyme of glycolysis, glyceraldehyde 3-phosphate dehydrogenase, is rapidly inhibited by toxic oxygen metabolites generated by leukocytes [12]. Mitochondrial enzymes of the citric acid cycle are less sensitive to extracellularly generated oxidants [12]. The loss of glycolytic activity in endothelial cells exposed to toxic oxygen metabolites decreases ATP levels intracellularly. Increasing ATP levels by furnishing endothelial cells with glutamine protects the cells and indicates that glycolytic-derived ATP is important for endothelial cell function [12].

The pentose cycle is the main source of reduced nicotinamide-adenine-dinucleotide phosphate (NADPH) in the lungs [13]. Synthesis of phospholipids and possibly other tissue components requires a supply of NADPH. NADPH is also required to maintain the supply of reduced glutathione, which may protect against damage to the lungs by oxidants. The latter function of NADPH has been paid some attention in the context of oxygen toxicity. The pentose cycle activity is high in alveolar type II cells, which synthesize surfactant. Type I alveolar cells, which only serve as lining cells, and endothelial cells seem to have low pentose cycle activity. This is also reflected by glucose-6-phosphate dehydrogenase activity, the key enzyme of the pentose cycle, in these cells. Oxygen toxicity may cause lung injury in critically ill patients depending upon respiratory support and high concentrations of oxygen. The mechanism of lung injury involves generation of toxic oxygen metabolites in the respiratory chain in mitochondria [3]. Alveolar type I cells and endothelial cells have increased susceptibility to the toxic effects of oxygen compared with type II alveolar cells. This may be related to high pentose cycle activity and production of NADPH in alveolar type II cells, and to the fact that high concentrations of oxygen increase activity of the pentose cycle, glucose-6-phosphate dehydrogenase, and concentrations of reduced glutathione in these cells.

Lipid Metabolism

Fatty acids are the major substrate for energy utilization in the lungs. Besides energy utilization, the main fate of fatty acids in the lungs is incorporation into phospholipids of surfactant. It has been estimated that phospholipids constitute 75% of the lipids in the lungs [14]. Surfactants are molecules that preferentially adsorb at a surface and act to lower interfacial tension as a function of their concentration. This property provides the underlying mechanism by which pulmonary surfactant allows for the variation of surface tension during lung expansion and deflation and thereby promotes the alveolar stability, minimal work of breathing, and lung inflation uniformity found during normal respiration in a system dominated by surface tension forces. Surfactant deficiency causes an increase in the surface tension across the blood–gas barrier leading to atelectasis, increased work of breathing, and decreased lung compliance. In addition, surfactant deficiency may promote the formation of pulmonary edema.

The majority of evidence to date indicates that the synthesis of surfactant occurs in the alveolar type II cells [14]. Surfactant secretions may be stimulated by a variety of agents including adrenergic agonists, prostaglandins, and cholinergic agonists. Although alveolar type II cells may tolerate high oxygen tension, surfactant function is impaired in acute lung injuries. The protein rich fluid of permeability edema impairs surfactant function in the lungs [14]. Both synthesis and secretion of surfactant in alveolar type II cells is impaired in acute lung injuries. Recently, it has been suggested that TNF inhibits synthesis of surfactant [15]. The role of surfactant dysfunction in acute lung injury is supported by the reported beneficial effect of surfactant replacement in neonatal respiratory distress syndrome, and some preliminary reports of potential therapeutic effects in patients with acute respiratory distress syndrome (ARDS) [14].

Amino Acid Metabolism

Although skeletal muscle is generally regarded as the primary producer of glutamine and alanine in normal and catabolic states, it has recently been suggested that the lungs may play a key role in the interorgan metabolism of glutamine. For example, in the postabsorptive rat, the lungs appear to release as much glutamine as skeletal muscle does [16]. Although the arteriovenous concentration difference of glutamin across the skeletal muscle is greater than the right ventricular-systemic arterial concentration difference, rat lung glutamine release is similar to the glutamine release in skeletal muscle because of the high flow of blood through the lungs. In septic patients without any signs of ARDS, there was reportedly a net release from the lungs of both alanine and glutamine [17]. This was not the case on postoperative day one in elective general surgical patients. However, in patients undergoing open heart surgery with cardiopulmonary bypass, the lungs exhibited net release of glutamine and alanine on postoperative day one [18]. When the pulmonary vascular endothelium is injured in rats, for example by endotoxin, TNF or interleukins, the concentration of glutamine flowing into the lungs (right ventricle) equals that flowing out of them (aorta), creating a net glutamine balance, within 12 h [19]. This is in accordance with a lack of net glutamine release in septic patients with concomitant ARDS [17].

Glutamine is the most abundant amino acid in blood and in the free amino acid pool in the body. It has multiple functions, one of the most important of which is as a vehicle for the transport of circulating nitrogen between tissues. In addition, glutamine is an essential precursor for nucleotide biosynthesis in all cells and a principal fuel for replicating cells such as small intestinal epithelial cells, fibroblasts, and cells in lymphoid tissue. Although the lung cells responsible for the uptake and release of glutamine have not been identified, it has been suggested that the vascular endothelial cells and the alveolar type II cells are most important. The specific transport system for glutamine in pulmonary endothelial cells and alveolar type II cells has been well-characterized [20]. The transport system is stimulated by agents known to mediate lung injury such as endotoxin, TNF, and interleukins [19]. This suggests that glutamine requirements may be increased during endotoxemia, and that the increase in glutamine transport may be an adoptive response designed to support maintenance of cell structure and function. The key enzymes of glutamine metabolism are glutaminase for energy utilization and glutamine synthetase for de novo synthesis of glutamine. The activity of glutaminase in pulmonary endothelial cells is 20-fold higher than that in lymphocytes, which is considered to possess a high activity of glutaminase [21]. This finding suggests that endothelial cells have a markedly high capacity for glutamine utilization. On the other hand, the activity of glutamine synthetase in endothelial cells is 16 times higher than the activity estimated in skeletal muscle [22]. The skeletal muscle is the principle site of free intracellular glutamine. The ability of the lungs to export large amounts of gluta-mine is, therefore, most likely secondary to accelerated de novo intracellular synthesis of glutamine rather than release of already existing intracellular stores.

Glucocorticoids cause a marked release of glutamine and alanine from the lungs, probably by stimulating glutamine synthetase activity [23]. It has, therefore, been suggested that these hormones are key mediators of the release of glutamine and alanine from the lungs in catabolic states.

The pulmonary endothelial cells also play an important role in the metabolism of arginine. Arginine is the exclusive precursor of nitric oxide (NO), a potent vasodilatator synthesized by vascular endothelium. NO production is elevated in sepsis despite decreased circulating arginine levels. This may be explained by the observation in pulmonary endothelial cells that endotoxin stimulates arginine trans-port into the cells, which is in keeping with the effect of endotoxin on glutamine transport [24].

Specific Metabolic Function of Pulmonary Endothelial Cells

In the last 25 years an increasing number of functions of the pulmonary vascular endothelium has been recognized. The endothelial cells have been shown to influence a number of critical functions, including the regulation of pulmonary and systemic vascular tone, hemofluidity, immunologic and inflammatory reactions, angiogenesis, and even vascular remodeling [25–29]. In recent years, it has also been found that the pulmonary vascular endothelium not only has a broad scope of constitutive functions, but is also capable responding to stimuli and injury to express a wide range of inducible functions. These functions alter the properties of the endothelial layer in ways that are relevant to a variety of pulmonary diseases, especially acute lung injury.

Important functional properties of pulmonary endothelial cells include he-mostatic, immunologic, and synthetic functions (especially with respect to synthe-sis of products involved in regulation of vascular tone and intercellular signaling), and their role as a biochemical filter [30].

It is known that the endothelium possesses a sophisticated, complex array of in-teractive factors that allow it to modulate all components of the hemostatic system: the platelet aggregation system, the blood coagulation system, and the fibrinolytic system. Under normal conditions the net effect of these factors is to render the en-dothelium antithrombogenic and anticoagulant. Pulmonary endothelial cells affect platelet function in many ways. One of the more important mechanisms is via the production of prostacyclin (PGI$_2$). PGI$_2$ is an extremely potent inhibitor of platelet aggregation. The release of PGI$_2$ from pulmonary and systemic endothelial cells can be induced by various stimuli including mechanical stimuli, hypoxia, bradykinin, serotonin thrombin, interleukin-1, and adenine nucleotides [2]. Conversely, toxic oxygen metabolites may interfere with the synthesis and release of PGI$_2$ by these cells. NO is another potent inhibitor of platelet aggregation, which has been reported to act synergistically with PGI$_2$ [31].

Aggregating platelets release adenosine diphosphate (ADP) and serotonin, which both produce further platelet aggregation. The pulmonary endothelial cells possess ADPase activity on the plasma membranes [30]. This enzyme converts ADP to adenosine monophosphate (AMP). Serotonin is effectively removed from the pulmonary circulation by a specific transport system in the plasma membrane of endothelial cells [30].

The major physiologic inhibitor of blood coagulation is believed to be antithrombin III that inhibits thrombin. The bulk of evidence suggests that endothelial cells possess heparin-like glycosaminoglycans and sulfated proteoglycans on their surface that promote an anticoagulant role by sequestering thrombin and antithrombin III from the circulation, thereby facilitating their reaction and subsequent thrombin inhibition [32]. Another anticoagulant factor associated with the endothelial cell surface is thrombomodulin, which binds to thrombin and accelerates its activation of protein C, a potent inhibitor of several coagulation factors [33].

Fibrinolysis, the final component of the hemostatic system, is also impacted upon by pulmonary endothelial cells [30]. The major physiologic effector of fibrinolysis is plasmin. Plasminogen, the inactive proenzyme form of plasmin is activated by endothelial cell-derived enzymes.

In catabolic states leading to acute lung injury, the endothelial cells may turn into a procoagulant state. The action of the cytokines TNF and interleukin-1 upon endothelial cells illustrates this. Both favor a state in endothelial cells more conductive to coagulation by: (1) causing the synthesis and expression of thromboplastin on the endothelial cell surface, (2) causing loss of thrombomodulin expression, and (3) inhibiting activation of plasmin [34]. Treatment of endothelial cells with TNF or interleukin-1 also promotes an inflammatory state in endothelial cells by increasing cell surface expression of endothelial cell adhesion molecules for leukocytes, leading to increased leukocyte adhesion [30].

The complex interaction between endothelial cells and cytokines is illustrated by the synthesis of endothelial cells of several cytokines including interleukin-1, granulocyte-macrophage colony-stimulating factor, interleukin-6, and interleukin 8, and chemotactic proteins in response to exogenous interleukin-1 or TNF [30].

A main synthetic property of pulmonary endothelial cells is the production of agents involved in the regulation of vascular tone. Both NO, PGI$_2$ and prostaglandin E$_1$ are potent vasodilators synthesized by endothelial cells. The principal physiologic pulmonary vasoconstrictor is hypoxia. HPV is important in matching ventilation and perfusion, thereby preventing arterial hypoxemia. Although first described nearly 50 years ago, the mechanism of HPV is still unknown. Endothelin-1, which is synthesized by the pulmonary endothelial cells, is the most potent pul-

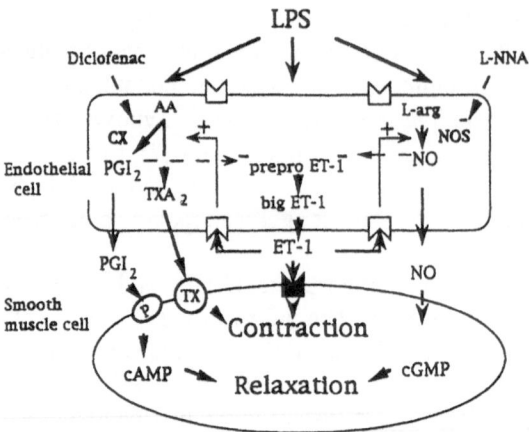

Fig. 1. Hypothetical interactions between endothelial cell derived vasoactive substances during endotoxin *(LPS)* challenge. For detailed explanation, see text. (Reprinted with permission from [35])

monary vasoconstrictor yet discovered [35]. It is present abundantly in human lungs. Probably both NO and endothelin-1 are important regulators of pulmonary vascular tone in physiologic and pathophysiologic conditions. Recently, inhaled NO was shown to reverse HPV in healthy human beings without causing a systemic vasodilation [31]. It has also been reported that NO has reduced pulmonary hypertension in humans with ARDS without any concomitant increased shunting of blood [31]. The pulmonary hypertension and ventilation/perfusion mismatching associated with acute lung injury indicate a dysfunction of vasomotor control. The regulation of vascular tone by endothelial cell products and the interactions between these products are illustrated in Fig. 1. The figure summarizes the complex hypothetical interactions between endothelin-1 (ET-1), endothelium-derived relaxing factor (NO) and arachidonic acid (AA) products from the cyclooxygenase (CX) pathway, prostacyclin (PGI_2) and thromboxane A_2 (TXA_2), during endotoxin lipopolysaccharide (LPS) challenge. LPS is a common stimulator for release of these products. Upon stimulation, ET-1 is synthesized and released mainly abluminally but also into the blood. ET-1 activates the ET_A receptor (filled symbol) on the vascular smooth muscle cells, which leads to contraction. ET-1 can also activate the ET_B receptor (open symbols), on the endothelial cell, which leads to production of NO and PGI_2/TXA_2. NO is produced from L-arginine (L-arg) by NO synthase (NOS), which exists in at least two principal forms: a constitutive Ca^{2+}-dependent NOS, probably regulating basal vascular tone, and an inducible Ca^{2+}-independent NOS which produces large amounts of NO in response to LPS, for example. NO easily diffuses into the vascular smooth muscle cell where it activates guanylate cyclase, which induces an elevation of cGMP, leading to relaxation. NOS is inhibited by N^G-nitro-L-arginine (L-NNA). PGI_2 acting via its receptor (P) elevates cAMP in the smooth muscle cell to induce relaxation, whereas TXA_2, via receptor activation (TX), induces contraction. Diclofenac inhibits the production of PGI_2 and TXA_2. NO and PGI_2 have been suggested to exert inhibitory effects on ET-1

Table 1. Handling of biologically active substances in the pulmonary circulation

---

Substances metabolized by the endothelial cells
  Bradykinin
  Adenine nucleotides
  Angiotensin I
  Serotonin
  Norepinephrine
  Prostaglandins E_2, D_2, F_{2a}
  Endothelin-1
Substances unaffected by transit through the pulmonary vascular bed
  Epinephrine
  Dopamine
  Angiotensin II
  Prostaglandin A_2
  PGI_2

---

synthesis, thereby creating a negative feedback mechanism. The relative distribution of ET_A and ET_B receptors may explain the different response to ET-1 between vascular beds and between species. Also the ET_B receptor mediated stimulation of NO, PGI_2 and/or TXA_2 seems to vary in different vessels and is not fully understood. The interaction described above probably occurs also in other cell types, such as macrophages upon endotoxin challenge.

A final functional metabolic property of lung endothelium is its role as a biochemical filter. Pulmonary endothelial cells metabolize biologically active substances in the circulation either by interiorizing the substance by specific plasma membrane transport processes or by enzymatic activity on the plasma membrane surface (Table 1). This function plays a part in the local regulation of vascular tone because most of the substances are vasoactive. Because the lungs receive nearly the entire cardiac output, the pulmonary endothelium is ideally suited to regulate the downstream concentration of vasoactive substances by means of its biochemical filter function. Impairment of the filter function may lead to altered concentrations of vasoactive substances both in the lungs and systemically. Impaired filter function has been demonstrated in acute lung injuries both experimentally and in humans [30].

Conclusion

Fatty acids are the most important substrate for energy utilization in the lungs. Both glucose and glutamine may have key functions in lung metabolism. Catabolic states have minor influence on energy utilization in the lungs. Sepsis, trauma, and major surgery may cause acute lung injury, which is characterized by damage to the pulmonary vascular endothelium and impaired gas exchange in the lungs. The endothelial cells have metabolic functions which are important for hemostatic functions, inflammatory reactions, and regulation of vascular tone in the pulmonary vascular bed. Noxious agents that are known to be released in catabolic states

154   J. Kjæve

impair these functions of the endothelium, thereby rendering the vascular bed procoagulant and proinflammatory, and causing vasomotoric dysfunction.

References

1. Hedenstierna G (1988) Mechanisms of postoperative pulmonary complications. Acta Chir Scand Suppl 550:152–158
2. McIntyre RC, Harken AH, Fullerton DA (1994) Mechanisms of pulmonary vascular control in normal and injured lungs. Surgery 115:273–275
3. Crapo JD, Barry BE, Foscue AA et al. (1980) Structural and biochemical changes in rat lungs occurring during exposures to lethal and adaptive doses of oxygen. Am Rev Respir Dis 122:123–143
4. Fisher AB (1976) Oxygen and energy utilization. In: Crystal RG (ed) The biochemical basis of pulmonary function. Marcel Dekker, New York, pp 75–104
5. Felts JM (1964) Biochemistry of the lung. Health Phys 10:973–979
6. Tierney DF, Levy SE (1976) Glucose metabolism. In: Crystal RG (ed) The biochemical basis of pulmonary function. Marcel Dekker, New York, pp 105–125
7. Ardawi MS (1991) Metabolism of glucose, glutamine, long chain fatty acids and ketone bodies by lungs of the rat. Biochimie 73(5):557–562
8. Date H, Matsumura A, Manchester JK et al. (1993) Evaluation of lung metabolism during successful twenty-four-hour canine lung preservation. J Thorac Cardiovasc Surg 101:1037–1043
9. Kerr JS, Fisher AB, Kleingeller A (1981) Transport of glucose analogues in rat lung. Am J Physiol 241:E191–E195
10. Wiener CM, Sylvester JT (1993) Effects of insulin, glucose analogues, and pyruvate on vascular responses to anoxia in isolated ferret lungs. J Appl Physiol 74(5):2426–2431
11. Rounds SS, McMarty, Reeves JT (1981) Glucose metabolism accelerates the decline of hypoxic vasoconstriction in rat lungs. Respir Physiol 44:239–249
12. Hinshaw DB, Benger JM (1990) Protective effect of glutamine on endothelial cell ATP in oxidant injury. J Surg Res 49:222–227
13. Bassett DJP, Fisher AB (1976) Pentose cycle activity of the isolated perfused rat lung. Am J Physiol 231:1527–1532
14. Holm BA, Matalon S (1989) Role of pulmonary surfactant in the development and treatment of adult respiratory distress syndrome. Anesth Analg 69:805–818
15. Arias-Diaz J, Vara E, Garcia C, Gomez M, Balibrea IL (1993) Tumor necrosis factor-α inhibits synthesis or surfactant by isolated human type II pneumocytes. Eur J Surg 159:541–549
16. Plumley DA, Austgen TR, Salloum RM et al. (1990) Role of the lungs in maintaining amino acid homeostasis. JPEN 14:569–573
17. Plumley DA, Souba WW, Hantamaki RD et al. (1990) Accelerated lung amino acid release in hyperdynamic septic surgical patients. Arch Surg 125:57–61
18. Herskowitz K, Plumley DA, Martin TD et al. (1991) Lung glutamine flux following open heart surgery. J Surg Res 51:82–86
19. Auslym TR, Chen MK, Salloum RM, Souba WW (1991) Glutamine metabolism by the endotoxin-injured lung. J Trauma 31:1068–1075
20. Herskowitz K, Bode BP, Block ER, Souba WW (1991) Characterization of L-glutamine transport by pulmonary artery endothelial cells. Am J Physiol 260:L241–L246
21. Leighton B, Curi R, Hussein A, Newsholme EM (1987) Maximum activities of some key enzymes of glycolysis, glutaminolysis, Krebs cycle and fatty acid utilization in bovine pulmonary endothelial cells. FEBS Letts 225:93–96
22. Sallek M, Ardawi M (1990) Glutamine-synthesizing activity in lungs of fed, starved, acidotic, diabetic, injured and septic rats. Biochem J 270:829–832
23. Sarantos P, Howard D, Souba WW (1993) Dexamethasone regulates glutamine synthetase expression in rat lung. Metabolism 42:795–800
24. Scott Lind D, Copeland EM, Souba WW (1993) Endotoxin stimulates arginine transport in pulmonary artery endothelial cells. Surgery 114:199–205

25. Ryan US, Ryan JW (1977) Correlations between the fine structure of the alveolar-capillary unit and its metabolic activities. In: Bakkle YS, Vane JR (eds) Metabolic functions of the lung. Marcel Dekker, New York, pp 197–232
26. Ryan US (1982) Structural bases for metabolic activity. Ann Rev Physiol 44:223–239
27. Ryan JW, Ryan US (1977) Pulmonary endothelial cells. Federation Proceedings 36:2683–2691
28. Fanberg BL (1988) Relationship of the pulmonary vascular endothelium to altered pulmonary vascular resistance. Chest 93:101S–105S
29. Ryan US (1987) Endothelial cell activation responses. In: Ryan US (ed) Pulmonary endothelium in health and disease. Marcel Dekker, New York, pp 3–33
30. Block ER (1992) Pulmonary endothelial cell pathobiology: Implications for acute lung injury. Am J Med Sci 304:136–144
31. Persson MG, Wiklund NP, Gustafsson LE (1993) Nitric oxide – more than a vasodilator. Läkartidningen 90:1365–1371
32. Crutchley DJ (1987) Hemostatic properties of the pulmonary endothelium. In: Ryan US (ed) Endothelium in health and disease. Marcel Dekker, New York, pp 237–273
33. Esmar CT, Owen W (1981) Identification of an endothelial cell co-actor for thrombin-catalyzed activation of protein C. Proc Natl Acad Sci USA 78:2249–2252
34. Nawroth PP, Handley DA, Esmar CT, Stern DM (1986) Interleukin-1 induces endothelial cell procoagulant while suppressing cell-surface anticoagulant activity. Proc Natl Acad Sci USA 83:3460–3464
35. Weitzberg E (1993) Circulatory responses to endothelin-1 and nitric oxide. Acta Physiol Scand 148(S611):5–13

Acute Metabolic Response to Skin Injury Following Burn and the Potential Use of Growth Hormone

D. A. Gilpin and D. N. Herndon

Introduction

The acute response to skin injury following burn is characterized by hypermetabolism, increased cardiac output, lipolysis, gluconeogenesis, and proteolysis. This review will describe the early responses to thermal trauma and potential methods for modulating deleterious consequences of these responses.

The Wound: Endocrinological and Physiological Aspects

The skin is a semipermeable barrier preventing water loss as well as contributing to temperature regulation and the prevention of entry of potentially pathological microbes. Severe thermal injury creates irreversible damage to this organ and interferes with all of the above functions, leading to fluid loss and an invitation to bacterial proliferation. Disruption of the vascular endothelium by wounding exposes collagen to blood, a situation which precipitates a cascade of events ultimately leading to clotting, inflammation, and repair. Platelet degranulation, endothelial damage, and leukocytes contribute to a pool of growth factors at a wound site which subsequently regulate enzymatic degradation, phagocytosis, chemotaxis, angiogenesis, and reepithelialization [1–4]. Reepithelialization, i.e., the migration by proliferation of epithelial cells from the wound edges, provides a protective roof over the wound under which repair can proceed away from abrasive forces, dehydration, and the risk of infection.

The wound site contains factors from multiple sources. Mediators produced locally at the wound site spill over into the circulation, where they are carried to distant organs or tissues. These tissues in turn secrete further growth factors which are then disseminated by the circulation of yet other target tissues. Mediators, including cytokines such as interleukin-6 (IL-6), interleukin-1 (IL-1), and tumor necrosis factor (TNF), growth factors, prostaglandins, and thromboxanes A_2 and B_2, all contribute to a chemical maelstrom. The physiological response to trauma and the processes of wound healing and repair are, in fact, intricately controlled and regulated by an interdependent network of chemical messengers [5–8]. Our understanding of these events is still, in many ways, rudimentary; however, with advances in molecular biology and the collaborative efforts of clinicians and scientists, the mechanisms can be described.

Evaporative fluid loss through the burn wound and extensive edema secondary to mediator-induced permeability changes lead to a substantial reduction in circulating blood volume and subsequent hypovolemia [9]. Systemic vasoconstrictors, such as thromboxane A_2 and B_2, catecholamines, and superoxide ions induce systemic vasoconstriction and increase heart rate in an attempt to preserve blood flow and hence oxygen delivery. Decreased renal perfusion along with circulating cellular debris, such as myoglobin released from damaged muscle, can precipitate oliguria and acute renal failure. Hypovolemia, in combination with gastrointestinal vasoconstriction, damages the normal mucosal barrier of the bowel, allowing bacteria and their toxic products to translocate into the lymphatic and circulatory systems, through which they become systemically disseminated.

Inhalation of hot poisonous gases induces an inflammatory response in distal airways, leading to excessive mucus secretion and damage to the columnar ciliated epithelium which lines the airways. Cellular debris and mucus pass downwards, blocking distal airways and producting air trapping, atelectasis, and an ideal culture medium for bacterial proliferation. Pneumonia, the result of this sequence of events, leads to reduced oxygenation, thereby exacerbating the effects of translocation, hypovolemia, and vasoconstriction.

Aspects of the Response to Trauma

Hypermetabolism: Etiology and Endocrinology

Over 60 years ago, Cuthbertson [10, 11] conducted careful studies on patients with limb fractures and discovered that soon after injury there followed a variable period of relative or absolute anura. This early period, or "ebb phase," preceded a more prolonged "flow phase" associated with increased urinary output, nitrogen loss, and a rise in body temperature and oxygen consumption. Thermally injured patients suffer a particularly severe and extended "flow" or hypermetabolic phase lasting weeks or even months. Massive protein catabolism and lipolysis result in peripheral muscle wasting and a redistribution of subcutaneous fat [7, 8]. The etiology of this condition is complex, and considerable efforts have been made to modulate its more harmful consequences. The initial response, the ebb phase, is focused on maintaining body function by selective preservation of essential organs. A huge increase in the hepatic synthesis of specific plasma proteins, the acute phase response, occurs at the same time as marked hormonal alterations [12]. Immediate endocrine changes during this period include a fall in plasma insulin and a marked increase in plasma catecholamines, cortisol, glucagon, antidiuretic hormone, and aldosterone. Initially, the cumulative effects of these hormones is to produce a decrease in metabolic rate, oxygen consumption, and cardiac output with a concomitant rise in blood levels of glucose, free fatty acids, and lactate. The hypermetabolic phase then follows, lasting weeks or months depending upon the severity of the injury (Fig. 1).

Persistently elevated catecholamine, adrenocorticotrophic hormone (ACTH), and cortisol level results in lipolysis, glycogenolysis, skeletal muscle proteolysis, and gluconeogenesis, culminating in significant hyperglycemia [13, 14]. Cortisol

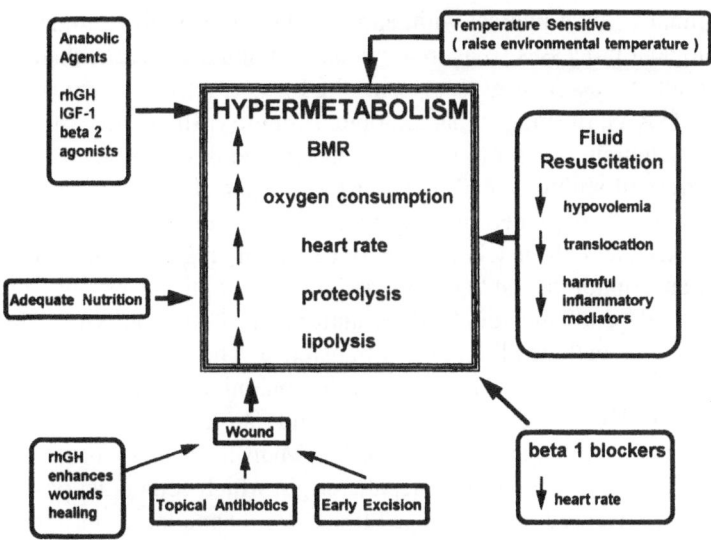

Fig. 1. Increased basal metabolic rate (BMR), oxygen consumption, heart rate, proteolysis, and lipolysis associated with hypermetabolism. Improvements in fluid resuscitation, antibiotic management of the wound, and the use of anabolic agents have helped to reduce the hypermetabolic response. *rhGH*, recombinant human growth hormone; *IGF*, insulin-like growth factor

and the catecholamines stimulate lipolysis directly. Epinephrine further stimulates lipolysis through β-receptor activation of glucagon. At the beginning of the flow phase, hepatic glycogenolysis results in an increase in blood glucose which causes a rise in insulin secretion. Gluconeogenesis of free fatty acids and amino acids further increases blood sugar. In the short term, these events may be viewed as the body attempting to provide fuel and molecular raw materials for tissue repair. The usual balance between the rates of synthesis and degradation for fat, protein, and gluconeogenesis favors degradation. When protracted, severe negative nitrogen loss occurs, along with urinary excretion of sulfur, potassium, and phosphorus [10], with the rise in metabolic rate and associated weight loss being proportional to the severity of injury. Clinical studies show that the metabolic rate rises to a plateau above which further stress precipitates death [13]. Investigations also indicate that a loss of weight equivalent to 20% of the ideal body weight for an individual is associated with a significant increase in mortality [15, 16]. In addition, chronically elevated catecholamine levels can induce pathological conditions such as myocarditis and cardiomyopathy and increase cardiac contractility and rate [13, 17]. Clinicians have therefore attempted to modulate these adverse effects of catecholamine stimulation.

Acute Phase Response

The term "acute phase response" refers to the sequence of early molecular events leading to the production of plasma proteins, cytokines, growth factors, and hormones which interact with, and facilitate, metabolic, immunological, and physiological processes so as to allow an individual to deal with stress regardless of its etiology. α_1-Acid glycoprotein (AGP), C-reactive protein (CRP), serum amyloid A (SAA), fibrinogen, haptoglobin, α_1-antitrypsin, α_2-macroglobulin, albumin, and prealbumin are some of the plasma proteins whose levels are altered following stressful stimuli [18–22]. The genes responsible for these proteins can be either positively regulated, leading to an increase in the synthesis of stable transcribed mRNA and ultimately protein, or negatively regulated, leading to a decrease in the transcription of stable mRNA and ultimately plasma protein levels. Positively regulated genes include AGP, α_1-antitrypsin, CRP, and SAA. Negatively regulated proteins include albumin and transferrin. The very marked and early decrease in plasma albumin levels seen after thermal injury cannot be accounted for purely on the basis of decreased transcription and translation. Losses due to increased vascular permeability are also responsible. Many acute phase proteins (APR) or reactants are protease inhibitors of hepatic origin which counteract potentially harmful proteases released from damaged tissue. For example, α_1-antitrypsin is a protease inhibitor with activity against chymotrypsin, elastase, and collagenase [18–22]. Although locally beneficial for degrading cell debris after injury, these enzymes could cause serious damage to normal cells should they become disseminated by the circulation. Others are antioxidants helping to decrease inflammation. The acute phase response is maximal during the ebb phase of the trauma response and appears to be one mechanism whereby the body attempts to localize damage. The APR are carried in the blood stream to areas of tissue injury, where they can neutralize harmful protease enzymes and superoxide ions. It is possible that within the liver, a decreased synthetic rate of negatively regulated genes "make way" for an increased synthetic rate of positively regulated genes. The huge rise in positively regulated APR should maintain the plasma oncotic pressure, despite the downregulation of albumin; however, the massive increase in vascular permeability and subsequent generalized edema associated with thermal injury prevents this from occurring. Some have suggested that a second tissue insult during the ebb phase, e. g., an additional injury, would overstress a host and lead to death.

Modulation of Hypermetabolism

Catecholamines, Basal Metabolic Rate, and Cardiac Function

The etiology of the rise in core temperature, oxygen consumption, and consequently metabolic rate remains unclear. Studies in thermally injured animals initially supported the view that the increased basal metabolic rate (BMR) of hypermetabolism was an attempt by the body to compensate for evaporative heat loss through the wound [23–27]. Wrapping the animal's wound in occlusive impermeable dressings reduced evaporative water loss and subsequently BMR [23–27]. Unfortunately, a similar approach in a clinical trial failed to support this hypothesis, suggesting that evaporative heat loss may be only one of multiple factors contributing to hypermetabolism. Both animal and clinical studies showed that a reduction in metabolic rate can be achieved by elevating the environmental temperature. The BMR has been shown to be temperature sensitive, but not temperature dependent [13, 23–25].

Since hyperthyroidism also produces weight loss and a rise in BMR, some suggested that changes in thyroid function may be the primary cause of hypermetabolism. Thyroidectomized rodents subjected to thermal injury failed to show any difference in BMR compared to similarly burned euthyroid animals [25]. In addition, clinical evaluation of thyroid function in burned patients indicates thyroid-stimulating hormone and T3/T4 levels to be normal or depressed [7, 8, 13]. Cytokines such as IL-6, IL-1, and TNF, released initially from a burn wound and later from organs such as the liver, were thought to be the mediators of the mysterious "endogenous pyrogen" which induced hypermetabolism. When these compounds were introduced into the hypothalamic area of laboratory animals, a rise in BMR was noted. The blood–brain barrier is thought to be impermeable to certain cytokines, indicating that if this mechanism were true, some form of secondary messenger must be the activator. Further, patients undergoing early burn wound excision, and hence excision of the proposed initial source of systemic cytokines, failed to show any difference in the degree of hypermetabolism compared to those treated by a more conservative approach [28, 29]. Several clinical studies suggested that hypermetabolism was due, at least in part, to the combination of hormones rather than any individual substance [13, 14]. Within the last ten years, it has been shown that an infusion of combined catecholamines into normal subjects can mimic aspects of the hypermetabolic response, therefore confirming clinical suspicions [30]. Prolonged plasma levels of catecholamines cause lipolysis, persistent tachycardia, and systemic vasoconstriction, which in turn lead to increased vascular smooth muscle tone and chronic elevation of blood pressure. These undesirable consequences can be reduced by β-blockade. Clinical trials did indeed show that β-blockade reduced BMR, cardiac rate, and blood pressure [13]. Free fatty acid levels were also diminished, suggesting a decrease in lipolysis. Another study in severely burned pediatric patients demonstrated that peripheral oxygen delivery and cardiac oxygen utilization were unaffected by β-blockade, whereas mean blood pressure, pressure work index, and rate pressure products were all reduced [31, 32]. Animal studies indicate that complete blockade of catecholamines could prevent subjects from responding appropriately to changes in environmental temperature, a potentially hazardous situation [33]. Clinical studies, however, verified that burned pediatric patients were still capable of responding to cold stress [29]. Further, an infusion of isoproterenol, a β-receptor agonist, indicated that β-blockade was incomplete at the dose of propranolol administered, therefore patients could still respond appropriately to catecholamine stimulation [34]. One drawback to the reduction in catecholamine-induced lipolysis was a pradoxical increase in the rate of proteolysis. Lipolysis provides fuel, in the form of free fatty acids, for gluconeogenesis, and therefore a reduction in the fuel supply is compensated for by an enhanced rate of proteolysis. Consequently, selective β_1-blockers, which affect only cardiovascular function and not lipid or protein kinetics, have been used successfully in preliminary clinical trials [35]. Further, β_2-agonists, such as clembuterol, stimulate protein synthesis [36]. Therefore, the combined action of a β_1-blocker along with a β_2-agonist could effectively dampen the deleterious consequences of excessive catechol-amines, while preserving the beneficial effects.

Eicosanoids

Vasoactive inflammatory mediators such as prostaglandins and thromboxanes are also produced in response to trauma. Prostaglandins, thromboxanes, and leu-kotrines belong to the eicosanoid family and share a common precursor, arachidonic acid, a dietary polyunsaturated fatty acid. The prostaglandins and thromboxanes share initial synthetic steps before diverging down different meta-bolic pathways. Prostaglandins, particularly PGE_2, are associated with beneficial effects in burned patients, including the attraction of neutrophils and vasodilatation [37–39]. Vasodilatation replenishes oxygen to previously ischemic or partially damaged tissues close to the burn wound, but it is frequently associated with in-creased vascular permeability and subsequent wound edema. The topical use of the cyclooxygenase inhibitor, ibuprofen, has been shown to reduce wound edema with-out adversely affecting systemic levels of these beneficial prostaglandins [37].

The thromboxanes, particularly thromboxane A_2, largely produce vasoconstric-tive effects, thereby reducing oxygenation and exacerbating tissue injury. Eico-sanoids have been found in burn wound blister fluid, lymphatic fluid, and in plasma [39–43]. Therefore, it has been suggested that circulating thromboxanes contribute to the reduced perfusion through the gastrointestinal vascular bed, lead-ing to gastrointestinal mucosal injury and bacterial translocation.

Attempts at reducing the vasoconstrictive effects of thromboxanes have shown encouraging results. Animal studies suggest that the systemic administration of ibu-profen reduced systemic vasoconstriction which followed pharmacological thermal injury [37]. Unfortunately, many pharmacological agents currently available, in-cluding ibuprofen, indomethacin, and aspirin, act by blockade of cyclooxygenase, an enzyme required for the synthesis of both prostaglandins and thromboxane. Fur-ther, all of these drugs can induce peptic ulceration when given orally over pro-longed periods. Selective thromboxane inhibitors are, at present, not in clinical prac-tice; however, the careful use of cyclooxygenase inhibitors, particularly topically or over short intervals, could limit some of the deleterious effects of eicosanoids.

Growth Hormone: An Agent with Multiple Effects

Although improvements in resuscitation, wound care, sepsis control, and β-block-ade all combine to reduce hypermetabolism, they have only a limited role individ-ually. For over 30 years, growth hormone has been recognized for its anabolic ac-tions. In the early 1960s, growth hormone obtained from postmortem pituitary glands was administered to burned patients and successfully reduced nitrogen loss [44, 45]. These initial studies had relatively small numbers and showed consider-able patient to patient variability. During the 1960s and early 1970s, clinical trials were sporadic due to difficulty in obtaining quantities of sufficiently pure human growth hormone [44–46]. A further setback occurred when some recipients of cadaveric growth hormone acquired Jacob-Creutzfeldt disease. Advances in molecular biology have made recombinant human growth hormone (rhGH) commercially available [47–50]. The earlier findings of growth hormone were confirmed in a variety of situations including healthy volunteers, burn victims, and cancer patients. It was also clearly demonstrated that for rhGH to be maximally effective at reducing or reversing nitrogen loss, adequate nutritional supplementation was required, either parenterally or preferably enterally [51–53].

Two forms of biosynthetic rhGH have been produced, and they differ only in the presence of a methionine molecule on the N-terminal which is absent from the second form [47–50]. They have been called Met rhGH and Met-less rhGH, respectively. The minor difference in sequence is due to a production technique. Met rhGH must be separated from other intracellular proteins, whereas the Met-less rhGH is obtained from a precursor protein secreted from the cell. Clinically, Met rhGH has been shown to be as effective as pituitary growth hormone in enhancing linear growth. So far, side effects from the use of Met rhGH have been minimal, although a few individuals have produced antibodies against the biosynthetic growth hormone [47–50]. Investigations suggest, however, that any antigenicity elicited may be due to minute quantities of bacterial protein remaining within the preparation. Several case reports have suggested a possible link between the administration of rhGH and leukemia. Supportive evidence is lacking and any link is tenuous [50].

Within the past 5 years, a number of detailed clinical trials have examined specific aspects of the use of rhGH in burned patients. One such investigation used a hyperinsulinemic euglycemic clamp in a pediatric population of burned victims and demonstrated that the administration of exogenous rhGH decreased glucose uptake, but did not affect glucose utilization compared to those not receiving rhGH [32, 34, 54, 55]. This study confirmed, therefore, that growth hormone induces insulin resistance. A consequence of insulin resistance is a rise in plasma glucose levels along with insulin itself, as it attempts to promote glucose uptake. The in some patients hyperglycemia resulting from the cumulative effects of cortisol, glucagon, and the catecholamines is therefore exacerbated by exogenous rhGH [14, 32, 33, 56]. Clinically, exogenous insulin is required in order to overcome the resistance and allow the entry of glucose and amino acids into cells [58]. The same study found that catecholamines and glucagon levels were also elevated in patients receiving rhGH compared to controls. It is possible that growth hormone is responsible directly for this or, alternatively, indirectly due to the increased insulin level stimulating catecholamine and glucagon release.

Insulin is well recognized as an anabolic hormone, and the use of this agent to control blood sugar may have an additive anabolic effect when given along with rhGH. To address this question, an investigation using a hyperinsulinemic euglycemic clamp measured the effects of insulin alone and in combination with rhGH on protein kinetics. The results showed that insulin along with rhGH was no more effective than insulin alone [54, 55]. This indicated that the addition of insulin would not increase further the anabolism produced by rhGH alone. In addition, the use of exogenous insulin required to control rhGH-induced hyperglycemia would not enhance the effectiveness of rhGH.

Growth hormone stimulates production of insulin-like growth factor I (IGF I), a somatomedin which is synthesized principally in the liver and known to have anabolic effects. Thermally injured rats showed a significant decrease in plasma IGF I levels 14 days after injury compared to unburned controls [60, 61]. When exogenous IGF I was administered to thermally injured animals, oxygen consumption was decreased and body weight was maintained or increased relative to untreated controls. Clinical studies show that the administration of exogenous rhGH is followed by an increase in plasma IGF I levels, and some suggest that the beneficial effects obtained with rhGH are in fact due to growth hormone inducing hepatic synthesis of IGF I [62, 63]. The synergistic action of rhGH, glucagon, insulin, IGF I, and the catecholamines seems more likely. Cell surface growth hormone and IGF I receptors are present in the liver and on various other cell types, including lymphocytes and fibroblasts, and it is possible that exogenous rhGH may have an autocrine and paracrine influence on these and other cells [64, 65]. IGF I produces hypoglycemia by some as yet unknown mechanism. Clinicians have suggested that a combined IGF I/rhGH regimen could counterbalance the deleterious effects on glucose kinetics of each agent given by itself. Recent clinical trials in normal subjects confirmed this hypothesis, indicating that IGF I and rhGH together produced a greater anabolic effect than IGF I alone. The results show that the synergistic effect is due to IGF I reducing the rate of protein degradation, whereas rhGH increases the rate of protein synthesis.

In addition to systemic anabolic effects, GH also influences collagen synthesis. Acromegalics have thick, tough skin due to extra collagen deposition, in contrast to individuals with growth hormone deficiency who have thin, delicate skin [66–68]. Tensile strength, the rate of collagen deposition, and wound healing are all enhanced following exogenous growth hormone administration. A recent study compared two forms of rhGH in their respective abilities to enhance donor site healing following split skin grafting. Both forms of biosynthetic rhGH were more effective than placebo [61, 69]. Patients with large cutaneous burns have a limited potential to supply donor sites from which to harvest autologous skin. Recombinant human growth hormone can therefore help to make previous sites more rapidly available for further harvest. The surgeon is, therefore, able to close the wound more rapidly, reducing hypermetabolism and the risk of infection. Other clinical studies did not show clinically beneficial effects on wound healing when patients received rhGH; however, this may have been due to the smaller dose used, indicating that maintenance of plasma levels within a therapeutic range is essential [56]. The clinical use of rhGH is expensive, particularly if given for long periods, as is sometimes required in patients with extensive burns. The cost may be $ 7000 per month for a 40-kg pediatric patient; however, this must be balanced against the tremendous saving in terms of patient suffering and hospital time. Naturally, rhGH is only required in patients with burns of sufficient size to require multiple skin grafting procedures.

The mechanism whereby growth hormone enhances donor site healing is unknown. A recent study from the Shriners Burns Institute Galveston compared the effect of systemic exogenous rhGH treatment on various histologic features within skin biopsies obtained from an initial graft donor site of patients with greater than

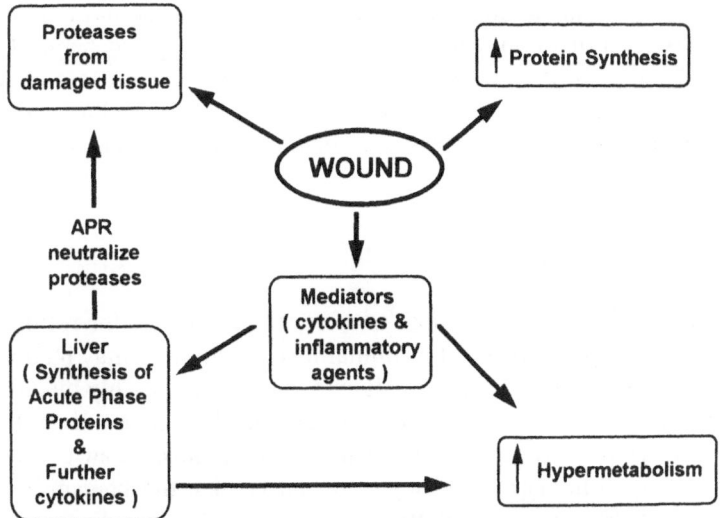

Fig. 2. Effect of the wound itself, contributing to protein synthesis and the acute phase response by indirectly inducing antiprotease production. *APR,* atrial natriuretic peptide

50% total body surface area burns. Skin biopsies were taken from the selected donor sites 7 days after harvesting the skin. The patients then received daily exogenous rhGH, and seven days later a second biopsy was obtained. The histologic findings for the patient population showed a significant increase in IGF I surface receptor expression along with increases in collagen (types IV and VII) and basal lamina formation. This confirms the work of others that rhGH administration induces an increase in IGF I receptor expression within a wound. In addition, it provides qualitative evidence that rhGH affects wound healing by influencing collagen synthesis in burn wounds.

Although hypermetabolism is associated with a net negative nitrogen balance caused mainly by proteolysis of peripheral skeletal muscle, it is possible that other areas of the body are in positive nitrogen balance (Fig. 2). An extensive wound in a severely burned patient is a voracious consumer of the raw materials needed to manufacture the large quantities of collagen and other proteins required for repair and healing. For example, initial investigations (data as yet unpublished) indicate that protein synthesis in a burn wound is significantly greater than in other areas of the body. The skin is therefore likely to be a significant, and thus far neglected, contributor to whole body protein kinetics. The wound may therefore be regarded from several perspectives. First, as a potential source of mediators and inflammatory agents which, should they seep into the circulation, contribute to triggering physiological and metabolic processes associated with hypermetabolism. Secondly mediators and oxidants from damaged tissue within a wound must be neutralized by APR before they leach into the circulation and become disseminated. Finally, as the processes of healing and repair gather momentum, the wound becomes a significant area for protein synthesis and therefore positive nitrogen balance.

Clearly, growth hormone has both local and systemic effects which influence both wound healing and systemic metabolic kinetics. Since rhGH can enhance the

166   D. A. Gilpin and D. N. Herndon

healing of donor site wounds after as little as seven days, it is not unreasonable to suggest that it may in some way affect the early biochemical events, or indeed the acute phase response and gene activation, which occur after trauma. Further studies are required, possibly using an in vitro tissue culture model, to see whether rhGH can affect the expression of genes involved with extracellular matrix formation.

Conclusion

The gross organ manifestations of severe trauma are the results of a sequence of earlier events initiated at a cellular level. Cytokines may interact with hormones and other mediators so as to affect metabolism, possibly by cross-reactivity with receptors. Cortisol, glucagon, insulin, catecholamines, IL-6, IL-1, and IL-2 are increased following trauma. Although their levels can be correlated with the severity of injury and the degree of sepsis, their mechanisms of action at the cellular level remain speculative. It is possible that a wide diversity of stimulatory agents affect metabolism and the acute phase response through a relatively small number of intracellular pathways. Through the action of pharmacological agents such as selective β-blockers and agonists, thromboxane inhibitors, and growth factors (IGF-1 and rhGH), beneficial modulation of the inflammatory and hypermetabolic responses can be achieved. Growth hormone is a particularly useful growth factor which influences systemic metabolism and local wound healing. It is possible which its beneficial effects are mediated at a cellular level, including gene expression.

References

1. McGrath MH (1990) Peptide growth factors and wound healing. Clin Plast Surg 17:421–432
2. Barbul A (1990) Immune aspects of wound repair. Clin Plast Surg 17:433–442
3. Martin PM, Wooley JH, McCluskey J (1992) Growth factors and cutaneous wound repair. Prog Growth Factor Res 4:25–44
4. Herndon DN, Nguyen TT, Gilpin DA (1993) Growth factors: local and systemic. Arch Surg 128(11):1227–1233
5. Dolecek R (1990) The endocrine and metabolic response to burn injuries: mechanisms and clinical applications. In: Dolecek R, Brizio-Molteni L, Molten A, Traber D (eds) Endocrinology of therma injury. Pathophysiologic mechanisms and clinical interpretation. Lea and Febiger, Philadelphia, pp 28–45
6. Sabiston DC (ed) (1991) Textbook of surgery. The molecular basis of modern surgical practice, 13th edn. Saunders, Philadelphia, pp 23–37 and pp 116–150
7. Wilmore DW, Aulick LH (1978) Metabolic changes in burned patients. Surg Clin North Am 58:1173–1187
8. Wilmore DW (1976) Hormone responses and their effect on metabolism. Surg Clin North Am 56:999–1018
9. Sevaljevic L, Glibetic M, Poznanovic G, Savic J, Petrovic M (1991) Effect of lethal scald on the mechanisms of acute-phase synthesis in rat liver. Circ Shock 33:98–107
10. Cuthbertson DP (1979) The metabolic response to injury and its nutritional implications: retrospective and prospective. JPEN J Parenter Enteral Nutr 3:108–130
11. Cuthbertson DP (1932) Observations on the disturbance of metabolism produced by injury to the limbs. Q J Med 3:233–246

12. Kushner I (1993) Regulation of the acute phase response by cytokines. Perspect Biol Med 36(4):611–622
13. Wilmore DC, Long JM, Mason AD, Skreen RW, Pruitt BA (1974) Catecholamines: mediators of the hypermetabolic response to thermal injury. Ann Surg 18(4):653–669
14. Fleming RYD, Rutan RL, Jahoor F, Barrow RE, Wolfe RR, Herndon DN (1992) Effect of recombinant human growth hormone on catabolic hormones and free fatty acids following thermal injury. J Trauma 32:698–703
15. Newsome TW, Mason AD, Pruitt BA (1973) Weight loss following thermal injury. Ann Surg 178:215–217
16. Kinney JM, Long CL, Gump FE, Duke JH (1968) Tissue composition of weight loss in surgical patients. I. Elective operations. Ann Surg 168:459–473
17. Joshi VV (1970) Effects of burns on the heart. JAMA 211:2130–2134
18. Sevaljevic L, Ivanovic-Matic S, Petrovic M, Glibetic M (1989) Regulation of plasma acute-phase protein and albumin levels in the liver of scalded rats. Biochem J 258:663–668
19. Sevaljevic L, Glibetic M, Poznanovic G, Petrovic M, Matic S, Pantelic D (1988) Thermal injury-induced expression of acute-phase proteins in rat liver. Burns 14(4):280–286
20. Sevaljevic L, Petrovic M, Bogojevic D, Savic J, Pantelic D (1989) Acute-phase response to scalding: changes in serum properties and acute-phase protein concentrations. Circ Shock 28:293–307
21. Dickson PW, Bannister D, Schreiber G (1987) Minor burns lead to major changes in synthesis rates of plasma proteins in the liver. J Trauma 27(3):283–286
22. Xia ZF, Coolbaugh MI, He F, Herndon DN (1992) The effect of burn injury on the acute phase response. J Trauma 32(2):245–251
23. Lieberman ZH, Lansche JM (1956) Effects of thermal injury on metabolic rate and insensible water loss in the rat. Surg Forum 7:83–88
24. Morgan HC, Andrews RP, Jurkiewicz MJ (1956) The effect of thermal injury on insensible water loss in the rat. Surg Forum 6:78–84
25. Caldwell FT, Osterholm JL, Sower ND, Moyer CA (1959) Metabolic response to thermal trauma of normal and thyroprivic rats at three environmental temperatures. Ann Surg 150:976–988
26. Zawacki BE, Spitzer KW, Mason AD, Johns LA (1969) Does increased evaporative water loss cause hypermetabolism in burned patients? Ann Surg 171:236–240
27. Neely WA, Petro AG, Holloman GH, Rushton FW, Turner MD, Hardy JD (1973) Researches on the cause of burn hypermetabolism. Ann Surg 179:291–294
28. Kowal-Vern A, Walenga JM, Hoppensteadt D, Sharp-Pucci M, Gamelli RL (1994) Interleukin-2 and interleukin-6 in relation to burn size in the acute phase response of thermal injury. J Am Coll Surg 178:357–362
29. Rutan TC, Herndon DN, Osten TV, Abston S (1986) Metabolic rate alterations in early excision and grafting versus conservative treatment. J Trauma 26(2):140–142
30. Bessey PQ, Watters JM, Aoki TT, Wilmore DW (1984) Combined hormonal infusion stimulates the metabolic response to injury. Ann Surg 200:264–280
31. Herndon DN, Barrow RE, Rutan TC, Minifeee P, Jahoor F, Wolfe RR (1988) Effect of propranolol administration on hemodynamic and metabolic responses of burned pediatric patients. Ann Surg 208:484–492
32. Gore DC, Honeycutt D, Jahoor F, Barrow RE, Wolfe RR, Herndon DN (1991) Propranolol diminished extremity blood flow in burned patients. Ann Surg 213:568–574
33. Estler CJ, Ammon HPT (1969) The importance of the adrenergic beta-receptors for thermogenesis and survival of acutely cold-exposed mice. Can J Physiol Pharmacol 47:427–433
34. Honeycutt D, Barrow RE, Herndon DN (1992) Cold stress response in patients with severe burns after beta-blockade. J Burn Care Rehabil 13:181–186
35. Maggi SP, Biolo G, Muller MJ, Barrow RE, Wolfe RR, Herndon DN (1993) Beta-1 blockade decreases cardiac work without affecting protein breakdown or lipolysis in severely burned patients. Surg Forum 75:1081
36. Choo JJ, Horan MA, Little RA, Rothwell NJ (1992) Anabolic effects of clenbuterol on skeletal muscle are mediated by beta 2 adrenergic activation. Am J Physiol 263:50–56
37. Demling RH, Lalonde C (1987) Topical ibuprofen decreases early postburn edema. Surgery 5:857–861

38. Haung YS, Li A, Yang ZC (1990) Roles of thromboxane and its inhibitor anisodamine in burn shock. Burns 4:249–253
39. Herndon DN, Abston S, Stein MD (1984) Increased thromboxane B2 levels in the plasma of burned and septic patients. Surg Gynecol Obstet 159:210–213
40. Arturson G, Hamberg M, Jonsson CE (1973) Prostaglandins in human burn blister fluid. Acta Physiol Scand 87:270–276
41. Lalonde C, Know J, Daryani R, Zhu D, Demling RH, Neumann M (1991) Topical flurbiprofen decreases burn wound induced hypermetabolism and systemic lipid peroxidation. Surgery 109:645–651
42. Heggers JP, Loy GL, Robson MC, Del Beccaro EJ (1980) Histological demonstration of prostaglandins and thromboxanes in burned tissue. J Surg Res 28:110–115
43. Heggers JP, Robson MC, Zachary LS (1985) Thromboxane inhibitors for the prevention of progressive dermal ischemia due to thermal injury. J Burn Care Rehabil 6:466–468
44. Soroff HS, Pearson E, Green NL, Artz CP (1960) The effect of growth hormone on nitrogen balance at various levels of intake in burned patients. Surg Gynecol Obstet 111:259–273
45. Liljedahl SO, Gemzell CA, Plantin LO, Birke G (1961) Effect of human growth hormone in patients with severe burns. Acta Chir Scand 122:1–14
46. Wilmore DW, Moylan JA, Bristow BF, Mason AD, Pruitt BA (1974) Anabolic effects of human growth hormone and high caloric feeding following thermal injury. Surg Gynecol Obstet 138:875–884
47. Goeddel DV, Heyneker HL, Hozumi T, Aretzen R, Itakura K, Yansura DG et al. (1979) Direct expression in Escherichia coli of a DNA sequence coding for human growth hormone. Nature 281:44–48
48. Watson JD, Gilman M, Witkowski J, Zoller M (1992) Recombinant DNA in medicine and industry. In: Watson JD Recombinant DNA. Freeman, New York, pp 455–458
49. Kaplin SL, August GP, Blethen SL, Brown DR, Hintz RL, Johansen A et al. (1986) Clinical studies with recombinant-DNA-derived methionyl human growth hormone in growth hormone deficient children. Lancet 1:697–700
50. Watanabe S, Tsunematsu Y, Fujimoto J, Komiyama A (1988) Leukaemia in patients treated with growth hormone (Letter to the editor). Lancet I:1159
51. Jiang ZM, He GZ, Zhang SY et al. (1989) Low dose growth hormone and hypocaloric nutrition attenuate the protein-catabolic response after major operation. Ann Surg 210:513–525
52. Ponting GA, Halliday D, Teale JD, Sim AJW (1988) Postoperative positive nitrogen balance with intravenous hyponutrition and growth hormone. Lancet 1:438–439
53. Ziegler TR, Young RD, McK Manson J, Wilmore DW (1988) Metabolic effects of recombinant growth hormone in patients receiving parenteral nutrition. Ann Surg 208:6–16
54. Gore DC, Honeycutt D, Jahoor F, Wolfe RR, Herndon DN (1991) Effect of exogenous growth hormone on whole-body and isolated limb protein kinetics in burned patients. Arch Surg 126:38–43
55. Wolfe RR, Herndon DN, Peter EJ, Jahoor F, Desai MH, Hollard OB (1987) Regulation of lipolysis in severely burned children. Ann Surg 206(2):214 221
56. Chance WT, Nelson JL, Foley-Nelson T, Kim M, Fischer J (1989) The relationship of burn induced hypermetabolism to central and peripheral catecholamines. J Trauma 29(3):306–312
57. Belcher HJCR, Mercer D, Judkins KC et al. (1989) Biosynthetic human growth hormone in burned patients: a pilot study. Burns 15:99–107
58. MacGorman LR, Rizza R, Gerich JE (1981) Physiological concentrations of growth hormone exert insulin like and insulin antagonistic effects on both hepatic and extrahepatic tissues in man. J Clin Endocrinol Metab 53(3):556–559
59. Fraser R (1960) Endocrine disorders and insulin action. Br Med Bull 16:242–246
60. Strock LL, Singh H, Abdullah A, Miller JA, Herndon DN (1990) The effect of insulin-like growth factor 1 on postburn hypermetabolism. Surgery 108:161–164
61. Herndon DN, Barrow RE, Kunkel KR, Broemeling L, Rutan RL (1990) Effects of recombinant human growth hormone on donor site healing in severely burned children. Ann Surg 211:424–431
62. Kupfer SR, Underwood LE, Baxter RC et al. (1993) Enhancement of the anabolic effects of growth hormone and insulin like growth factor 1 by use of both agents simultaneously. J Clin Invest 91:391–396

63. Clemmons DR, Smith-Banks A, Underwood LE (1992) Reversal of the diet-induced catabolism by infusion of recombinant insulin-like growth factor (IGF-1) in humans. J Clin Endocrinol Metab 75:234–238
64. Lee PDK, Rosenfeld RG, Hintz RL, Smith SD (1986) Characterization of insulin-like and growth hormone receptors on human leukemic lymphoblasts. J Clin Endocrin Metabol 62(1):28–35
65. Weigent DA, Blalock JE (1989) Expression of growth hormone by lymphocytes. Int Rev Immunol 4:193–211
66. Jorgenson PH, Andreassen TT, Jorgensen KD (1989) Growth hormone influences collagen deposition and mechanical strength of intact rat skin. A dose response study. Acta Endocrinol (Copenh) 120:767–772
67. Jorgenson PH, Andreassen TT (1987) A dose response study of the effects of biosynthetic growth hormone on formation and strength of granulation tissue. Endocrinology 121:1637–1641
68. Jorgenson PH, Andreassen TT (1988) The influence of biosynthetic human growth hormone on biomechanical properties and collagen formation in granulation tissue. Horm Metab Res 20:490–493
69. Gilpin DA, Barrow RE, Rutan RL, Broemling L, Herndon DN (1994) Recombinant human growth hormone accelerates wound healing in children with large cutaneous burns. Ann Surg (in press)

The Endothelium

J. R. Bradley and D. Rubenstein

Introduction

The acute catabolic state represents a response to a diverse range of injurious stimuli, including trauma, sepsis, surgery and haemorrhagic shock. Each of these conditions may lead to haemodynamic collapse, disturbed coagulation, leucocytic infiltration into tissues, and ultimately multiple organ failure. Vascular endothelium is uniquely positioned at the interface between the tissues and the circulation and is thus able to directly influence the development of pathophysiological responses in these conditions.

When endothelial cells are ischaemic, injured or exposed to inflammatory mediators, they undergo a number of functional and morphological changes. These changes, which have been collectively termed activation [1], include the modulation of vascular tone, and hence control of local blood flow, changes in structure which allow vascular leakage, the local accumulation and subsequent extravasation into the tissues of leucocytes and the synthesis of both surface molecules and soluble factors involved in leucocyte activation and coagulation (Fig. 1). Endothelial cells can thus modify the development of the catabolic state, not only by serving as targets for injury, but by undergoing a number of functional changes which enable them to determine the response of tissues to injury.

Understanding the mechanisms by which the endothelium is able to regulate vascular structure, vasomotor tone, coagulation and inflammatory responses may thus increase our appreciation of how haemodynamic instability, coagulopathy and tissue injury develop in the catabolic state. Furthermore, recognition of the pivotal role of endothelial cells in the development of these events increases the potential of the endothelium as a target for therapeutic intervention.

Endothelial Cells as Regulators of Vascular Tone

The observation that the action of many known vasodilators depends on the integrity of the vascular endothelium overlying smooth muscle cells led to the realisation that endothelial cells themselves can modulate vascular tone by the release of vasoactive substances [2]. Several families of endothelial-derived compounds which influence vasomotor function have now been identified, of which the most extensively studied are the arachidonic acid metabolite, prostacyclin (prostaglan-

172   J. R. Bradley and D. Rubenstein

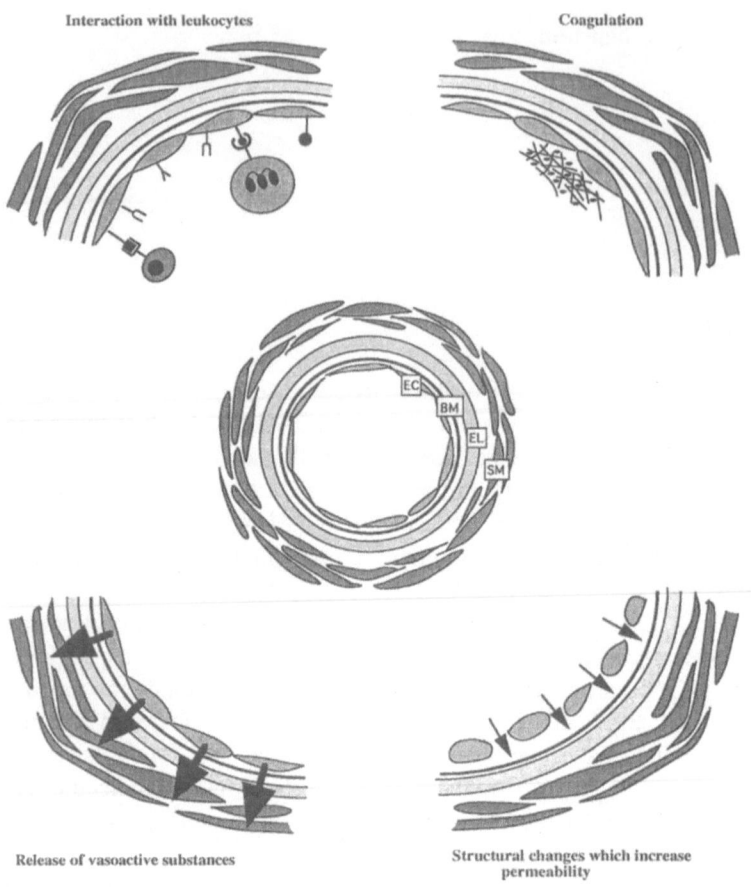

Interaction with leukocytes   Coagulation

Release of vasoactive substances   Structural changes which increase
                                              permeability

Fig. 1. Endothelial cell activation. Endothelial cells *(EC)* respond to inflammatory mediators by undergoing a number of structural and functional changes. *BM,* basement membrane; *EL,* elastic layers; *SM,* smooth muscle

din I_2, PGI_2), nitric oxide (NO) and NO-containing compounds, and the endothelins.

Prostacyclin and NO both cause vasodilatation and hence increase local blood flow, leading to increased delivery of plasma proteins and leukocytes at sites of production. Both prostacyclin and NO are synthesised in response to inflammatory mediators such as thrombin, histamine, bradykinin, serotonin and leukotriene C_4 which raise cytoplasmic free calcium [3]. Prostacyclin is produced by endothelial cells, platelets and monocytes via a phospholipase A_2 (PLA_2)-dependent pathway and causes smooth muscle cell relaxation, and also inhibition of platelet aggregation, via intracellular increases in cyclic 3,5-adenosine monophosphate (cAMP). Interleukin (IL)-1 and tumour necrosis factor (TNF) increase the activity of the enzymes mediating prostacyclin generation.

NO (originally named "endothelial-derived relaxing factor") is produced by endothelial cells from arginine by oxidation of the guanidine-nitrogen terminal of L-arginine [4]. Production of NO is regulated via activity of NO synthase, a predominantly cytosolic calcium–calmodulin-requiring enzyme which is similar in structure to cytochrome P-450 enzymes [5]. In addition to agents which raise intracellular calcium levels, enzyme activity is also increased by mechanical forces such as shear stress. Analogues of L-arginine such as L-NG-monomethyl arginine (L-NMMA) and L-nitroarginine methyl ester (L-NAME) act as inhibitors of NO production. Endothelin is a 21-amino acid peptide which is produced by vascular endothelium [6]. Four different isoforms (endothelin-1, endothelin-2, endothelin-3 and endothelin-4) have been described [7], of which endothelin-1 is produced by vascular endothelial cells. It is synthesized as preproendothelin, which is converted to big (pro)endothelin and subsequently to endothelin, which possesses the biological activity. Although recognised as a potent vasoconstrictor, endothelin can also induce transient vasodilatation.

Endothelial Leucocyte Adhesion Molecules

Endothelial leucocyte adhesion molecules belong to two families of cell surface glycoproteins, the selectins and the immunoglobulin superfamily (Fig. 2).

Selectins

Selectins are characterised by a carbohydrate-binding (lectin) domain at the amino terminal, an epidermal growth factor-like domain, multiple short consensus repeats that are structurally related to proteins involved in complement activation, a transmembrane segment and a short cytoplasmic tail.

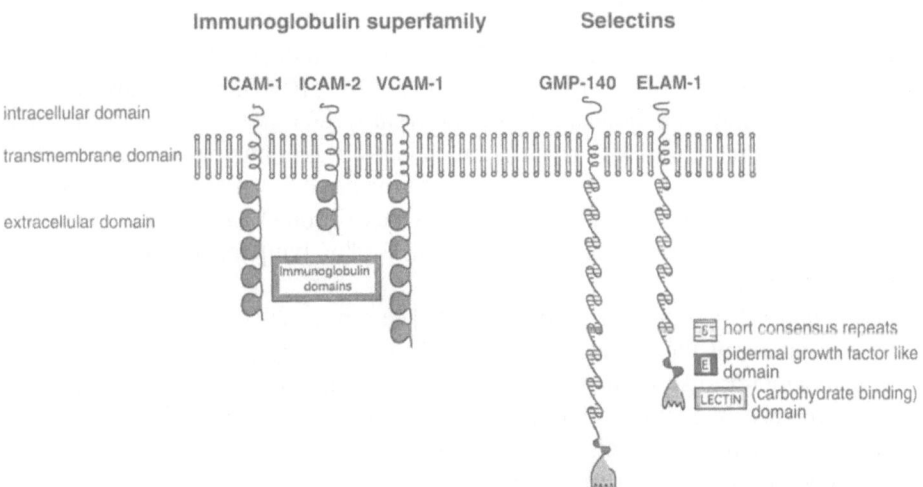

Fig. 2. Endothelial leucocyte adhesion molecules. *ICAM,* intercellular adhesion molecule; *VCAM,* vascular cell adhesion molecule; *GMP,* granule membrane protein; *ELAM,* endothelial cell adhesion molecule

Granule membrane protein-140 (GMP-140, also known as P-selectin, LECAM-3 or CD62) is induced by inflammatory mediators which increase intracellular calcium such as histamine and thrombin, phorbol esters [8] and free oxygen radicals. These agents cause translocation within minutes of GMP-140, a constitutive membrane protein of the Weidel-Palade body (endothelial cell secretory organelle), to the cell surface, where it acts as an adhesion molecule for neutrophils. GMP-140 is also found in granules of platelets, where it is referred to as platelet activation-dependent granule-external membrane protein (PADGEM).

Endothelial cell adhesion molecule-1 (ELAM-1, also known as E-selectin or LECAM-2) is a 115-kDa transmembrane glycoprotein which is synthesised and expressed in response to IL-1 or TNF [9]. ELAM-1 mRNA appears within 1 h of treatment with either cytokine and is followed by surface expression, which peaks at 4–6 h. ELAM-1 increases adhesiveness for neutrophils, and the ligands which have been identified for ELAM-1 are all sialylated polylactosamine structures with fucose linked to the 3-hydroxyl of at least one N-acetylglucosamine residue [10]. The fucose and sialic acid residues are both required for recognition.

GMP-140 and ELAM-1 are both similar in structure to a third leucocyte adhesion molecule, leucocyte adhesion molecule-1 (LAM-1, also known as L-selectin or LECAM-1), which is preferentially expressed on T cells and mediates binding to the specialised high endothelial cell venules of lymph nodes through interaction with a constitutive ligand. It has also been implicated in the binding of neutrophils and lymphocytes to cytokine-stimulated endothelial cells [11].

Together GMP-140, ELAM-1 and LAM-1 form the three known members of the selectin family of transmembrane proteins. All three proteins are encoded by closely linked genes on the long arm of chromosome 1 [12].

Immunoglobulin Superfamily

Vascular Cell Adhesion Molecule-1. In addition to inducing ELAM-1, IL-1 and TNF also induce the synthesis and expression of the 110-kDa surface glycoprotein vascular cell adhesion molecule-1 (VCAM-1, also referred to as inducible cell adhesion molecule-110, INCAM-110), a member of the immunoglobulin supergene family [13]. Induction occurs over a slower time period than ELAM-1, peaking at 24 h. The ligand for VCAM-1 is the very late activation (VLA) antigen, VLA-4, a member of the integrin family, which is expressed on lymphocytes and monocytes but not neutrophils.

Intercellular Adhesion Molecule-1 and -2. These molecules (ICAM-1 and -2) are also members of the immunoglobulin supergene family [14]. ICAM-1 has five immunoglobulin-like domains, whereas ICAM-2 has two. ICAM-1 is expressed constitutively on a wide variety of cells, including endothelial cells. ICAM-1 expression on endothelial cells increases in response to IL-1, TNF and also to a lesser extent interferon-γ, reaching a plateau by about 24 h. In contrast, ICAM-2 has a more restricted distribution, being expressed mainly on endothelial cells and certain interstitial cells [15]. Although ICAM-2 is basally expressed to a greater extent than ICAM-1 on endothelial cells, it does not appear to be regulated by inflammatory mediators [16]. ICAM-1 and ICAM-2 are both ligands for leucocyte function-associated antigen-1 (LFA-1), a member of the integrin family of adhesion receptors, also known as the β_2- or leucocyte integrins. This family consists of three high molecular weight heterodimeric glycoproteins that share a common β-subunit (CD18), which is non-covalently associated with related α-subunits (CD11a, b and c). LFA-1 (CD11a/CD18) is broadly distributed on leucocytes, whereas Mac-1 (CD11b/CD18) and p150/95 (CD11c/CD18) are mainly expressed on NK cells and cells of the myeloid lineage. Mac-1 has been identified as a ligand for ICAM-1 [17], and p150/95 has been implicated in leucocyte binding to endothelium, possibly through epitopes of ICAM-1 or ICAM-2. In addition, ICAM-1 has been identified as a ligand for CD43, which is expressed on all T cells, a subset of B cells and other haematopoietic cells [18]. CD43 is a single chain molecule, not structurally related to the integrin family.

The low basal expression and inducibility of ICAM-1 has led to speculation that it may be important during inflammatory or immune responses, whereas ICAM-2 may be more important in the unstimulated resting state or early stages of an inflammatory response.

A third member of the intercellular adhesion molecule family, ICAM-3, does not appear to be expressed on endothelium.

Platelet/Endothelial Cell Adhesion Molecule-1. This molecule (PECAM-1, CD31) [19], a further member of the immunoglobulin supergene family, is concentrated at apposing endothelial cell borders, where it is thought to contribute to endothelial–endothelial interactions. It may also influence endothelial transmigration of leucocytes.

Upregulation of endothelial adhesion molecule expression by inflammatory mediators thus occurs in a time-dependent manner. Expression of GMP-140 and ELAM-1, which promote neutrophil adhesion, occur transiently and at an early stage (within minutes and hours, respectively), whereas more sustained stimulation with cytokines may favour mononuclear cell accumulation as a result of increased VCAM-1 and ICAM-1 expression.

Endothelial Cells as Regulators of Coagulation

Endothelial cells constitutively express thrombomodulin and secrete protein S [20, 21], which both catalyse the activated protein C pathway, and also express heparan [22], which catalyses the anti-thrombin III pathway. In addition, the endothelium acts as a barrier separating intravascular coagulation factors (factor VIIa) from tissue factor, which is localised predominantly in the subendothelium, and preventing the exposure of platelets to matrix proteins, such as collagen, which promote their aggregation. Basally, the endothelial cell surface is thus anticoagulant. Exposure of endothelial cells to tumour necrosis factor or IL-1 induces expression of tissue factor which binds factor VIIa, thereby initiating the extrinsic clotting pathway, and decreases the expression of thrombomodulin [23–26].

Endothelial cells also regulate the fibrinolytic process. Fibrinolysis requires the activation of plasminogen to plasmin, which degrades fibrin and so breaks up throm-

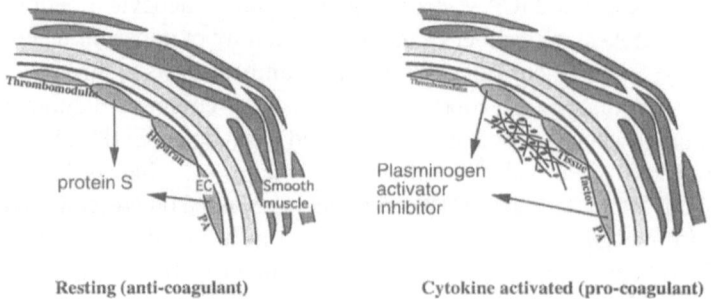

Resting (anti-coagulant)   Cytokine activated (pro-coagulant)

Fig. 3. Anti- and procoagulant activities of endothelial cells *(EC); PA,* plasminogen activator

bi. Plasminogen activators, which are serine proteases, and inhibitors of plasminogen activators are both synthesized by endothelium. Normally, endothelial cells express tissue plasminogen activator (tPA), which is most active when bound to fibrin. In response to inflammatory cytokines, endothelial cells preferentially synthesise urokinase-type plasminogen activator (uPA) [27], which is active in the fluid phase, and increase their synthesis of plasminogen activator inhibitor [28, 29].

In response to inflammatory mediators such as TNF and IL-1 there is therefore both loss of basal endothelial cell surface anticoagulant activity and induction of new procoagulant functions (Fig. 3).

Vascular endothelial cells thus respond to various stimuli by undergoing a number of alterations which endow them with new functional capacities. This capacity of vascular endothelial cells to influence the pathophysiological response to clinical conditions has largely been defined in vitro. However, there is increasing evidence that alterations in endothelial cell function play a critical role in defining the response to such conditions, including the acute catabolic state, in vivo.

Endothelium in the Acute Catabolic State: In Vivo Studies

Critical illnesses, including trauma, major surgery, sepsis and haemorrhagic shock, are associated with an increased catabolic rate which, if prolonged, is associated with increased morbidity and mortality. Each of these processes results in a complex response in which reduced haemodynamic stability, alterations in metabolism, production of toxins and release of inflammatory mediators occur to a variable extent depending on the underlying cause.

For example, the catabolic state is associated with elevation in the level of circulating cytokines, including TNF and IL-1, which have direct effects on endothelial cell function. However, the pattern and magnitude of cytokine production varies according to the precipitating factor. Thus, levels of TNF have been shown to be higher in haemorrhagic shock than following trauma in both patients [30] and in animal studies [31]. In addition, massive cytokine release has been reported in septic but not traumatic shock in baboons [32].

Septic shock is often further complicated by the presence of bacterial products, such as lipopolysaccharide, which have been implicated as important mediators of tissue injury. Studies have shown that extracts of bacterial cell walls such as lipopolysaccharide (endotoxins) can activate endothelium in a manner which promotes endothelial cell procoagulant and inflammatory functions. In this respect endotoxin mimics many of the actions of TNF and IL-1 on endothelium, although quantitatively endotoxin appears less efficient than cytokines [33, 34].

It is not surprising, therefore, that the pattern of endothelial cell activation also appears to vary according to the precipitating cause in the acute catabolic state. Baboons subjected to septic shock by injection of live *Escherichia coli* develop widespread de novo ELAM-1 expression throughout the vascular tree of most organs, whereas baboons with hypovolaemic or traumatic shock have minimal focal expression of ELAM-1 [35]. In addition, evidence of neutrophil activation, measured by granulocyte elastase levels in plasma, is much more pronounced in animals with septic shock. The potential role of endotoxin in the development of endothelial activation has been confirmed by studies in which endotoxin was infused into cytomologus monkeys [36]. Serial skin biopsies showed increases in ELAM-1 expression peaking at 4 h after the start of the infusion.

Vasomotor Responses

Critical illness, regardless of the cause, is frequently complicated by hypotension, modulated by either reduced cardiac output, vasodilatation or both. Whilst mechanisms leading to hypotension in the acute catabolic state are undoubtedly complex, endothelial cell production of vasodilators is likely to be an important contributor to the low systemic vascular resistance which is characteristic. 6-Keto PGF1a (the stable metabolite of prostacyclin) levels increase following administration of endotoxin to dogs [37] or infusion of live *E. coli* into baboons [38]. Furthermore, cyclooxygenase inhibitors have been shown to have a protective effect in models of endotoxic shock [39, 40]. In addition, L-NG-monomethyl arginine (L-NMMA), an inhibitor of endogenous NO synthesis, reverses endotoxin-induced hypotension in rats [41]. The observation that NO synthase inhibitors can exert a dose-dependent increase in blood pressure and systemic vascular resistance in patients with septic shock raises the possibility that such agents may form a novel therapy in the management of resistant hypotension [42, 43]. Thus, both prostacyclin and NO production by vascular endothelial cells have been implicated in the development of hypotension during septic shock. Endothelin-1 levels are elevated in conditions such as acute myocardial infarction, surgery, haemorrhage and cardiogenic shock, perhaps as a protective mechanism to maintain blood pressure and perfusion of vital organs [44].

Vascular Leakage

In addition to alterations in vasomotor responses, critical illnesses are often associated with vascular leakage, which contributes to the haemodynamic collapse characteristic of the acute catabolic state. This vascular leakiness may be due to endothelial injury or the direct effects of leucocyte-derived products such as TNF and hydrogen peroxide, which increase transendothelial permeability [45].

Endothelial Cell–Leucocyte Interactions in the Acute Catabolic State

The response to shock and ischaemia is improved in animals depleted of leucocytes [46]. Vascular endothelium is likely to play a key role in mediating leucocyte-dependent tissue injury under such circumstances, by promoting their local recruitment, activation and transmigration. These interactions have been found to be of particular importance during the resumption of organ blood flow following a period of ischaemia.

Reperfusion Injury

Reduced tissue perfusion as a consequence of hypotension, often in association with regional vasoconstriction, leads to impaired cellular functions and ischaemic injury. However, restoration of blood flow often leads to further cellular injury, which is characterised by vascular leakage and leucocytic infiltration. The mechanisms of this reperfusion-induced tissue injury are not fully understood, although the local generation of free oxygen radicals may be an important factor.

Endothelial cells contain xanthine dehydrogenase and xanthine oxidase in addition to a number of mechanisms for reducing free radicals, including superoxide dismutase, catalase and the glutathione redox cycle. Although initially studied principally as mediators of endothelial injury, recent observations suggest that free radicals may directly increase the pro-inflammatory capacity of vascular endothelium. Such changes include alterations in endothelial cell cytoskeletal structure that influence vascular permeability [45], increased synthesis of platelet-activating factor [47] and tissue plasminogen activator, increased platelet adherence and prostacyclin release [48], increased translocation of P-selectin to the endothelial cell surface [49], increased expression of ICAM-1 and major histocompatibility complex (MHC) class I and increased adhesiveness for leucocytes [45].

Coagulation

Disseminated intravascular thrombosis frequently complicates critical illness, and the endothelium is thought to play a major role in the widespread disturbance of coagulation. One of the earliest studies providing evidence for increased procoagulant activity of the endothelium in response to sepsis was provided by Shwartzman [50], who described an animal model in which an intradermal injection of lipopolysaccharide and other bacterial products is followed 24 h later by an intravenous injection. Tissue necrosis, associated with thrombotic occlusion of local vessels, occurs at the original injection site. Leucocytes appear essential to the development of the response, thus implicating both the coagulation system and the development of an inflammatory response. More recent studies have confirmed that both proco-agulant and inflammatory functions of the endothelium are increased during septic shock, but emphasise the heterogeneity of activation responses. Thus, although widespread expression of ELAM-1 occurs in baboons exposed to lethal infusion of *E. coli*, endothelial expression of tissue factor is only increased in the splenic microvasculature, reinforcing the complexity of the endothelial activation process [51].

Vascular Endothelium as a Target for Therapeutic Intervention

Increasing evidence that the vascular endothelium plays a key role in modifying responses to the acute catabolic state has led to a search for endothelium-directed therapies. Although intervention studies aimed at neutralising inflammatory mediators with effects on vascular endothelium have shown beneficial effects in animal studies, results of clinical trials in patients with septic shock have been less encouraging. Neutralizing anti-sera to TNF can reduce toxicity to endotoxin in mice [52] and protect primates against the effects of gram-negative infection [53]. Furthermore, mice lacking the p55 TNF receptor (TNFR1, which can mediate the cytotoxic effects of TNF) are resistant to the lethal toxicity of endotoxin which follows sensitisation with the hepatotoxin D-galactosamine [53]. In addition to raising the possibility of anti-TNF-directed therapies, these observations also suggest that TNF, released in response to endotoxin, may be the principal mediator of the response to sepsis.

However, TNF may under certain circumstances act as a host defence against invading micro-organisms. Interfering with the actions of TNF may thus have harmful as well as beneficial effects. Indeed, both neutralising antibodies to TNF and deletion of the TNFR1 suppress the ability of mice to control infection with *Listeria monocytogenes* [53–55].

The results of clinical trials in patients provide less optimism that neutralisation of inflammatory mediators will provide a useful therapy. Antibodies against TNF did not improve survival in human subjects with septic shock [56, 57], although neutralising antibodies directed against endotoxin have been shown to be of benefit in a subset of patients. However, it may not be possible to predict which patients will benefit from therapy prospectively, and these agents have not yet entered routine clinical practice [58–60].

The possibility of inhibiting the actions of endothelial-derived vasoactive substances has also received attention [42], although therapy aimed at interfering with leucocyte–endothelial cell interactions may offer the most hope for the future. Recent studies have shown that therapies which interfere with the function of endothelial adhesion molecules can suppress tissue injury in a number of experimental models [61, 62]. Of particular interest is the observation that oligosaccharides which bind to the lectin domain of selectin molecules can be used to protect against acute tissue injury [63, 64], suggesting that sialyl-Lewis X carbohydrates may provide a novel anti-endothelium-directed therapy.

Conclusion

Vascular endothelial cells respond to various stimuli by undergoing a number of changes, collectively called activation, which endow them with new functional capacities. These changes include the production of vasoactive substances, vascular leakage, increased adhesiveness for leucocytes and the induction of procoagulant activities. There is increasing evidence that activation of vascular endothelium is central to the pathophysiological response in the acute catabolic state, raising the possibility that therapies aimed at limiting the cause or consequences of endothelial activation may prove beneficial.

Acknowledgements. JRB is the recipient of a National Kidney Research Fund Senior Fellowship.

References

1. Pober J (1988) Cytokine-mediated activation of vascular endothelium: physiology and pathology. Am J Pathol 133:426–433
2. Brenner B, Troy J, Balterman B (1989) Endothelium dependent vascular responses: mediators and mechanisms. J Clin Invest 84:1373–1378
3. Pober J, Cotran R (1990) The role of endothelial cells in inflammation. Transplantation 50:537–544
4. Palmer R, Ferrige A, Moncada S (1987) Vascular endothelial cells synthesize nitric oxide from L-arginine. Nature 333:524–526
5. Bredt D, Hwang P, Glatt C et al. (1991) Cloned and expressed nitric oxide synthase structure resembles cytochrome P-450 reductase. Nature 351:714–718
6. Yanagisawa M, Kurihara H, Kimura S et al. (1988) A novel potent vasoconstrictor peptide produced by vascular endothelial cells. Nature 332:411–415
7. Sessa W, Kaw S, Hecker M et al. (1991) The biosynthesis of endothelin-1 by human polymorphonuclear leukocytes. Biochem Biophys Res Commun 174:613–618
8. Geng JG, Bevilacqua MP, Moore K et al. (1990) Rapid neutrophil adhesion to activated endothelium mediated by GMP-140. Nature 343:757–760
9. Bevilacqua MP, Pober JS, Wheeler ME et al. (1987) Identification of an inducible endothelial-leukocyte adhesion molecule. Proc Natl Acad Sci USa 84:9238–9242
10. Tyrell D, James P, Rao N et al. (1991) Structural requirements for the carbohydrate ligand of E-selectin. Proc Natl Acad Sci USA 88:10372–10376
11. Speritini O, Luscinskas F, Kansas GM et al. (1991) Leukocyte adhesion molecule-1 (LAM-1, L-selectin) interacts with an inducible endothelial ligand to support leukocyte adhesion. J Immunol 147:2565–2573
12. Watson M, Kingsmore S, Johnston G et al. (1990) Genomic organization of the selectin family of leukocyte adhesion molecules on human and mouse chromosome 1. J Exp Med 172:263–272
13. Osborn L, Hession C, Tizard R et al. (1989) Direct expression cloning of vascular cell adhesion molecule 1, a cytokine induced endothelial protein that binds to lymphocytes. Cell 59:1203–1211
14. Springer T (1990) Adhesion receptors of the immune system. Nature 346:425–434
15. De Fougerolles A, Stacker S, Schwarting R et al. (1991) Characterization of ICAM-2 and evidence for a third counter-receptor for LFA-1. J Exp Med 174:253–267
16. Nortamo P, Li R, Renkonen R et al. (1991) The expression of human intercellular adhesion molecule-2 is refractory to inflammatory cytokines. Eur J Immunol 21:2629–2632
17. Diamond M, Staunton D, de Fougerolles A et al. (1990) ICAM-1 (CD54): a counter-receptor for Mac-1 (CD11b/CD18). J Cell Biol 111:3129–3139
18. Rosenstein Y, Park J, Hahn W et al. (1991) CD43, a molecule defective in Wiskott-Aldrich syndrome, binds ICAM-1. Nature 354:233–235

19. Newman PJ, Berndt MC, Gorski J et al. (1990) PECAM-1 (CD31) cloning and relation to adhesion molecules of the immunoglobulin gene superfamily. Science 247:1219–1222

20. Esmon C, Owen W (1981) Identification of an endothelial cofactor for thrombin-catalyzed activation of protein C. Proc Natl Acad Sci USA 78:2249–2252

21. Stern D, Brett J, Harris K et al. (1986) Participation of endothelial cells in the protein C-protein S anticoagulant pathway: the synthesis and release of protein S. J Cell Biol 102: 1971–1978

22. Rosenberg R, Rosenberg J (1984) Natural anticoagulant mechanisms. J Clin Invest 74:1–5

23. Bevilacqua M, Pober J, Majeau G et al. (1984) Interleukin-1 (IL-1) induces biosynthesis and cell surface expression of procoagulant activity in human vascular endothelial cells. J Exp Med 160:618–623

24. Nawroth P, Handley D, Esmon C et al. (1986) Interleukin-1 induces endothelial cell procoagulant while suppressing cell surface anticoagulant activity. Proc Natl Acad Sci USA 83: 3460–3464

25. Schorer A, Kaplan M, Rao G et al. (1986) Interleukin-1 stimulates endothelial cell tissue factor production and expression by a prostaglandin independent mechanism. Thromb Haemost 56:256–259

26. Nawroth P, Stern D (1986) Modulation of endothelial cell haemostatic properties by tumor necrosis factor. 163:740–745

27. Biasi F, Vassalli J-D, Dang K (1987) Urokinase type plasminogen activator: proenzyme, receptor and inhibitors. J Cell Biol 104:801–804

28. Nachman R, Hajjar K, Silverstein R et al. (1986) Interleukin 1 induces endothelial cell synthesis of plasminogen activator inhibitor. J Exp Med 163:1595–1600

29. Bevilacqua M, Schleef R, Gimbrone MJ et al. (1986) Regulation of the fibrinolytic system of cultured human vascular endothelium by interleukin 1. J Clin Invest 78:587–591

30. Roumen R, Hendricks T, van der Ven-Jongekrijg J et al. (1993) Cytokine patterns in patients after major vascular surgery, hemorrhagic shock, and severe blunt trauma. Ann Surg 218:769–776

31. Ayala A, Wang P, Ba Z et al. (1991) Differential alterations in plasma IL-6 and TNF levels after trauma and hemorrhage. Am J Physiol 260:R167–R171

32. Redl H, Schlag G, Paul E et al. (1989) Monocyte/macrophage activation with cytokine release after polytrauma and sepsis in baboon. Circ Shock 27:308

33. Bevilacqua M, Pober J, Majeau G et al. (1986) Recombinant tumor necrosis factor induces procoagulant activity in cultured human vascular endothelium; characterization and comparison with the actions of interleukin 1. Proc Natl Acad Sci USA 83:4533–4537

34. Bevilacqua M, Pober J, Wheeler M et al. (1985) Interleukin 1 (IL-1) activation of vascular endothelium: effects on procoagulant activity and leukocyte adhesion. Am J Pathol 121:393–403

35. Redl H, Dinges H, Buurman W et al. (1991) Expression of endothelial leukocyte adhesion molecule-1 in septic but not traumatic shock. Am J Pathol 139:461–466

36. Engelberts I, Samyo S, Leeuwenberg J et al. (1992) A role for ELAM-1 in the pathogenesis of MOF during septic shock. J Surg Res 53:136–140

37. Hales C, Sonne L, Peterson M et al. (1981) Role of thromboxane and prostacyclin in pulmonary vasomotor changes after endotoxin in dogs. J Clin Invest 68:497–505

38. Camporesi E, Oda S, Fracica P et al. (1989) Eicosanoids and the haemodynamic course of live E. coli-induced sepsis in baboons. Circ Shock 29:229–244

39. Jacobs E, Soulsby M, Bone R et al. (1982) Ibuprofen in canine endotoxin shock. J Clin Invest 70:536–541

40. Halushka P, Wise W, Cook J (1983) Studies on the beneficial effects of aspirin in endotoxic shock. Am J Med 74:91–96

41. Nava E, Palmer R, Moncada S (1991) Inhibition of nitric oxide synthesis in septic shock: how much is beneficial? Lancet 338:1555–1557

42. Petros A, Bennet D, Vallance P (1991) Effect of nitric oxide synthase inhibitors on hypotension in patients with septic shock. Lancet 338:1557–158

43. Geroulanos S, Schilling J, Cakmacki M et al. (1992) Inhibition of NO synthesis in septic shock. Lancet 339:434–435

44. Chang H, Wu G-J, Wang S-M et al. (1993) Plasma endothelin level changes during hemorrhagic shock. J Trauma 35:825–833
45. Bradley J, Johnson D, Pober J (1993) Endothelial activation by hydrogen peroxide: selective increases of ICAM-1 and MHC class I. Am J Pathol 142:1598–1609
46. Vedder N, Fouty B, Winn R et al. (1989) Role of neutrophils in generalized reperfusion injury associated with resuscitation from shock. Surgery 106:509–516
47. Lewis M, Whatley R, Cain P et al. (1988) Hydrogen peroxide stimulates synthesis of platelet activating factor by endothelium and induces endothelial cell dependent neutrophil adhesion. J Clin Invest 82:2045–2055
48. Shatos M, Doherty J, Hoak J (1991) Alterations in human vascular endothelial cell function by oxygen free radicals; platelet adherence and prostacyclin release. Arteriosclerosis Thromb 11:594–601
49. Patel K, Zimmerman G, Prescott S et al. (1992) Oxygen radicals induce human endothelial cells to express GMP-140 and bind neutrophils. J Cell Biol 112:749–759
50. Shwartzman G (1928) Phenomenon of local skin reactivity to B. typhosus culture filtrate. J Exp Med 48:247–268
51. Drake T, Cheng J, Chang A et al. (1993) Expression of tissue factor, thrombomodulin, and E-selectin in baboons with lethal E. coli sepsis. Am J Pathol 142:1458–1470
52. Beutler B, Milsark I, Cerami A (1985) Passive immunization against cachectin/tumor necrosis factor protects mice from lethal effects of endotoxin. Science 229:869–871
53. Tracey K, Fong Y, Hesse D et al. (1987) Anti-cachectin/TNF monoclonal antibodies prevent septic shock during lethal bacteraemia. Nature 330:662–664
54. Havell E (1987) Production of tumor necrosis factor during murine Listeriosis. J Immunol 139:4225–4231
55. Nakane A, Minagawa T, Kato K (1988) Endogenous tumor necrosis factor (cachectin) is essential to host resistance against Listeria monocytogenes infection. Infect Immun 56:2563–2569
56. Fisher C, Opal S, Dhainaut J et al. (1993) Influence of an anti-tumor necrosis factor monoclonal antibody on cytokine levels in patients with sepsis. Crit Care Med 21:318–327
57. Bone R (1993) Monoclonal antibodies to tumor necrosis factor in sepsis: help or harm? Crit Care Med 21:311–312
58. Ziegler E, Fisher C, Sprung C et al. (1991) Treatment of gram-negative bacteraemia and septic shock with HA-1A human monoclonal antibody against endotoxin. N Engl J Med 324:429–436
59. Wortel C, von der Möhlen M, van Deventer S et al. (1992) Effectiveness of a human monoclonal anti-endotoxin antibody (HA-1A) in gram-negative sepsis: relationship to endotoxin and cytokine levels. J Infect Dis 166:1367–1374
60. Greenman R, Schein R, Martin M et al. (1991) A controlled trial of E5 murine monoclonal IgM antibody to endotoxin in the treatment of gram-negative sepsis. JAMA 266:1097–1102
61. Nishikawa K, Guo Y, Miyasaka M et al. (1993) Antibodies to ICAM-1/LFA-1 prevent crescent formation in rat autoimmune glomerulonephritis. J Exp Med 177:667–677
62. Yednock T, Cannon C, Lawrence C et al. (1992) Prevention of experimental autoimmune encephalomyelitis by antibodies against α4β1 integrin. Nature 356:63–66
63. Buerke M, Weyrich A, Zheng Z et al. (1994) Sialyl Lewis x-containing oligosaccharide attenuates myocardial reperfusion injury in cats. J Clin Invest 93:1140–1148
64. Mulligan M, Paulson J, De Frees S et al. (1993) Protective effects of oligosaccharides in P-selectin-dependent lung injury. Nature 364:149–151

Aspects of Bone Tissue in Relation to Catabolic States

O. Reikeraas

Introduction

The metabolic response to injury is related to the extent of the trauma; the greater the trauma, the greater the response, which generally increases until it plateaus at a maximum level [1]. The signals that stimulate the response are mixed. Nervous afferent signals play a significant role in the early phase after injury, and circulating and local humoral factors act as major mediators for homeostatic adjustments. Pyrogens may serve as circulating afferent signals to the brain to stimulate the output of an integrated hormonal response.

The metabolic changes are characterized by a shift to fat oxidation with an accelerated consumption of energy and a negative nitrogen balance – the catabolic state [2]. Muscle tissue serves as a protein reservoir, and critical illness is followed by a generalized and progressive breakdown of skeletal muscle proteins. Furthermore, in most injuries the musculoskeletal system is involved. Much interest has been focused on skeletal muscles in catabolic states, but less attention has been paid to bone tissue.

Modern therapy aims to provide nutritional support for the tissues in catabolic situations, but protein breakdown in skeletal muscles is only marginally influenced by conventional nutritional therapy. It is a challenge to develop therapeutic strategies that involve mobilizing the critically ill patient in the early stages of catabolism. In order to develop such strategies, it is first necessary to describe bone pathophysiology at the tissue level. In this presentation some aspects of bone tissue that might be relevant for catabolic situations are presented. The overview describes present states of knowledge concerning physiology and pathophysiology and effects that hormonal and humoral factors involved in catabolic changes in the critically ill patient might have on bone tissue.

Bone Physiology

Bone has two major functions; it provides mechanical stability and it serves as a reservoir for calcium homeostasis. Bone volume is determined by the relative rates of bone formation by osteoblasts and bone resorption by osteoclasts. Bone remodeling is influenced by hormones and local humoral as well as biomechanical factors [3]. There is a clear correlation between strain and structure of bone, but the mechanism of such functional adaptations is far from clear. Bone metabolism is systematically activated by growth, thyroid, and parathyroid (PTH) hormones, and it is inhibited by calcitonin and cortisone. In the human skeleton, about 90% of the total bone surface is in a resting state, i.e., the cells are resting and not subjected to any remodeling activity.

The cellular and biochemical events that occur during bone healing are complex and highly variable and depend on a number of physiological and mechanical conditions.

The repair process after fracture is characterized by at least three distinct stages: inflammation, reparation, and remodeling [4]. Similar to that of tissue wounds in general, the inflammatory phase may be the most critical. At this stage there is a particular activation of cellular mechanisms that are necessary for repair, but also for protecting the healing bone tissue from infection. During the first few days of inflammation, the injury is translated into waves of chemical messengers, such as kinins, complement factors, histamine, serotonin, and leukotrienes. The messengers mediate the inflammatory reaction by causing vasodilatation, migration, and chemoattraction, thus initiating the next step in repair. The coagulation cascade contributes fibrin. Platelets involved in the fibrin clot are critical for production and secretion of specific growth factors to initiate and control the healing process of the bone. Macrophages and, to a lesser extent, lymphocytes aid in the destruction of bacteria, but also stimulate repair by releasing angiogenesis and cell growth factors which initiate angiogenesis and mesenchymal cell proliferation [5]. The inflammatory response has a triggering role in activating a cascade of cellular mechanisms necessary for the subsequent events of repair.

The reparative phase involves a rapid cellular activity with fundamental periosteal and external soft tissue responses. Over a period of weeks early bridging callus tissue that enhances stability develops, which is essential for the biological events to proceed. Angiogenesis involves migration and proliferation of endothelial cells. This process appears to be stimulated by growth factors [6]. Hypoxia is essential for the maintenance of angiogenesis in healing tissue, and fracture callus shows low oxygen tension [7]. At this stage there is a close coupling phenomenon between osteoblastic and osteoclastic cells in the callus, and ultimately there is a remodeling phase in which reactions in the endosteum and bone marrow replace the callus tissue by bone formations. Over a period of months, then, bone is rebuilt to its original shape, depending on the physical stresses present.

Bone Ischemia

In skeletal development and healing, bone tissue differentiation is considered to be sensitive to blood supply and tissue oxygen tension. Osteogenetic precursor cells in poorly vascularized or oxygenated regions tend to develop in a chondrogenetic rather than an osteogenetic pathway, which favors fibrous healing and nonunion at the fracture site. However, the minimal metabolic demands of bone tissue do not necessitate good vascularity, and the critical dependence upon vascularity in the viciently of a fracture site is more or less unknown.

In a recent thesis [8] a model for skeletal muscle ischemia of the hindlimb in rat was developed. Ischemia was transient, and the leg was reperfused for 3 days be-

fore the animals were killed. Ischemic necrosis of the muscles could be characterized by a central zone of no resorption, an intermediate zone of resorption necrosis, and an outer zone of intact muscle fibers. The degrees of necrosis were dependent on time and temperature. This model was used to investigate the tolerance of
bone to ischemic damages after 4.5 h ischemia at 27° C [9]. Such ischemia induces about 100% necrosis of the leg muscles. In the cortical bone of the tibia there
was no visible necrosis; all the histological specimens showed living bone with
normal osteocytes in the lacunas. The histopathological changes of the osteogenetic layer were characterized by hypertrophy and hyperplasia of the cells, with differentiation into osteoblasts in the deeper part of the periosteum. This distinct cellular
response was similar to that of external callus production seen in fracture healing.
The results indicate that transient hypoxia may be a factor in initiating activation of
the periosteum. Fracture healing after complete arrest of blood flow to the leg for
4.5 h at 27° C was then studied [10]. At 6 weeks after such transient tissue
hypoxia, the animals were killed and the healing fractures were evaluated. It was
found that the repair of the ischemic bones followed the same pattern as the control
bones, at least regarding mechanical characteristics at the fracture site.

General Reactions to Bone Trauma

A skeletal trauma in the form of total hip replacement is followed by changes in the
plasma proteolytic cascade system involved in coagulation, fibrinolysis, and kallikrein–kinin production [11]. Activations of the coagulation system are found as
early as 4 h after the trauma, while the fibrinolytic and kallikrein–kinin systems
seem to be maximally engaged at 1 day after the trauma (Fig. 1 a–c). In general,

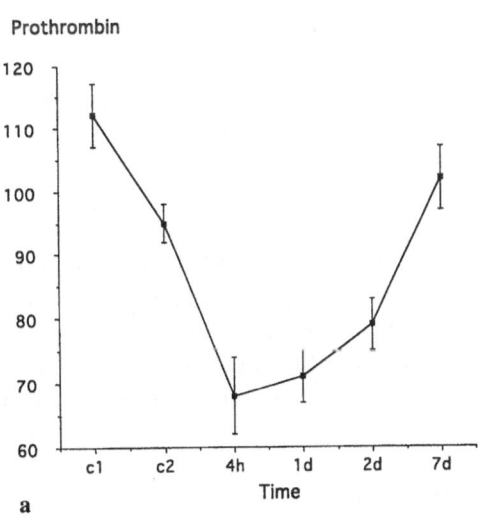

a

Fig. 1. Analyzed values of prothrombin **a**, plasminogen **b**, and prekallikrein **c** as a percentage of
standard plasma pool in patients undergoing total hip replacement. Means and standard error of the
means ($c1$, control before anesthesia; $c2$, control after anesthesia)

Plasminogen

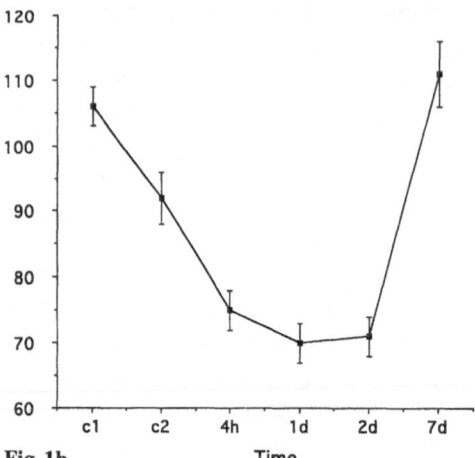

Fig. 1b

Prekallikrein

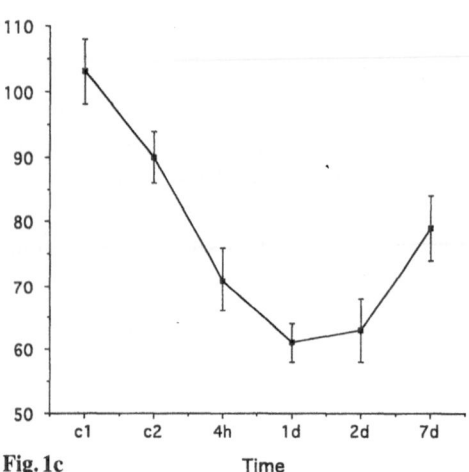

Fig. 1c

there is an imbalance towards a more thrombotic stage [12]. Furthermore, such skeletal trauma is associated with increases in concentrations of acute phase proteins and interleukins [13]. The increases in concentrations of interleukin-6 (Fig. 2) precede the changes in acute phase proteins, and there was a significant correlation between interleukin-6 and acute phase proteins. These observations reflect a possible role of interleukin-6 in the regulation of expression of acute phase protein genes in the hepatic cells in skeletal trauma situations.

Hormones

A number of hormones are important in the metabolism of the skeleton, partly by regulating calcium homeostasis and partly by direct effects on bone tissue. The

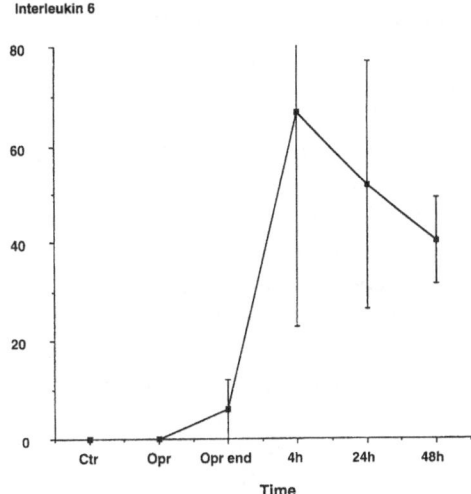

Fig. 2. Plasma concentrations (pg/ml) of interleukin-6 in patients undergoing total hip replacement. Means and standard error of the means. *Ctr,* control; *Opr,* operation

main regulators of bone metabolism are PTH and vitamin D and its metabolites. PTH has early as well as late effects on bone. The early effects occur within 1 h by release of bone minerals from the endosteal surface, while the late effects can be detected within hours by increased resorption activity of the osteoclasts [14].

Thyroid hormones are necessary for normal growth and development of the skeleton [15], but the exact mechanism by which thyroxin acts is far from clear. Calcitonin reduces the concentrations of calcium and phosphate in serum through inhibition of bone resorption. The osteoclasts are the predominant cells affected by calcitonin.

Growth hormone has general stimulatory effects on bone tissue and is necessary for the normal development of the skeleton [16]. Likewise, androgens have a general stimulatory action on bone, possibly by a direct inhibitory effect on prostaglandin E_2 production.

Estrogens act as protectors of bone against resorption by making bone more resistant to the effects of PTH and interleukin-6 [17]. The onset of menopause is associated with changes in calcium metabolism, with a negative calcium balance and loss of bone. In oophorectomized rats, loss of ovarian function caused a significant loss of trabecular bone of the tibia during 8 weeks [18]. In the cortical bone, however, there were only modest reductions at this time, and the mechanical characteristics of the tibial cortex were hardly affected. The results indicate that postmenopausal bone loss is primarily trabecular and that there is far less loss in cortical regions.

Long-term use of corticosteroids induces severe loss of bone mass. The effects of short-term use in trauma situations have therefore been questioned. In a recent study, the effects of short-term therapy with high doses of steroids were studied on the healing of femoral fractures in rats [19]. No inhibitory effects on the repair of the fractures were seen following corticosteroid treatment, neither under stable nor unstable healing conditions.

Proteins and Enzymes

In connective tissue, 11 genetically different types of collagen are known to be involved. Types I, II, I, V, IX, and X appear to be of importance for bone development and healing. During the initial stage of fracture repair, types III and V predominate [20], and at the beginning of the second week types II and IX are present. During vascularization and mineralization, synthesis of type X occurs [21]. Type I collagen is expressed at the end of the second week, when the activities of the osteoblastic and osteoclastic cells produce a granulation tissue that is mechanically competent.

At fracture sites extracellular matrix proteins are synthesized. By activation in the cell nucleus, specific messenger ribonucleic acid (mRNA) is transcribed from the genes, and proteins are translated from these mRNA templates. In the mineralization and bone formation stages of fracture healing, 17 families of noncollagenous proteins have been identified by in vivo localization studies and in vitro testing of their ability to either enhance or retard development of calcium in a matrix system [22]. Furthermore, different enzymes and their inhibitors, primarily alkaline phosphatases, metalloproteinases, and tissue inhibitors of metalloproteinases, are involved. Structural proteins lay the foundation of fracture callus tissue, and the enzymes catalyze the transformation of the tissue. Growth factors and cytokines may further regulate the development of these processes.

Growth Factors

Bone cells produce substantial quantities of growth factors. These may have acute effects on the osteoblasts in an autocrine manner, they can act on the cells in the near vicinity in a paracrine manner, or they are stored in the matrix by binding proteins that have a strong affinity for hydroxylapatite [23–25]. Bone matrix, then, may be considered a storehouse for growth factors. In bone, growth factors may provide an efficient autoregulatory feedback system to modulate metabolism by different biological actions.

According to their main biological action, growth factors can be classified as competence factors, progression factors, mitogenic factors, or differentiation factors [26]. Platelet-derived growth factor (PDGF) and fibroblast-derived growth factor (FDGF) are involved in cell cycle regulation in the initial stages of bone healing. These factors make the mesenchymal cells competent to respond to other growth factors, for instance progression factors such as transforming growth factor (TGF)-β which commits the cells to replicate. The mitogenic factors such as epidermal growth factor (EGF), insulin-like growth factor (IGF) I and II as well as FGF, PDGF, and TGF-β maintains the dividing cells in a proliferative state. Finally, other members of the TGF-β family act as differentiation factors on proliferating pluripotent stem cells. In this way they are stimulated to mature and differentiate into the various specialized cell types involved in bone healing.

Since multiple growth factors are contained in bone matrix, an interaction between these on cell proliferation and differentiation in bone tissue has been suggested. In vitro studies in cultures of bone cells have shown that IGF interacts synergistically with FGF and TGF-β [27]. Similarly, a synergistic interaction between TGF-β and FGF has been reported for isolated bone cells [28]. Furthermore, there is evidence to suggest an interdependence of growth factors and anabolic/catabolic hormones in a self-regulating network of bone homeostasis. PTH causes release of IGF, and these then feed back to inhibit the bone-resorbing effects of PTH [29]. A common pathway in the coupling of both resorption and formation of bone, then, appears to be induction of IGF production, stimulated by both PTH and prostaglandins.

The exact physiological significance of growth factors in the modulation of bone cell proliferation and differentiation in local milieus remains to be determined, however. In vitro studies indicate that they might induce periosteal cell proliferation, and exogenous administration indicates periosteal cell mitogenesis in vivo [30]. Since exogenous growth factors result in callus enlargement by modifying cell proliferation and differentiation, growth factors may modulate the fracture repair process. In a recent study we postulated that growth factors might improve the healing of fractures under instable conditions [31]. Local medication with platelet extract containing different growth factors such as PDGF and TGF-β as well as monoclonal antibodies to PDGF were applied to healing femoral fractures in rats. The effects were evaluated 6 weeks after fracture. As compared to the control group, there were no improvements in fracture healing in the rats given platelet extracts. Treatment with anti-PDGF, however, significantly improved bone healing. These results might indicate that trauma situations such as bone fractures give rise to an overshoot of endogenously locally produced growth factors, resulting in excessive formation of granulation tissue and fibrogenesis without time-related osteogenetic potential. Additional exogenous administration of growth factors locally at the fracture site appears to be unnecessary. However, when the growth factors are reduced or modulated by antibodies, a level of expression may be obtained that is more optimal for a proper osteogenetic healing response.

Cytokines

Cytokines are postulated to be of importance as mediators in bone metabolism and remodeling [26, 32, 33]. The central role of interleukin-1 (IL-1) in mediating pathological processes, especially inflammation and the acute phase response, is well known. Osteoblastic cells produce interleukin-1, suggesting an autocrine/paracrine function of IL-1 in bone tissue [34]. This cytokine has biphasic effects on bone formation, i.e., it is a potent stimulator of bone resorption and, under certain conditions, it can stimulate bone formation [35]. It has been shown that IL-1 synergizes its bone-resorbing activity with PTH [36]. The effects of IL-1 on osteoblastic cells have in part been attributed to the stimulation of prostaglandin formation in a dose-dependent manner, especially the E type [37], and modulation of gene expression of several proteins.

Tumor necrosis factor (TNF) acts on bone in a similar fashion to IL-1, with increased mitogenesis and stimulation of resorption [38, 39]. TNF is a potent stimulator of osteoclastic recruitment, proliferation, and activity [40]. It has been suggested that IL-1 and TNF act in a synergistic way under certain conditions [39].

Interleukin-6 is assumed to be an important mediator of systemic effects to local inflammatory events [39]. IL-6 can stimulate the production of IL-1, and it has been suggested that IL-6 has important overlapping activities with IL-1 and TNF [39]. It is felt that IL-1 and TNF may depend on IL-6 to exert their bone-resorbing activities [41]. IL-6, then, may be a central factor involved in cytokine-mediated bone resorption, but further information is needed to clarify this.

Cytokines have not been shown to be directly implicated in the regulation of fracture healing, but cell types resident in the fracture callus are known to secrete and respond to specific cytokines. IL-1 and -6 actively participate in the regulation of fracture callus matrix synthesis and its subsequent degradation during the healing stages. In fracture callus organ cultures, levels of IL-1 and IL-6 expression have been identified, and the peak time of expression of IL-1 in fracture callus organ cultures is identical to that for metalloendoproteinase activity [42]. This indicates that IL-1 may induce metalloproteinase activity at the most critical stages of the healing process. Furthermore, IL-1 and IL-6 play a role in the replication of extracellular matrix of connective tissue, and IL-1 stimulates the production of collagenase and proteoglycanase [26, 43].

Prostaglandins

Several stimulators, including neural, inflammatory, anaphylactic, hormonal, and mechanical stimuli, induce the release of prostaglandins [44]. Mechanical stimuli may be of special importance in the response of the skeleton to mechanical forces. Prostaglandins are not stored, and their site of action is therefore at or near their site of synthesis. Thus they must be considered local hormones [45]. The release of prostaglandins by bone has been known for years, but the differential roles on the distinct bone cells, osteoblasts, osteocytes, and osteoclasts remain relatively unexplored. The prostaglandins may act as biphasic mediators of bone metabolism and homeostasis; in certain doses they stimulate bone formation, while at other concentrations they stimulate bone resorption [46]. The resorptive activity of the prostaglandins is associated with their ability to induce osteoclastic differentiation [47]. Prostaglandins of the E type are the most effective stimulators of bone resorption, but a prolonged exposure of bone to prostaglandins is required.

Under certain circumstances prostaglandins induce bone formation. In vitro bone collagen production is altered by adding prostaglandin E, and bone remodeling induced by physical stress has been shown to be mediated by prostaglandin E_2 [48]. Furthermore, exogenously added prostaglandins have been found to stimulate bone formation, both in vitro and in vivo, but this seems to be dependent on the presence of cortisol [49]. At physiological concentrations of cortisol, prostaglandins stimulate type I collagen synthesis in bone tissue. Bone formation effects of prostaglandins may also be attributed to increased production of cyclic adenosine monophosphate (AMP), which in turn stimulates the production of IGF-1 [50].

Prostaglandins have both pro- and anti-inflammatory actions, and they are released locally from bone and surrounding soft tissues during the immediate postfracture period [51]. The in vivo effects of prostaglandins on fracture repair are somewhat mixed, but in general appear to favor healing. In rats treated systematically with anti-inflammatory drugs which inhibit prostaglandin synthesis, such as indomethacin, fracture repair is significantly delayed [52]. On the other hand, prostaglandins administered to the periosteum have been shown to enhance periosteal callus formation [53].

Macrophages

Much attention has been paid to the role of macrophages in wound healing of soft tissues, but there is less information available on their role in bone healing. The reported effects of macrophages in soft tissue wounds include increased fibroblastic collagen synthesis, increased collagen synthesis, increased collagen cross-linking, stimulation of angiogenesis, and improved wound strength [54]. These effects have been attributed to the production of IL-1 by macrophages [55]. By this mechanism macrophages also might influence bone tissue.

Macrophages have been identified in fractures, and their presence in the early stages of repair has been suggested to be of importance in laying down the groundwork for the healing events to proceed [56]. Furthermore, we postulated that stimulation of macrophages might enhance the acute inflammatory response in fracture healing [57], possibly through the release of humoral factors, especially IL-1 and prostaglandin E_2, effects that might be opposite to those of anti-inflammatory drugs. This hypothesis was studied in fractured femoral bones in rats. The animals were subjected to aminated glucan, which is known to stimulate the macrophages. Groups of animals were killed at 4, 8, and 12 weeks after fracture. At each time interval, it appeared that stimulation of the macrophages induced a hypertrophic and immature callus response that caused a negative effect on the fracture repair. The effects were more pronounced by local than by systemic activation of the macrophages.

Conclusion

There is little exact knowledge of the role of bone in catabolic situations, either as an effector or affector organ. As bone tissue may be considered a storehouse for growth factors, bone injury may cause the release of significant amounts of these factors, which may act in concert with the systemic metabolic changes following trauma. Bone seems to tolerate severe ischemic injury better than any other tissues. Bone repair is characterized by a cascade of cellular and biochemical events in which there are several requirements for a well-balanced development. Both systemic and local factors may influence the processes. Theoretically, different interventions might be used to enhance the cascade events. Recognizing the proper cell mediators and the physical means to stimulate these may develop therapeutic strategies to increase precursor elements. Control of macrophage function and production of chemoattractant substances for endothelial cells may help to promote angiogenesis and cell proliferation. Furthermore, as bone cells produce and respond to different growth factors, these may be used systemically or locally as therapeutic agents to modulate bone healing.

References

1. Wilmore DW (1977) The metabolic management of the critically ill. Plenum, New York
2. Mgiuid MM, Brennan, Aoki TT, Muller WA, Ball MR, Moore FD (1974) Hormone-substrate interrelationship following trauma. Arch Surg 109:776–783
3. Frost HM (1963) Bone remodeling dynamics. Thomas, Springfield
4. McKibbin B (1978) The biology of fracture healing in long bones. J Bone Joint Surg [Br] 60:105–162
5. Hunt TK (1984) Can repair processes be stimulated by modulators without adversely affecting normal processes? J Trauma 24:S39–S46
6. Glaser BM, D'Amore PA, Seppa H, Schiffmann E (1980) Adult tissues contain chemoattractants for vascular endothelial cells. Nature 288:483–484
7. Heppenstad RB, Grislis G, Hunt TK (1975) Tissue gas oxygen consumption in healing bone defects. Clin Orthop 106:357–365
8. Skjeldal S (1994) Acute skeletal muscle ischemia. Microcirculation and histological changes in rat hindlimbs. Thesis, University of Oslo
9. Skjeldal S, Svindland A, Nordsletten L, Kase T, Torvik A, Reikeras O (1993) Tourniquet ischemia induces periosteal hyperplasia in the rat tibia. Trans Scand Orthop Res Soc 1:11 (abstract)
10. Kase T, Skjeldal S, Nordsletten L, Reikeras O (1993) Healing of tibial fractures after acute ischemia in the rat hindlimb. Trans Scand Orthop Res Soc 1:10 (abstract)
11. Hogevold HE, Aasen AO, Kierulf P, Garred P, Mollnes TE, Reikeras O (1989) High dose of corticosteroids in total hip replacement. Effects on components of coagulation, fibrinolytic, plasma kallikrein-kinin and complement systems. Acta Chir Scand 155:247–250
12. Hogevold HE, Lyberg T, Kierulf P, Reikeras O (1991) Generation of procoagulant (thromboplastin) and plasminogen activation activities in peripheral blood monocytes after total hip replacement surgery. Effects of high doses of corticosteroids. Thromb Res 62:449–457
13. Hogevold HE, Kierulf P, Ovstebo R, Reikeras O (1992) Acute phase reactants and interleukin 6 after total hip replacement. Effects of high dose corticosteroids. Eur J Surg 158:339–345
14. Rosenblatt M, Kroneneberg HM, Potts JT (1989) Parathyroid hormone: physiology, chemistry, biosynthesis, secretion, metabolism and mode of action. In: DeGroot LJ et al. (eds) Endocrinology, vol 2. Grune and Stratton, New York, pp 848–891
15. Adams PH (1979) Calcium regulating hormones: general. In: Nordin BEC (ed) Human nutritional reviews: calcium in human biology. Springer, Berlin Heidelberg New York, pp 68–91
16. Isaksson OGP, Edens S, Jansson JO (1985) Mode of action of pituitary growth hormone on target cells. Annu Rev Physiol 47:483–499
17. Jilka RL, Hangoc G, Girasole G, Passeri G, Williams D, Abrams JS, Boyce B, Broxmeyer H, Manolagas SC (1992) Increased osteoblast development after estrogen loss: mediation by interleukin-6. Science 257:88–91
18. Kaastad TS, Reikeras O, Narum S, Madsen JE, Haug E, Obrand KJ, Nordsletten L (1993) Intensive training of oophorectomized rats does not affect the in vivo structural strength of the lower leg during muscle contraction (Abstr). Trans Nor Surg Soc 157
19. Hogevold HE, Grogaard B, Reikeras O (1992) Effect of short-term treatment with corticosteroids and indomethacin on bone healing. A mechanical study of osteotomies in rats. Acta Orthop Scand 63:607–611
20. Mueller-Glauser W, Hunbel B, Glatt M, Straeuli P, Winterhalter KH, Bruckner P (1986) On the role of type IX collagen in the extracellular matrix of cartilage: type IX collagen is localized to intersections of collagen fibrils. J Cell Biol 102:1931–1939

21. Grant WT, Wang GJ, Balian G (1987) Type X collagen synthesis during enchondral ossification. J Biol Chem 262:9844–9849
22. Boskey AL (1989) Noncollagenous matrix proteins and their role in meralization. Bone Miner 6:111–123
23. Canalis E, McCarthy T, Centrella M (1988) Growth factors and the regulation of bone remodeling. J Clin Invest 81:277–285
24. Linkhart TA, Mohans S, Jennings JC, Farley JR, Baylink DJ (1984) Skeletal growth factors. In: Li CH (ed) Hormonal proteins and peptides. Academic, New York, pp 279–296
25. Urist MR, De Lange RJ, Finermann GAM (1983) Bone cell differentiation and growth factors. Science 220:680–689
26. Goldring MR, Goldring SR (1990) Skeletal tissue response to cytokines. Clin Orthop 258:245–278
27. Kasperk C, Wergedal JE, Mohan S, Long DL, Lau KHW, Baylink DJ (1990) Interaction of growth factors present in bone matrix and bone cells: effects on DNA synthesis and alkaline phosphatase. Growth Factors 3:147–155
28. Globus RK, Patterson-Buckendahl P, Gospopdarowicz D (1988) Regulation of bovine bone cells synthesize basic fibroblast growth factor and transforming growth factor beta. Endocrinology 123:98–105
29. McCarthy TL, Centrella M, Raisz LG, Canalis E (1989) Parathyroid hormone enhances the transcript and polypeptide levels of insulin-like growth factor 1 in osteoblasts-enriched cultures from fetal rat bone. Endocrinology 124:1247–1254
30. Joyce ME, Jinguish S, Roberts SA, Sporn MB, Bolander ME (1989) Transforming growth factor beta initiates cartilage and bone formation in vivo. J Bone Miner Res 4:S259–S265
31. Hogevold HE, Grogaard B, Reikeras O (1994) Local treatment with platelet extract and anti-PDGF in fracture healing in rats. Eur J Exp Musculoskel Res 3 (in press)
32. Kennedy RL, Jones TH (1991) Cytokines in endocrinology: their roles in health and in disease. J Endocrinol 129:167–178
33. Rodan GA (1992) Introduction to bone biology. Bone 13:53–56
34. Hanazawa S, Amano S, Nakuda K, Ohmori Y, Miyoshi T, Hirose K, Kitano S (1987) Biological characterization of interleukin-1 cytokine produced by cultured bone cells from newborn mice calvaria. Calcif Tissue Int 41:31–37
35. Gowen M, Mundy GR (1986) Actions of recombinant interleukin-1, interleukin-2 and interferon gamma on bone resorption in vitro. J Immunol 136:2478–2482
36. Dewhirst FA, Age JM, Peros WJ, Stashenko P (1987) Synergism between parathyroid hormone and interleukin-1 in stimulating bone resorption in organ culture. J Bone Miner Res 2:127–134
37. Klein-Nulend J, Pilbeam CC, Harrison JR, Fall PM, Raisz LG (1991) Mechanism of regulation of prostaglandin production by parathyroid hormone, interleukin-1 and cortisol in cultured mouse parietal bone. Endocrinology 128:2503–2510
38. Bertolini DR, Nedwin GE, Bringman TS, Smith DD, Mundy GR (1986) Stimulation of bone resorption and inhibition of bone formation in vitro by human tumor necrosis factor. Nature 319:516–518
39. Russell RGG (1990) Bone cell biology: the role of cytokines and other mediators. In: Smith R (ed) Osteoporosis. Royal College of Physicians, London, pp 9–33
40. Thompson BM, Mundy GR, Chambers TJ (1987) Tumor necrosis factors alpha and beta induce osteoblastic cells to stimulate osteoclastic bone resorption. J Immunol 138:775–779
41. Mundy GR (1991) Mechanism of osteolytic bone destruction. Bone 12:S1–S6
42. Einthorn TA, Majeska RJ, Bosch CG, Rusch EB, Horowitz MC (1991) The production of cytokines by fracture (Abstr). Trans Orthop Res Soc 16:117
43. Gowen M, Wood DD, Ihrie EJ, Meats JE, Russel GG (1984) Stimulation by human interleukin-1 of cartilage breakdown and production of collagenase and proteoglycase by human chondrocytes, but not by human osteoblasts in vitro. Biochim Biophys Acta 797:186–193
44. Flower RJ, Blackwell GJ (1976) The importance of phospholipase A2 in prostaglandin biosynthesis. Biochem Pharmacol 25:285–291
45. Zor V, Lamprecht SA (1977) Mechanism of prostaglandin action in endocrine glands. Biochem Actions Horm 4:85–133

46. Raisz LG, Fall PM (1990) Biphasic effects of prostaglandin E2 on bone formation in cultured fetal rat calvariae: interaction with cortisol. Endocrinology 126:1654–1659
47. Collis DA, Chambers TJ (1991) Effect of prostaglandins E1, E2 and F2 alpha on osteoclast formation in mouse bone marrow cultures. J Bone Miner Res 6:157–164
48. Crawford A, Atkins D, Martin TJ (1978) Rat osteogenetic sarcoma cells: comparisons of the effect of prostaglandins E1, E2, I2, 6 keto F1 and thromboxane B2 and cyclic AMP production and adenyl cyclase activity. Biochem Biophys Res Commun 82:1195–1201
49. Somsen D, Binderman I, Berger EI, Havell A (1980) Bone remodeling induced by physical stress is PGE2 mediated. Biochem Biophys Acta 267:91–100
50. McCarthy TL, Centrella M, Raisz LG, Canalis E (1991) Prostaglandin E2 stimulates insulin-like growth factor 1 synthesis in osteoblast enriched cultures from fetal rat bone. Endocrinology 128:2895–2900
51. Dekel S, Lenthall G, Francis MJO (1981) Release of prostaglandins from bone and muscle after tibial fracture. An experimental study in rabbits. J Bone Joint Surg [Br] 63:185–189
52. Hogevold HE, Gragaard B, Reikeras O (1993) The effects of short-term and long-term treatment with indomethacin on primary and secondary fracture healing in rats. Eur J Exp Musculoskel Res 2:3–8
53. Norrin RW, Jee WSS, High WB (1990) The role of prostaglandins in bone in vivo. Prostaglandins Leuko Essent Fatty Acids 41:139–149
54. Browder W, Williams D, Lucore P, Pretus H, Jones E, Mc Namee R (1988) Effect of enhanced macrophage function on early wound healing. Surgery 104:224–230
55. Schmidt JA, Mizel SB, Cohen D, Green I (1982) Interleukin-1, a potential regulator of fibroblast proliferation. J Immunol 128:2177–2182
56. Horowitz MC, Coleman DL, Ryaby JT, Einthorn TA (1989) Osteotropic agents induce the differential secretion of granulocyte-macrophage colony-stimulating factor by the osteoblast cell line MC3T3-E1. J Bone Miner Res 4:911–921
57. Reikeras O, Grundnes O, Seljelid R (1993) The effects of macrophage activation on bone healing (Abstr). Trans Eur Orthop Res Soc 3:79

Catabolism and Tumor – Could a General Catabolic Reaction Be Useful in Treatment of Solid Tumors?

K.-E. Giercksky and H. Qvist

Introduction

Treatment of cancer, the disease complex due to uncontrolled tissue growth, is in urgent need for more effective therapeutic modalities. An increasing population age combined with successful development of treatments against a number of important infectious diseases have moved cancer to the forefront of human health problems in developed countries. Tremendous efforts have been made in "the war against cancer," but an improvement in cure rates comparable to those of most infectious diseases has not materialized. On the other hand, allocation of resources to basic and clinical research has provided extremely important knowledge of the molecular basis for the development of malignant cells and general cellular biology.

The demonstration of oncogenes and tumor suppressor genes as normal contents of the human genome fortified the hypothesis of "multiple hits" in development of cancer. The tricky question of why a normal cell should harbor genes with such a disasterous potential was answered when oncogenes were found to be mutated forms of genes, so-called proto-oncogenes, with important functions during development, growth, and repair processes. Tumor suppressor genes inhibit cancer development because their protein products among other things also have a key role in the control of replication fidelity [1]. The development of a malignant cell type is today presumed to be due to a number of viable mutations within proto-oncogenes leading to uncontrolled growth and disturbed maturation and apoptosis. This process is greatly facilitated by the lack of replication fidelity induced by mutated or absent tumor suppressor gene products [2].

The treatment problems in the majority of clinical cases are not posed by the primary malignant tumor but by the metastases. Modern surgery is usually capable of handling most primary tumors regardless of size and localization, but it lacks the biological potential to treat disseminated disease. Not all tumors will give rise to metastases. It is now believed that the capability to settle down in other organs and develop new tumors is independent of the malignant transformation itself, needing further mutations but being closely linked to malignant cells due to their unstable genome. Following this putative order of events, a number of malignant cells will not be able to metastasize even if they have access to blood or lymphatic vessels. Indeed, in a significant number of clinical cases of solid tumors, finding tumor cells in circulating blood does not correlate well with the development of metastatic disease [3].

A biologically important differentiation between the development of malignant growth and metastasis is good news for surgeons as well as for all other disciplines engaged in cancer treatment, because at least outlines of potential new therapeutic targets appear. Prophylaxis against all forms of malignant development is not a realistic target. Early removal or destruction of the main tumor combined with an effective inhibition or killing of metastatic cells seems to be a more realistic strategy to improve survival for cancer patients. This should be the rationale behind the much touted "multimodal cancer treatment."

Can Catabolism Be a Part of Multimodal Cancer Treatment?

The catabolic state is characterized by severe disturbancies of tissue metabolism and is a general reaction to trauma and infection. Over a limited timespan (days) it may be an efficient reactive pattern for securing necessary substrate for vital organs and biochemical reactions, but prolonged catabolism (weeks or months) will lead to impaired organ functions and eventually death of the organism.

Catabolism is often followed by injuries to tissues with a high turnover rate (such as small-bowel mucosa) and could therefore also be hostile to rapidly growing tumor tissue. This assumption seems to be considerably oversimplified, as it is difficult to draw a distinction between the direct effect on tumor tissue of catabolic inducers and the effect of a general catabolic state. This distinction would, of course, not be of great practical importance if solid evidence for tumor or metastatic regression was evident. As long as such evidence is at best only cursory and highly unpredictable, mechanisms that can be further developed have to be discovered.

The dearrangement of substrate due to rapid resolution of certain tissue and increased production of certain proteins (the acute phase reaction) might deprivate tumor cells of some essential nutrients. Even though the malignant cells have undergone a series of mutations which is likely to have influenced their metabolic pathways, it is very unlikely that such cells are superior to normal cells in every metabolic aspect, even if their genotype has let them escape normal growth control. Cancer cells are often classified as immortal, which is an exaggeration. The malignant cells themselves are not immortal. They have growth patterns, maturation, and organizations that are different from their normal progenitors, but after a number of cell cycles they will die. However, before death they will have divided a number of times and given life to more cells that are organized into highly irregular and infiltrating structures. If cancer cells are deprived of nutritious substrate and oxygen, they will die just as any other tissue cells do. The expression "immortal cells" is derived from their ability to keep their progeny going in cell cultures, i.e., although the cancer cells themselves are certainly not immortal, their cell line is. Two of the main general cancer treatment modalities, radiation and chemotherapy, are actually based on increased vulnerability of cancer cells compared to their normal counterparts.

So far starvation of the host has not led to a clinically significant reduction in tumor growth. The autonomous nature of malignant growth often results in continuous tumor expansion with even less substrate available to normal cells and increased deterioration of the host. Molecular biology has provided new and important insights into the mechanisms of the catabolic reaction to different stimuli. Tumor necrosis factor/cachectin (TNF) and interleukins (IL-1 and IL-6) are important early participants that can be blocked, inhibited, or injected to study their different roles in the process. More or less well founded expectations of their possible antitumor effects, based on cell culture and animal studies, led to clinical trials with these substances either alone or in combination with other so-called biological response modifiers (BRM) such as interferons and IL-2 [4]. In spite of some highly encouraging clinical pilot studies, their general potential for increasing the cure rate of most solid tumors has not materialized [5]. These clinical trials, however, have amply demonstrated their ability to induce a severe catabolic reaction leading to serious side effects and even lethal complications [6]. Other BRM participants of the catabolic reaction are being isolated and made available for experimental and clinical studies at an impressive speed. The numerous putative combinations and dosages of different BRM may result in future discoveries of important antitumor effects. This line of research has not yet been exhausted, but needs some serious strategic refinement instead of a seemingly endless number of crude, time-consuming, and exprensive clinical trials unable to answer decisive questions.

Is the Antitumor Effect of Catabolic Inducers Dependent on General or Local Mechanisms?

Interest in the catabolic reaction is due to the long-standing claim that certain cancer patients who developed concurrent bacterial infections would also experience concomitant remissions of their malignant disease. Fever was at one time regarded as the important part of this general catabolic reaction and was ingenuously imitated by means as different as injections of mixtures of milk and blood, malaria parasites, and crude bacterial toxins [7]. There is actually a number of ancient reports containing evidence of tumor regression in the course of a general infection, the most frequent combination reported being erysipelas in sarcoma patients [8].

The New York surgeon William B. Coley found such a case and became deeply interested in the possibilities of using bacteria in cancer treatment. Considering the almost nonexistent knowledge of BRM at that time and limited biochemical resources, it is remarkable how he managed to make such intricate observations and even achieve clinical results that are not without interest today [8]. Being a practical man, he tried to reproduce his observations in a stepwise fashion. After visiting various libraries and finding a substantial number of publications reporting corresponding observations, he carefully began a deliberate induction of erysipelas, using live bacteria, in some of his cancer patients. (Critics of such a direct approach involving patients should remember that suitable animal models and transformed cell lines were not available and efficient chemotherapy for cancer was virtually nonexistent). Using at first this crude and direct approach, he actually managed to achieve complete tumor regression in a few patients, but also found that erysipelas was sometimes difficult to induce and, when successfully induced, difficult to control in a preantibiotic era. In 1892, using a heat-killed version of the bacteria com-

Table 1. Summary of patients treated with Coley's toxin before 1940

Type of cancer	Total patients (n)	Group (n)				
		A	B	C	D	E
Soft tissue sarcomas	104	38	12	17	15	22
Lymphosarcomas (lymphomas)	50	24	7	4	7	8
Osteosarcoma	3	2	1	0	0	0
Ovarian carcinoma	4	1	2	0	0	1
Cervical carcinoma	2	0	1	0	0	1
Testicular	18	10	2	3	2	1
Renal	6	3	0	1	1	1
Multiple myeloma	1	0	0	1	0	0
Colorectal carcinoma	2	1	1	0	0	0
Breast carcinoma	14	8	4	2	0	0
Melanoma	6	2	3	0	1	0

Evaluation was restricted to those patients considered inoperable at the time of treatment who had received no therapy other than the vaccine. Group A, patients with no beneficial response to treatment; B, those with an initial response but either known to relapse or lost to follow-up at 5 years; C, those rendered free of disease but lost to follow-up between 5 and 10 years; D, those rendered free of disease but lost to follow-up between 10 and 20 years; E, those rendered free of clinical evidence of disease for at least 20 years. (Source of data is a series of articles by H. C. Nauts and G. A. Flower in the *Cancer Research Institute Monograph* between 1969 and 1975. From [8])

bined with *Serratia marcescens,* he solved the problem of controlling a dangerous infection and achieved a more reproducible reaction in the patients.

The combination of gram-positive heat-killed *Streptococcus* and gram-negative heat-killed *S. marcescens* is referred to as "Coley's toxin." The clinical description of symptoms following injection of Coley's toxin includes a typical catabolic state with shaking shills and fever. No metabolic studies were done on these patients 100 years ago, but the clinical reaction was almost identical to that described and carefully combined with metabolic investigations and studies of BRM using purified endotoxin a century later by Mitchie et al. [9]. It should be remembered that Coley's toxin was given daily for weeks and sometimes months compared to the usual one-injection studies of endotoxin today. The results of using Coley's toxin are shown in Table 1. Two things are obvious from the survey: a successful antitumor effect was more common in tumors of mesodermal origin (sarcomas) than in epithelial cancers, and given the disseminated state of the disease some of the results are indeed remarkable. Daily injections of Coley's toxin must have led to a severe and prolonged catabolic state, and the results could be taken as evidence for a general antitumor effect of catabolism. After Coley's death in 1936, clinical interest in his toxin treatment more or less vanished due to the advent of modern radiotherapy and chemotherapy. (In retrospect and considering the comparatively small number of toxin-treated patients, radiotherapy and chemotherapy have not convincingly given superior results).

Other lines of research do not support general catabolism as the most important active antitumor principle in Coley's toxin:

1. Injection of foreign material results in a complex immune reaction, and repeated injections lead to the production of neutralizing antibodies in the majority of patients; the effect and symptoms taper off just as described by Coley. Production of such antibodies is a slow and complicated process, involving different subsets of lymphocytes and antigen-presenting cells. Some bacteria and their toxins are able to circumvent this slow and gradual process and activate subsets of killer cells directly by so-called superantigens. The best-known source of superantigen is streptococcus, and today this method of inducing killer cell attack on experimental tumors is considered to be of major importance [10]. Indeed, one major pharmaceutical company has just started a clinical trial in patients based on this principle. Toxin-induced production of BRM with or without superantigen, and not the induction of catabolism, seems to be an alternative explanation of the effect of Coley's toxin.
2. TNF is central to the development of catabolism, but cancer treatment with TNF either alone or in combination with other BRM has given disappointing tumor effect (but severe catabolism) when given intravenously (systemic therapy); the tumor effect markedly improved when high local concentrations were achieved. Such localizing treatment has been carried out with regional perfusion (with minimal systemic overflow and symptoms of catabolism) or tumor-seeking TNF-producing cells using gene therapy, monoclonal antibodies, or tumor-infiltrating host cells. The results following isolated limb perfusion with TNF in the treatment of regional metastases from melanoma have been very promising and considerably more efficient than systemic TNF treatment [11].

Even if no definite conclusion can be drawn from such indirect lines of evidence, they lend considerable support to the hypothesis that the inducers and reactants of catabolism represent the effectors of the antitumor activity and not the catabolic derangement of nutritional substrates. This does not mean that the mechanisms for the tumor regression sometimes observed during catabolic situations are fully understood. It is possible that inducers of catabolism such as Coley's toxin contain uncharacterized substances with direct or indirect effects on malignant cells. The molecular understanding of catabolic induction as well as its local counterpart, inflammation, is far from complete, and important reactants are regularly being discovered. The recent cloning of IL-12 and the demonstration of its in vitro effect on tumor cells rapidly led to approval for its inclusion in clinical trials starting this year.

Search for Specific Endogenous Anticancer Defense Mechanisms: From Holy Grails to Foreign Bodies

The discovery of specific endogenous human defense reactions to tumors has been the ultimate challenge to cancer immunology. After characterizing such putative reactions, escalation and strengthening of specific mechanisms would seem to be a more trivial task. This would certainly change and improve our strategy of cancer treatment, driving the field away from distinctly harmful and unpleasant radiation and chemotherapy regimens towards treatment that is highly specific for malignant cells, leaving normal tissue unharmed. Because of its enormous economic potential and its easily advocated and intellectually inspiring principles, funding and recruitment for this research have been easily obtained. This has given the field of biology an enormous boost, rapidly expanding our knowledge of both general and tumor immunology. There is no reason to doubt that this has had important consequences for both the understanding and treatment of a number of diseases (including a small number of rare cancers), but specific endogenous cancer defense mechanisms are still shrouded in mist. There could be two reasons for this: either the specific endogenous cancer defense mechanism is based on principles that elude detection with our present state of methods or it simply does not exist. At first glance it would seem unlikely that man should lack host defense mechanisms against cancer when we are equipped with complex and effective defense mechanisms against far more trivial problems.

The development of elaborate and costly vital mechanisms is inevitably governed by the general rules of evolution, with its driving force being random mutation and its directional force positive selection. For man to have obtained a specific defense mechanism against malignant tumors, cancer must have represented a significant evolution pressure. We believe that cancer as a population problem does not represent a strong stimulus for evolutionary changes. Cancer is mainly a disease of the elderly. There is a small but significant peak in childhood compared to adolescence, but the overwhelming number of symptomatic cancer patients are not in the reproductive age. The incidence of childhood and adolescent cancer is low and almost insignificant when compared to the frequency of serious diseases due to virus, bacteria, and parasites experienced within the time frame of human evolution. It is only because of the advent of effective anti-infectious therapy and the rapid increase in the average life-expectancy of humans that cancer now plays a major part in health problems. The fundamental changes in longevity and effective treatment of infections have taken place within a century and therefore have had no evolutionary impact.

This does not mean that man is unable to react to a growing tumor, as can be seen in any hospital ward, but the reaction is not highly specific or very effective. Instead of a specific cancer defense mechanism, we believe that the organism reacts to a growing tumor using parts of its well-established anti-infectious and inflammation mechanisms. This is not an exceptional biological strategy. A complex organ or defense reaction is not created de novo out of the blue, but slowly develops from modifications of already existing or duplicated genes. Duplicated genes or ones that are no longer necessary can, following mutation, be used for new purposes, but their homology will give their origin away, as recently illustrated by Ulevitch for a MAP kinase targeted by endotoxin and now an important part of the infectious host defense reaction. The origin of the gene is convincingly demonstrated in yeast, in which it serves as part of the single cell's defense against potentially lethal changes in the surrounding osmolarity [12].

Depending on the degree of nonself interpretation by the host, the reaction to growing tumors varies from a simple, foreign body reaction (no antigenes recognized) to a full-blown catabolic reaction with increased temperature and rapid weight loss when tumor cells are interpreted as virulent introducers (antigene cross-reaction).

The unstructured growth of tumors with more or less uncoordinated relations between nonparenchymal support tissue (e.g., blood vessels, nerves, fibroblasts) frequently leads to partial tumor necrosis. Such tissue necrosis is a strong stimulus for inflammatory reactions compared to the controlled cell death of apoptosis in the life cycle of normal tissue cells in which no inflammatory reaction can be found. The principal reactions to a growing tumor in man are based on variations within the inflammatory host defense reactive system dependent upon the degree of non-self within the tumor cell population and the degree of tumor necrosis.

If No Specific Endogenous Tumor Defense Mechanism Exists, Why Does Not Everyone Get Cancer?

It is mandatory to understand the difference between transformation of a normal cell into a potentially malignant cell and the growth of a malignant tumor, because the all-important endogenous prophylaxis against cancer is based on the fidelity of DNA replication. Elaborate exclusion and repair mechanisms of faulty replication have been developed in the evolution from a RNA world to a DNA world. In the human genome, an infidelity factor of 10^{-9} has been estimated [13]. DNA replication in man is an astonishing feat of perfection with only a minuscle failure rate. Even if they are very small due to the large number of replications in multicellular organisms, these mutations are the reasons for the origin of malignant cells (the frequency of faulty replication can be considerably increased by external stimuli such as radiation, carcinogens, and inherited or acquired defects in control genes). Why is there not a 100% efficient fidelity mechanism? The small error in fidelity of DNA has an all-important task, being the molecular basis of random mutation and therefore the driving force of evolution and adjustment. Sexual reproduction is merely an accelerator or promotor of this process. Without mutations, the same genetic blueprints would only be endlessly reshuffled, giving rise to a large but fixed number of combinations. This is no longer an esoteric hypothesis entertained by molecular evolutionists, but can be experimentally tested under controlled conditions, as recently demonstrated using so-called sexual polymerase chain reaction [14]. We postulate that man does not have a very effective endogenous defense mechanism against a growing tumor, but the control and defense mechanisms against the malignant transformation of normal cells are indeed impressive and very efficient.

It can, of course, be argued that DNA replication fidelity is our specific tumor defense mechanism. Given the general nature of repair and exclusion mechanisms following faulty replication, it seems to us better classified as a global control mechanism against possible harmful and nonviable cells than a specific antitumor mechanism. Semantics aside, the implications for the treatment of cancer patients would be that endogenous prophylaxis is highly effective and directed towards avoiding potentially carcinogenic mutations. Endogenous treatment against established, symptomatic tumors is lacking or conspicuously ineffective. The sporadic appearance of tumors is the result of unrepaired changes in the genes (usually in genes with growth and signal functions), resulting in clones with a local growth advantage in that organism only.

It should be remembered that most mutations lead to serious defects and an early cell death. Cancerogenic mutations may be regarded as successful mutations for the cell, but due to their disturbance of the body as a whole they do not represent an advantage in terms of increased production of offspring and survival and ultimately lead to the death of the organism, making the process self-limiting (with the exception of nonlethal mutations of the germ cells). Transfer of the cancer process between different individuals is practically impossible due to complex histocompatibility checks that result in rejection, but not because of reaction to tumor antigens. Some of the growth mutations leading to cancer in multicellular organisms could, under particular circumstances, have given single cell organisms an advantage in terms of positive selection. Mutations in "corresponding" genes leading to death in man and other multicellular organisms very likely resulted in important virulence capabilities for bacteria.

Development of symptomatic cancer is an extremely unpleasant experience for a single individual and his relatives, but before nature is condemned for its extreme brutality it should be remembered that mutations represent the possibility for future adjustments; they are perhaps even more impressive if we are able to admit that they constitute the principal mechanism behind evolution from prokaryotic *Archaeobacteria* to man. Even in an age in which genetic tinkering has taken its first fumbling steps, it would be devastingly irresponsible and outright foolish to believe that we can relieve nature from this task and take care of our planet's future alone. However, mastering the molecular nuts and bolts of mutations could give us extremely powerful methods for the early detection of malignant cells, means to avoid the effect of most carcinogens and to repair potentially harmful germ cell mutations.

Cancer and Metabolism: Is There a Relationship that Can Be Therapeutically Exploited?

Our treatment methods of disseminated solid cancers are often unsuccessful, and weight loss in such patients is a prominent symptom heralding the inevitable demise of the patient. This weight loss is a regular and obvious accompaniment to disseminated cancer and is sometimes the patient's only symptom, leading both professional and lay people to believe that its reversal would cure the patient. Others, however, have interpreted this weight loss as a metabolic defense mechanism aimed at denying or reducing the flow of nutritional substrates to the tumor. The absolute contradiction between these two interpretations should in theory make it relatively easy to find a solution to the problem, and some are still puzzled why even today no single definite answer can be given. Both clinical and experimental data have given a mixture of more or less well founded answers.

We believe one important reason for this discrepancy is the interchange between two (or even more) different metabolic disturbancies leading to weight loss in cancer patients. There are at least two major and in many respects different metabolic reactions to cancer. One is a simple adaption to starvation due to mechanical or psychological blocking of food intake. This can be illustrated by a small intraluminally growing esophageal tumor blocking the passage of food. In such situations, resting energy expenditure is not increased above normal and a typical fasting biochemical profile can be demonstrated. The other is due to the inflammatory nature of tumor defense and represents a more or less "continous acute phase reaction" that is characterized by increased resting energy expenditure, increased production of inflammation inducers, and acute phase proteins. The first situation can often be easily reversed, at least for a while, with feeding procedures bypassing the blockade; the patients react with the expected weight gain. This is not the case with the other group. In spite of more than adequate protein and caloric feeding, either parenterally or by the use of feeding tubes, they do not gain the expected weight or achieve a normal biochemical profile. They behave in a similar way to catabolic patients following severe infections or trauma. If these two groups of patients could be easily identified, it would facilitate finding a satisfactory solution to the problem, but with increasing growth of the tumor a mixture of these two patterns is regularly found. This dynamic interchange between catabolism and adaption to starvation has made the metabolic reaction to cancer difficult to characterize and modulate. The possibility cannot be excluded that some tumors can produce inducers of catabolism directly (without having to stimulate host defence mechanisms) or substances able to interfere with appetite, satiety, or biochemical substrate handling. Such putative mechanisms will blur the view, but not change the basic picture of a dynamic interchange between catabolism and starvation as the basic metabolic problem in patients with symptomatic solid cancers.

In April 1994, Mullen [15] of Philadelphia, a distinguished researcher of catabolism, ends his editorial article in *Annals of Surgery* with the following remark: "… finally more global questions remain unanswered: Why is this hypermetabolic state triggered in some cancer patients but not in others? Why are some tumor types implicated more frequently than others?"

The important clinical observation that some patients lose weight in a hypermetabolic state while in others the weight loss is clearly related to fasting finally brings us back to a defense mechanism against growing tumors. There is no effective, specific antitumor mechanism. Depending on the degree of nonself, necrosis, and production of inflammation inducers, a graded local or more general inflammatory reaction pattern evolves without strict borders. With none or very modest antigens, a localized inflammatory foreign body reaction would be the result, and more (but still moderate) antigens would result in a less circumscript inflammatory reaction similar to some autoimmune diseases, with metabolic reactions varying from mild infection to the typical fully developed catabolic state. It should not be forgotten that the genomes of tumor cells are defined as unstable and are as such themselves subject to frequent mutations which, during the course of tumor growth and spread, could change the metabolic reaction towards catabolism, as can sometimes be observed in clinical cases.

How does this help us answer the question of whether we should use fasting or feeding as a therapeutic measure in the treatment of cancer patients? Westin found that starvation led to a slowing of tumor growth and partially inhibited tumor growth in the G0–G1 phase, arguing that, in spite of being detrimental to cancer patients, loss of appetite may be looked upon as an appropriate adaption to the tumor-bearing state [16]. The effects of cytokines that are central to the development of catabolism and that form part of both local and general inflammatory reactions (IL-1, TNF) include loss of appetite. The anorectic effect of inflammatory cytokines has been proposed as an explanation for tumor regression in animal studies. In vivo inhibition using IL-1 led to reduced tumor growth, but did not increase survival. As expected from observations in man, thinner animals died with smaller tumors and no benefit was found [17].

We are inclined to interpret these results differently. Catabolic states and anorectic reactions to tumors are part of the nonspecific inflammatory reaction directed against the tumor. This is considerably strengthened by recent controlled studies of patients demonstrating that nonsteroidal anti-inflammatory drugs (indomethacin) significantly improve nutritional status [18]. Further manipulations intended to reduce food intake as such have never satisfactorily been demonstrated to cure patients or prolong their lives. Intentional overfeeding has never been proved to normalize catabolism either in infectious or in malignant diseases. Catabolism or anorexia are not tumor-specific or tumor-eradicating reactions. Patients should be encouraged to have a normal intake of nutrients, possibly supplemented when specific deficiencies are demonstrated or suspected; blocked intake should be treated appropriately without fear of feeding the tumor and killing the patient.

References

1. Lewin B (ed) (1994) Genes V. Oxford University Press, Oxford, pp 1205–1209
2. Levine AJ, Perry ME, Chang A et al. (1994) The 1993 Walter Hubert Lecture: the role of p53 tumour-suppressor gene in tumorigenesis. Br J Cancer 69:409–416
3. Riethmüller G, Schneider-Gädicke E, Schlimok G et al. (1994) Randomized trial of monoclonal antibody for adjuvant therapy of resected Duke's C colorectal carcinoma. Lancet 343:1177–1183
4. Rosenberg SA, Lotze MT, Muul LM et al. (1987) A progress report on the treatment of 157 patients with advanced cancer using lymphokine activated killer cells and interleukin-2 or high dose interleukin-2 alone. N Engl J Med 316:889–905
5. Demetri GD, Spriggs DR, Sherman ML et al. (1989) A phase I trial of recombinant human tumor necrosis factor and interferon-gamma: effects of combination cytokine administration in vivo. J Clin Oncol 7:1545–1553
6. Thompson JA, Benyunes MC, Bianco JA, Fefer A (1993) Treatment with pentoxifylline and ciprofloxacin reduces the toxicity of high-dose interleukin-2 and lymphokine-activated killer cells. Semin Oncol 20:46–51
7. Nauts HC, Fowler GA, Bogatko FH (1953) Review of the influence of bacterial infection and of bacterial products (Coley's toxins) on malignant tumors in man. Acta Med Scand Suppl 276
8. Starnes CO (1992) Coley's toxins in perspective. Nature 357:11–12
9. Michie HR, Manogue KR, Spriggs DR et al. (1988) Detection of circulating tumor necrosis factor after endotoxin administration. N Engl J Med 318:1481–1486
10. Johnson HM, Russell JK, Pontzer CH (1992) Superantigens in human disease. Sci Am 266:42–74
11. Lienard D, Ewalenko P, Delmotte J-J, Renard N, Lejeune FJ (1992) Highdose recombinant tumor necrosis factor alpha in combination with interferon gamma and melphalan in isolation perfusion of the limbs for melanoma and sarcoma. J Clin Oncol 10:52–60

12. Han J, Lee J-D, Bibbs L, Ulevitch RJ (1994) A MAP kinase targeted by endotoxin and hyperosmolarity in mammalian cells. Science 265:808–811
13. Alberts B, Bray D, Lewis J et al. (eds) (1989) Molecular biology of the cell. Garland, New York, p 97
14. Smith GP (1994) Applied evolution: the progeny of sexual PCR. Nature 370:324–325
15. Mullen JL (1994) Hypermetabolism and advanced cancer. Ann Surg 219:323–324
16. Westin T (1990) Ornithine decarboxylase activity in malignant tumours. An experimental and clinical study with reference to cell proliferation and nutrition. Thesis, University of Gothenburg, p 155
17. Gelin J, Andersson C, Lundholm K (1991) Effects of indomethacin, cytokines and cyclosporin A on tumor growth and the subsequent development of cancer cachexia. Cancer Res 51:880–885
18. Lundholm K, Hyltander A (1994) Anemia, a promotor behind elevated energy expenditure in cancer patients. First Nordic EPREX (epoetin alfa) symposium on the management of anemia in cancer patients. Cilag Biotech, Stockholm, p 8

Effect of Neural Blockade in the Acute Catabolic State

H. Kehlet

Introduction

Surgical injury represents a catabolic state, characterized by changes in the endocrine milieu with increased secretion of catabolically acting hormones and decreased secretion and/or effect of anabolically acting hormones, with additional modification from various humoral cascade systems. The subsequent clinically relevant sequelae for the surgical patient are pain, nausea, vomiting and ileus, loss of muscle tissue contributing to postoperative fatigue, increased demands on the heart and lung, thereby the increasing risk of cardiac and pulmonary complications, and changes in blood flow, coagulation, and fibrinolysis contributing to thromboembolic complications. It has been hypothesized that such nonspecific, surgeon-unrelated complications may be reduced by modifying various aspects of the surgical stress response [1]. Unfortunately, we have no clear picture of which responses are of importance for various organ functions in the hospitalized surgical patient and which responses may have detrimental effects. This especially applies to the various humoral cascade systems, which may be important for wound healing, resistance to infections, etc. On the other hand, a prolonged and amplified humoral mediator response may have detrimental effects on several body organs, contributing to multiple organ failure.

This chapter summarizes the effect of neural blockade techniques on clinically relevant surgical responses such as the endocrine metabolic response, pain, and gastrointestinal paralysis; we conclude that utilization of afferent neural blockade techniques represents an important part of the integrated approach to control in the postoperative period.

Effect of Central Neural Blockade (Epidural and Spinal Anesthesia) on Perioperative Endocrine Metabolic Function

The important role of the peripheral and central nervous system in mediating the adrenocortical response to clean trauma was demonstrated in early studies by Hume and Egdahl [2]. Subsequently, several studies on various neural blockade techniques have documented that various parts of the classical hormonal response to surgical injury may be inhibited, while humorally mediated responses (most immunological changes, most changes in coagulation and fibrinolysis) are not or

Table 1. Effect of epidural analgesia on endocrine responses to surgery (data compiled from [1] and [4])

Technique	Surgical site	Degree of inhibition
Lumbar epidural local anesthetic	Lower body	++++
Thoracic epidural local anesthetic	Abdominal/thoracic	++
Lumbar epidural opioid	Lower body	++
Thoracic epidural opioid	Abdominal/thoracic	+
Combined epidural local anesthetic and opioid		
Lumbar	Lower body	?
Thoracic	Abdominal/thoracic	++

only slightly inhibited by neural blockade (for reviews see [1, 3, 4]). Since major endocrine metabolic changes and clinically relevant morbidity mainly occur in relatively large procedures in which central blockade techniques with epidural or spinal anesthesia are necessary, studies on afferent blockade techniques with local infiltration anesthesia, intercostal blocks, or other peripheral neural blocks will not be discussed here. Their effects on the surgical stress response has been reviewed elsewhere [1, 3–5].

Effect of Epidural Analgesia on Classical Hormonal Responses

Several studies have demonstrated that the classical hormonal responses such as the increase in cortisol, aldosterone, catecholamines, growth hormone, and renin are inhibited by epidural analgesia [1, 3, 4]. The effect is most pronounced in lower body procedures involving lumbar epidural analgesia with local anesthetics (Table 1), where operations can be performed without significant alterations in these hormones. In contrast, epidural analgesia with opioids provides a more selective nociceptive blockade, with some pain relief, but without major inhibition of the endocrine metabolic responses [1, 3–5]. Subsequently, and due to the inhibition of the various endocrine responses, hyperglycemia, lipolysis, and impairment in glucose tolerance are reduced.

In contrast to the pronounced endocrine metabolic effects in lower body operations, epidural analgesia has a smaller effect when used with the thoracic technique during abdominal or thoracic operations [1, 3, 4] (Table 1).

Effect of Epidural Analgesia on Nitrogen Economy

Subsequent to the inhibition of the catabolic endocrine responses, nitrogen balance has been demonstrated to be improved by continuous epidural analgesia in several operations (Table 2). It appears that with lumbar epidural anesthetics in lower body surgery, nitrogen balance and changes in the muscle amino acid pattern are improved. During thoracic epidural local anesthetic regimens, a similar, albeit less

Table 2. Effect of epidural or spinal anesthesia on postoperative nitrogen economy

	Surgery	Comment	Author
Lumar epidural local anesthetic	Hysterectomy	Improvement (24-h block)	Brandt et al. [6]
	colonic	Improvement (48-h block)	Vedrinne et al. [7]
	Hip surgery	No effect (single dose)	Carli and Emmery [8]
	Hip surgery	Improvement (24-h block)	Christensen et al. [9]
Thoracic epidural local anesthetic	Colonic	Improvement (24-h block)	Carli et al. [10]
	Gastric	Improvement (48-h block)	Tsuji et al. [11]
	Aortic	No effect (24-h block)	Smeets et al. [12]
	Abdominal	Improvement (~6-h block)	Shaw et al. [13]
	Abdominal and thoracic	No effect (96-h block)	Seeling et al. [14]
	abdominal	No effect (single dose)	De Lalande et al. [15]
		Improvement (24-h block)	De Lalande et al. [15]
Lumbar or thoracic epidural opioid	Colonic	No effect (48-h block)	Vedrinne et al. [7]
	Gastric (72-h block)	Improvement	Tsuji et al. [11]
Lumbar epidural locar anesthetic and opioid	Abdominal	No effect (24-h local anesthesia and 72-h opioid)	Hjortsø et al. [16]

pronounced effect is obtained. With epidural opioid administration, there is less effect on nitrogen balance. No conclusion can be made about epidural combination regimens because of insufficient data. Apparently, the block has to be continued at least for 24 h, since a single-dose block has no effect (Table 2). The data do not allow conclusions to be made as to the optimal local anesthetic dose regimen.

The data on protein economy with different epidural techniques are in accordance with the findings in hormonal responses, where the inhibitory effect of neural blockade is most pronounced with lumbar epidural local anesthetic techniques and less pronounced with thoracic techniques or epidural opioid administration [1, 3–5, 17, 18]. Combination of epidural analgesia with growth hormone administration further improved nitrogen balance [19]. Since thoracic epidural analgesia may be less efficient on cortisol and glucagon responses, but reasonably effective on sympathetic responses, a combined regimen of thoracic epidural analgesia to inhibit the sympathetic response, etomidate to inhibit the cortisol responses, and somatostatin to inhibit glucagon response was investigated [20]. This study showed that urea production and functional hepatic nitrogen clearance could be maintained at normal levels compared to control patients operated on with general anesthesia and systemic opioids for postoperative pain management after classical cholecystectomy [20]. These results therefore suggest that, following clean surgery, the neural component may be the more important than humoral mediators in releasing catabolic responses and negative postoperative nitrogen economy.

Effect of Type and Duration of Neural Blockade

The modifying effect of neural blockade on surgical stress responses is highly dependent on the type and duration of the block. Thus, as mentioned above, lumbar epidural local techniques are more effective than thoracic blocks, in accordance with a more efficient afferent blockade measured by evoked potentials to peripheral electrical stimulation [3, 5, 21].

The optimal duration of the afferent blockade has not been elucidated in systematic studies, but it is well documented that a single-dose block with a 2- to 4-h duration has no major prolonged endocrine metabolic effects [1, 3–5]. In contrast, studies using blockade from 24 to 72 h have demonstrated metabolic effects for several days [1, 3–5] (Table 2). The block probably has to be extended as long as significant afferent traffic persists from the periphery, although the duration and intensity of this traffic has yet to be determined.

Pre- Versus Post-traumatic Neural Blockade

Recently, pronounced neuroplastic changes in the spinal cord have been demonstrated following noxious injury, and these changes have been assumed to be important for the magnitude and duration of postoperative pain [22]. Subsequently, and based upon experimental studies, it has been hypothesized that a preemptive neural blockade may be more effective than a postinjury blockade on pain patterns. However, clinical studies have not confirmed the timing of neural blockade to be of major importance in the treatment of postoperative pain [23]. Nevertheless, the only metabolic study comparing the modifying effect of an identical pre- versus postincisional epidural local anesthetic blockade showed a more pronounced reduction of the stress response with the preemptive blockade [24]. This suggests that endocrine metabolic responses may be more difficult to modify after the nociceptive stimulus has led to activation of various neural and enzymatic responses as well as of different humoral cascade systems, etc. The role of timing of the neural blockade may therefore be of importance in our understanding of measures to modify postinjury metabolism and should be further explored.

Pain

The significance of neural blockade in postoperative pain management is well established, and following all major operations continuous epidural analgesia

techniques are necessary to provide sufficient pain relief to allow early mobilization [25]. The optimal technique for epidural analgesia is a combined regimen
according to the "balanced analgesia" concept [26]. Similarly effective pain relief
allowing early mobilization cannot be achieved by other pain treatment modalities
such as systemic opioids or treatment with nonsteroidal anti-inflammatory drugs
(NSAID) [25, 26].

Effect of Neural Blockade on Postoperative Ileus

Postoperative gastrointestinal paralysis continues to be a clinical problem, with relatively few improvements in the understanding of its pathogenesis and therapy
[27]. The most important mechanism is probably neurogenic, since reflex mechanisms leading to the activation of inhibitory efferent sympathetic pathways will inhibit gastrointestinal motility [27, 28]. Early restoration of normal gastrointestinal
integrity following major operative procedures is of obvious importance, because
it avoids the conventional semistarvation period which may amplify catabolism.
Furthermore, reduction of ileus may allow early nutrition, which may be important
in the maintenance of mucosal integrity and barrier function.

Continuous epidural analgesia combined with local anesthetics is therefore a rational technique to shorten postoperative gastrointestinal ileus [4, 28]. The indication is further strengthened by the additional positive effects in postoperative patients such as improved pain relief, reduced thromboembolism, improvement of
pulmonary function, etc. (see below). Several controlled trials have documented
that neural blockade improves postoperative gastrointestinal motility after abdominal procedures (Fig. 1) as well as in neurosurgical intensive care patients [29]. The
same positive effect cannot be obtained by epidural opioid treatment [4, 28].
Although initial studies during combined epidural local anesthetic and opioid

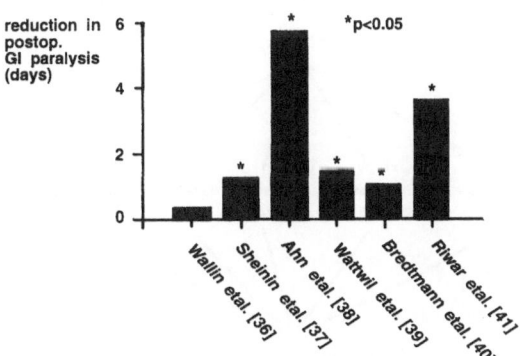

Fig. 1. Effect of continuous epidural bupivacaine (24–76 h) versus systemic opioid treatment on
gastrointestinal (*GI*) function after abdominal surgery (controlled studies)

treatment are positive [30], further studies are needed to evaluate whether the advantageous effect of epidural local anesthetics on gastrointestinal motility can be maintained by the addition of small doses of epidural opioids.

Integration of Neural Blockade Techniques in the Control of the Postoperative Period

It has generally been assumed that adequate postoperative pain relief may reduce pulmonary, cardiovascular, thromboembolic, and other complications and improve the general postoperative outcome. However, data from several controlled studies in major abdominal and thoracic procedures [1, 4, 5, 25] have not been able to demonstrate important general clinical effects on outcome using epidural opioids, local anesthetics, or combinations thereof. In contrast, the use of neural blockade with local anesthetics in lower body procedures (major orthopedic surgery) has been shown to significantly improve outcome by reducing blood loss and thromboembolic and pulmonary complications [1, 4, 5, 25]. The explanation for the disapointing findings in major abdominal and thoracic procedures during effective epidural analgesia regimens is most probably that the achieved pain relief was not utilized to enhance mobilization and intake of oral nutrition. Thus, a conservative approach with gastrointestinal tubes and restrictions on oral intake is still common, despite evidence that tubes have no advantage [31] and that early enteral nutrition is advantageous [32]. A multimodal approach to improve postoperative morbidity has therefore been proposed [33] (Fig. 2), based upon the fact that no single treatment modality will have a pronounced positive effect. Instead, several approaches have to be combined, parallel to the principles for the optimization of postoperative pain relief [26].

Preliminary data from our group have shown major improvements in postoperative convalescense and a reduction in the duration of hospital stay following hip replacement [34] and open colonic surgery [30] with such a combined approach involving enforced preoperative patient information, optimal pain relief with

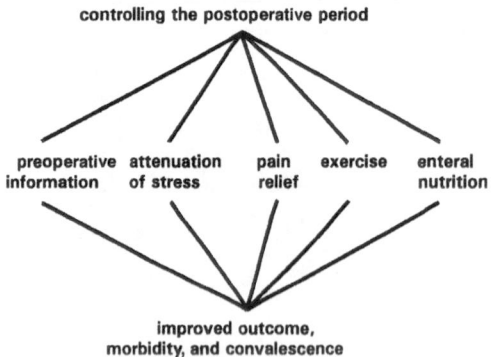

Fig. 2. Multimodal approach to control the postoperative period

multimodal pain therapy, enforced postoperative exercise and mobilization, and immediate enteral nutrition. A further step towards reduction in the duration of hospital stay and prevention of surgery-induced organ dysfunction has been the combination of minimally invasive laparoscopic surgery, combined with epidural local anesthetic blockade, enforced early oral nutrition and mobilization, and avoidance of opioids to reduce their potential side effects on the gastrointestinal tact (nausea, vomiting, ileus). Our preliminary data from eight patients with a mean age of 79 years undergoing colonic cancer surgery suggest that such an approach is of major clinical importance. Thus, gastrointestinal function was reestablished within the first 24–48 h and hospital stay reduced to 2 days; convalescense after discharge was normal, without the need for additional health service and with reduced fatigue [35].

In summary, neural blockade may be a very effective, although not optimal technique to reduce various aspects of the surgical stress response. Furthermore, neural blockade is able to diminish postoperative organ dysfunction, to enhance recovery, and to provide effective pain relief. However, the neural blockade techniques need to be further improved during thoracic and abdominal procedures due to insufficient afferent blockade. In order to achieve important, clinically advantageous effects on catabolism and outcome, the neural blockade has to be integrated into a multimodal postoperative care system, utilizing the achieved pain relief for early mobilization and enteral nutrition. Preliminary data suggest that such an approach is of major significance, but this needs to be confirmed in larger patient series after several procedures. This is especially true for the reduction of causes of severe morbidity such as cardiopulmonary, thromboembolic, and septic complications. Most importantly, future studies should evaluate whether such relatively stress-free patients emerging from major surgery handle a surgical complication ("second hit") more easily and with less organ dysfunction, since they never responded to the "first hit" (the operation). If this hypothesis is true and is confirmed, such patients may be in a more favorable position to avoid transition into multiple organ failure syndromes, should a serious postoperative complication occur.

References

1. Kehlet H (1987) Modification of responses to surgery and anesthesia by neural blockade: clinical implications. In: Cousins MJ, Bridenbaugh PO (eds) Neural blockade in clinical anesthesia and management of pain. Lippincott, Philadelphia, pp 145–188
2. Hume DM, Egdahl RH (1959) The importance of the brain in the endocrine response to injury. Ann Surg 150:697–704
3. Kehlet H (1992) Role of neural stimuli and pain. In: Lamy M, Thijs LG (eds) Mediators of sepsis. Springer, Berlin Heidelberg New York, pp 196–205
4. Kehlet H (1993) General vs. regional anesthesia. In: Rogers M, Tinker J, Covino B, Longnecker DE (eds) Principals and practice of anesthesiology. Mosby, St Louis, pp 1218–1234
5. Kehlet H (1994) Effect of postoperative pain on surgical outcome. In: Stanley TH, Ashburn MA (eds) Anesthesiology and pain management. Kluwer, Amsterdam, pp 99–103
6. Brandt MR, Fernandes A, Mordhorst R, Kehlet H (1978) Epidural analgesia improves postoperative nitrogen balance. Br J Med 1:1106–1108
7. Vedrinne C, Vedrinne JM, Guiraud M, Patricet MC, Bouletreau P (1989) Nitrogen sparing effect of epidural administration of local anesthetics in colon surgery. Anesth Analg 69:354–359

8. Carli F, Emmery PW (1990) Intraoperative epidural blockade with local anesthetics and post-operative protein break down associated with hip surgery in elderly patients. Acta Anaesthesiol Scand 34:263–266

9. Christensen T, Waaben J, Lindeburg T, Vesterberg K, Vinnars E, Kehlet H (1986) Effect of epidural analgesia on muscle amino-acid pattern after surgery. Acta Chir Scand 152:407–411

10. Carli F, Webster J, Pearson M, Pearson J, Bartlett S, Bannister P, Halliday D (1991) Protein metabolism after abdominal surgery: effect of 24-h extradural block with local anaesthetic. Br J Anaesth 67:729–734

11. Tsuji H, Shirasaka C, Asoh T, Uchida I (1987) Effects of epidural administration of local anesthetics and morphine on postoperative nitrogen loss and catabolic hormones. Br J Surg 74:421–425

12. Smeets HJ, Kievit J, Dulfer FT, van Kleef JW (1993) Endocrine metabolic response to abdominal aortic surgery: a randomised trial of general anesthesia versus general plus epidural anesthesia. World J Surg 17:601–607

13. Shaw JHF, Galler L, Holdaway IM, Holdaway CM (1987) The effect of extradural blockade upon glucose and urea kinetics in surgical patients. Surg Gynecol Obstet 165:260–266

14. Seeling W, Altemeyer K-H, Berg S, Feist H et al. (1982) The influence of continuous epidural analgesia on the metabolic response to abdominal surgery. Anaesthesist 31:439–448

15. Delande JP, Page JL, Peramant M, Lozach P, Tanguy RL (1984) Influence of epidural anesthesia on protein sparing major visceral surgery. Ann Fr Anesth Reanim 3:16–21

16. Hjortsø N-C, Christensen NJ, Andersen T, Kehlet H (1985) Effects of extradural administration of local anesthetic agents and morphine on the urinary excretion of cortisol, catecholamines and nitrogen following abdominal surgery. 57:400–406

17. Watters JM, March RJ, Desai D, Munteith K, Hurtig JB (1993) Epidural anesthesia and analgesia do not affect energy expenditure after major abdominal surgery. Can J Anaesth 40:314–319

18. Naito Y, Tamai S, Shingu K et al. (1992) Responses of plasma adrenocorticothropic hormone, cortisol and cytokines during and after upper abdominal surgery. Anesthesiology 77:426–431

19. Mjaaland M, Unneberg K, Hotvedt R, Revhaug A (1991) Nitrogen retention caused by growth hormone in patients undergoing gastrointestinal surgery with epidural analgesia and parenteral nutrition. Eur J Surg 157:21–27

20. Heindorff H, Schulz S, Mogensen T, Almdal T, Kehlet H, Vilstrup H (1992) Hormonal and neural blockade prevents the postoperative increase in amino-acid clearance and urea synthesis. Surgery 111:543–550

21. Lund C (1993) Somatosensory evoked potentials in the assessment of neural blockade. Dan Med Bull 40:266–272

22. Woolf CJ, Chong M-S (1993) Preemptive analgesia – treating postoperative pain by preventing the establishment of central sensitisation. Anesth Analg 77:362–379

23. Dahl JB, Kehlet H (1993) The value of preemptive analgesia in the treatment of postoperative pain. Br J Anaesth 70:434–439

24. Møller IW, Rem J, Brandt MR, Kehlet H (1982) Effect of posttraumatic epidural analgesia on the cortisol and hyperglycemic response to surgery. Acta Anaesthesiol Scand 26:56–60

25. Kehlet H (1994) Postoperative pain relief – what is the issue? Br J Anaesth 72:375–378

26. Kehlet H, Dahl JB (1993) The value of multi-modal or balanced analgesia in postoperative pain relief. Anesth Analg 77:1048–1056

27. Livingston EH, Passaro EP (1990) Postoperative ileus. Dig Dis Sci 35:121–130

28. Wattwill M (1988) Postoperative pain relief and gastrointestinal motility. Acta Chir Scand Suppl 550:140–145

29. Weinstabel C, Porges P, Pleiner B, Werba A, Spiss CK, Seitz H (1993) Coeliac plexus block with bupivacaine reduces intestinal dysfunction in neurosurgical ICU patients. Anaesthesia 48:162–164

30. Møiniche S, Bülow S, Hesselfeldt P, Hestbæk A, Kehlet H (1995) Convalescence and hospital stay after colonic surgery during balanced analgesia, enforced oral feeding and mobilization. Eur J Surg (in press)

31. Sagar PM, Kruegenar G, MacFie J (1992) Nasogastric intubation and elective abdominal surgery. Br J Surg 79:1127–1131

32. Moore FA, Feliciano DV, Andrassy REJ et al. (1992) Early enteral feeding compared with par-enteral, reduces postoperative septic complications. The results of a meta-analysis. Ann Surg 216:172–183
33. Kehlet H (1994) Postoperative pain relief. A look from the other side. Reg Anesth 19:369:377
34. Møiniche S, Hansen BN, Christensen S-E, Dahl JB, Kehlet H (1992) Activity of patients and duration of hospitalization following hip-replacement with balanced treatment of pain and early mobilization Ugeskr Læger 154:1495–1499
35. Bardram L, Jensen PF, Jensen P, Crawford M, Kehlet H (1995) Accelerated recovery after laparoscopic colonic surgery with epidural analgesia, enforced oral nutrition and mobilisation. Lancet (in press)
36. Wallin G, Cassuto J, Högström S, Rimbäck G, Faxén A, Tollesson P-O (1986) Failure of epidural anesthesia to prevent postoperative paralytic ileus. Anesthesiology 65:292–297
37. Sheinin B, Asantila R, Orku R (1987) The effect of bupivacaine on pain and bowel function after colonic surgery. Acta Anaesthesiol Scand 31:161–164
38. Ahn H, Bronge A, Johansson K, Ygge H, Lindhargen J (1988) Effect on continuous postoperative epidural analgesia on intestinal motility. Br J Surg 75:1176–1178
39. Wattwill M, Thorén T, Hennerdal S, Garvill J-E (1989) Epidural analgesia with bupivacaine reduces postoperative paralytic ileus after hysterectomy. Anesth Analg 68:353–358
40. Bredtmann RD, Herden RN, Teichmann W, Moecke HP, Kniesel B, Batdgen R (1990) Epidural analgesia in colonic surgery: results of a randomized prospective study. Br J Surg 77:1897–1903
41. Riwar A, Schär B, Grötzinger U (1991) Effekt von kontinuierlicher postoperativer Analgesie mit Bupivacain peridural auf die Darmmotilität nach colorectalen Resektionen. Helv Chir Acta 58:729–733

Use of Cyclooxygenase Inhibitors in the Acute Catabolic State

A. Revhaug

Introduction

In the early phases of an acute catabolic state, different cascades in the inflammatory process are activated. Among the many important mediators involved in the acute catabolic state are the eicosanoids. These substances are generated from phospholipids in response to a great variety of stimuli. After the discovery of prostaglandin in the 1930s, later work with these substances has elucidated the knowledge of a great diversity of eicosanoids with different properties.

Over the years it has become evident that the different eicosanoids are heavily involved in the production of the inflammatory processes. Because the generation of these inflammatory substances is dependent to a great extent on the action of cyclooxygenase, a diversity of inhibitors of the latter has been investigated and used as anti-inflammatory therapeutic agents.

Cyclooxygenase Inhibitors

Most of the cyclooxygenase inhibitors belong to the group of nonsteroid anti-inflammatory drugs (NSAID). Deriving from the phospholipids by actions of phospholipase, arachidonate gives origin to the eicosanoids. Arachidonate can be metabolized either by cyclooxygenase, giving rise to various prostanoids, or by 5-lipo-oxygenase, giving rise to various leukotrienes. Cyclooxygenase is found bound to the endoplasmic reticulum and is present in every cell type in the body. However, the different steps in the arachidonate metabolism vary in different cells. Thus, it may lead to thromboxane, A_2 (TXA_2) synthesis in the platelets, to prostacyclin synthesis in the vascular endothelium, or to the synthesis of prostaglandin E_2 in the macrophages (Fig. 1).

Cyclooxygenase acts on arachidonate to produce cyclic endoperoxides, i.e., prostaglandin (PG) G_2, PGH_2, which in turn can give rise to PGI_2, TXA_2, PGE_2, PGF_2, and PGD_2. The NSAID include a variety of agents belonging to different chemical classes (Table 1). The major effects of these drugs, namely antipyretic, analgesic, and anti-inflammatory effects, are related to the primary action of the drugs by the inhibition of arachidonate cyclooxygenase and thus the inhibition of prostataglandin and thromboxane production.

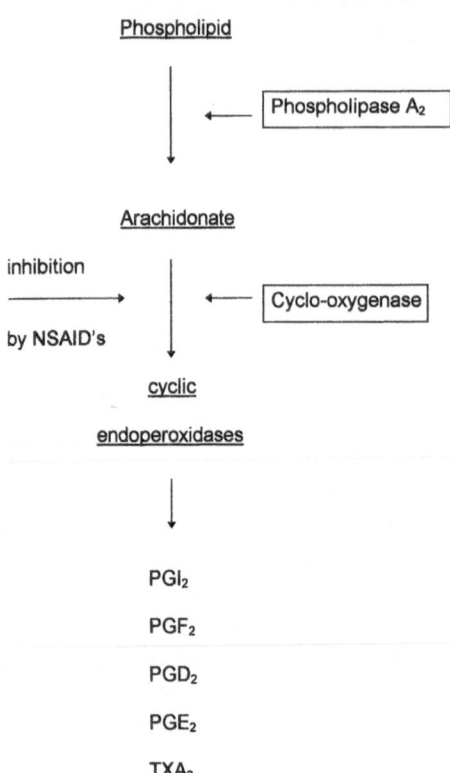

Fig. 1. Biosynthesis of prostaglandins and the interaction by nonsteroidal anti-inflammatory drugs (*NSAID*). *PG,* prostaglandin; *TX,* thromboxane

Table 1. Comparison of some commonly used nonsteroidal anti-inflammatory drugs (NSAID) with respect to their actions as analgesic, antipyretic, and anti-inflammatory drugs

NSAID group	Analgetic	Antipyretic	Anti-inflammatory
Salicylic acids	+	+	+
Propionic aicds	+	+	+
Acetic acids	+	+	++
Oxicams	+	+	++
Pyrazolones	±	+	++
Paracetamol	+	+	−

±, weak action; +, medium action; ++, strong action; −, no action

Cyclooxygenase exists in at least two isoforms. Cyclooxygenase-1 is expressed constitutively and was first characterized and cloned from sheep vesicular glands [1]. Cyclooxygenase-2 is induced in cells exposed to proinflammatory agents, e.g., cytokines and endotoxin [2, 3]. The prevailing theory is that the ability of NSAID to inhibit cyclooxygenase-2 explains their anti-inflammatory actions, whereas the inhibition of cyclooxygenase-1 explains their unwanted side effects [4].

Accordingly, the ideal anti-inflammatory cyclooxygenase inhibitor should inhibit the activity of cyclooxygenase-2, thereby inhibiting the production of proinflammatory prostanoids without affecting the production of substances produced by cyclooxygenase-1, which have cytoprotective and other positive effects.

Accordingly, there are differences in the actions of the more than 50 different NSAID currently on the market [5]. Even in the most analgesic drugs, the degree of action may vary, as does the anti-inflammatory activity. Some of these drugs may present very little anti-inflammatory activity [6].

The antipyretic effect of these drugs is probably due to an effect on the liberation of prostaglandins of the E series in the hypothalamus as a response to macrophage-released interleukin-1 (IL-1) in response to bacterial endotoxins during a inflammatory reaction. It is noteworthy that a normal temperature is not affected by the NSAID [7].

The NSAID are effective against certain types of pain, e.g., those in which prostaglandins amplify the basic pain mechanisms. In general these drugs are mainly effective against pain associated with inflammatory processes. The anti-inflammatory action is mainly due to the decrease in the vasodilator prostaglandins (PGE_2, PGI_2), leading to less vasodilatation and accordingly decreasing the edema [8].

Experimental Experience

Animal Studies

Over many years different cyclooxygenase inhibitors have been investigated in acute septic and endotoxin models. In animals, these cyclooxygenase inhibitors have improved survival rate [9–11]. The lung injury in sepsis and after reperfusion can be markedly attenuated with these substances [12–14].

When investigating the possible effects of cyclooxygenase inhibition on the tumor necrosis factor (TNF)-induced effects in dogs using ibuprofen, which inhibits cyclooxygenase by substrate competition with arachidonic acid [15], Evans et al. demonstrated that many of the TNF effects are mediated via cyclooxygenase pathways [16]. In this study dogs were pretreated with ibuprofen and one dose of ibuprofen was also administered after the administration of TNF. Ibuprofen reversed the hemodynamic effects of TNF. The febrile response and stress hormone elaboration were blunted. Changes in respiratory gas exchange were restored toward baseline. However, ibuprofen did not prevent other changes associated with the infusion of TNF (Table 2).

In experimental burn injury studies, Hansbrough and coworkers [17, 18] demonstrated improved immune functions in mice which were given ibuprofen following burn injury.

When investigating the effects of cyclooxygenase inhibitors on IL-1 effects, Okusawa et al. demonstrated that ibuprofen attenuated these IL-1 effects [19]. The inadequate mesenteric perfusion seen in endotoxin pigs was attenuated by the use of a cyclooxygenase inhibitor [20].

Positive effects have thus been observed with several of the cyclooxygenase inhibitors in different animal models which resemble several of the acute catabolic situations.

Table 2. Summary of the physiologic responses to tumor necrosis factor (TNF) infusion and the effect of ibuprofen pretreatment

Physiologic responses	TNF	TNF + IBP
Hemodynamics		
Blood pressure	↓	Blocked
Heart rate	↑	Partially blocked
Central venous pressure	↓	Blocked
Pulmonary artery pressure	↓	Blocked
Wedge pressure	↓	Blocked
Cardiac index	No effect	↑
SVR	No effect	↑
Temperature, urine output, and hematology		
Urinary output	↑	Blocked
Rectal temperature	↑	Partially blocked
Hematocrit	↑	↑↑
White blood cells	↓	↓
Respiratory indices		
Minute ventilation	↑	Partially blocked
Oxygen consumption	↑	Blocked
pH	No effect	No effect
Base excess	↓	↓
Hormones		
ACTH	↑	Partially blocked
Cortisol	↑	Partially blocked
Glucagon	↑	Partially blocked
Insulin	No effect	↓
Epinephrine	↑	Partially blocked
Norepinephrine	↑	Partially blocked
Substrates		
Glucose	↓	↓↓
Lactate	↑	Partially blocked
Pyruvate	↑	Partially blocked
Free fatty acids	No effect	No effect
Serum triglycerides	No effect	No effect

IBP, ibuprofen; SVR, systemic vascular resistance; ACTH, adrenocorticotrophic hormone. ↓, significant decrease over time; ↑, significant increase over time; no effect, no change over time; partially blocked, the response observed with TNF was attenuated; blocked, the response observed with TNF was no longer observed.

Human Studies

After years of experience with different animal studies using a diversity of models and drugs, investigative human studies followed. To determine the effects of cyclooxygenase inhibition on metabolic and acute phase responses, we studied subjects after endotoxin administration who had been pretreated with ibuprofen given orally [21]. The administration of endotoxin produced a response similar to an acute illness, with flu-like symptoms, fever, tachycardia, increased metabolic rate, and stimulation of stress hormone release. These changes were markedly attenuated by cyclooxygenase inhibition. However, the leukocytosis, hypoferremia, and elevation of the C-reactive protein level induced by endotoxin were unaffected. The liberation of TNF-α to the circulation in response to endotoxin administration in humans is not affected by cyclooxygenase inhibition [22].

In the acute catabolic state, a typical hormonal response involving the stress or counterregulatory hormones is taking place. This increased elaboration of cortisol, catecholamines, and glucagon is believed to be critical for the maintenance of cardiovascular stability during critical illness and is also important for the stimulation of gluconeogenesis and lipolysis [23]. However, for the adverse metabolic state seen in the acutely ill patient [24], the induction of hypothalamic factors represents the first step in the afferent pathway leading to the neuroendocrine response. Different afferent stimuli interact with the hypothalamus to initiate the neuroendocrine response [24, 25]. The release of the corticotropin-releasing hormone (CRH) leads to the induction of adrenocorticotropic hormone (ACTH) by the anterior pituitary gland [23]. In addition, products of the cyclooxygenase pathway and the original vasopressin (AVP) are also important in the induction of ACTH [23, 26].

When ibuprofen was administered in humans subjected to endotoxinemia, the neuroendocrine elaboration was abolished [27]. This indicates that products of the cyclooxygenase pathway are proximal mediators of the stress response. Noteworthy, though, is the demonstration that this cyclooxygenase-dependent step is bypassed by noninflammatory stimuli such as pain, hypoxia, hypotension, and hypoglycemia. Accordingly, in most acute catabolic states cyclooxygenase inhibition may attenuate, but not abolish the stress response [16].

The cytokine interleukin-2 (IL-2) is a primary modulator of the immune response in the acute catabolic state. The administration of IL-2 to humans resulted in symptoms very similar to those seen after endotoxin stimulation in humans [28]. When ibuprofen was administered prior to the IL-2 infusion, the fever and neuroendocrine responses were greatly attenuated. The general symptoms, including headaches, myalgias, chills, and nausea, were almost totally abolished with the ibuprofen pretreatment (Fig. 2).

Early clinical studies also demonstrated that cyclooxygenase inhibitors markedly attenuated the stress response occurring after major abdominal surgery [29]. During the investigation of immune responses in humans, Rodrick et al. treated healthy volunteers with ibuprofen alone or with ibuprofen prior to endotoxin administration. Ibuprofen pretreatment completely restored the peripheral blood mononuclear cell response to phytohemagglutinin to normal and caused a significant decrease in the endotoxin-induced suppression of IL-2 production. However, the decrease in circulating peripheral blood mononuclear cell number and adherent cell secretion of IL-1 were not affected by inhibition of the cyclooxygenase pathway [30].

When giving indomethacin to patients following major surgical trauma, similar augmentation of the cellular immune response was observed by Faist et al. [31].

The ketorolac tromethamine, which belongs to the pyrrolo-pyrrole NSAID group, has been shown to inhibit several of the inflammatory functions of human neutrophils [32]. It must, however, be supposed that some of the effects mediated by the NSAID are not necessarily mediated through the cyclooxygenase pathways [33].

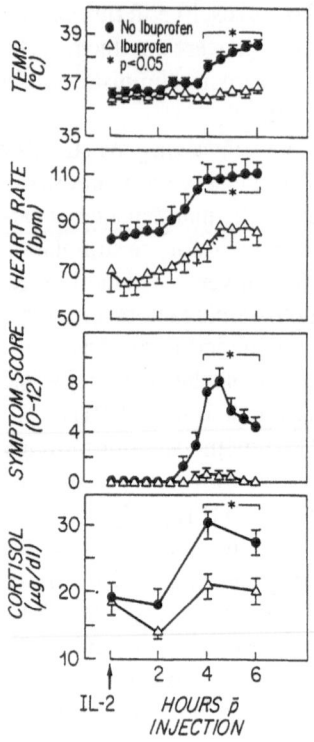

Fig. 2. The effect of pretreatment with ibuprofen (1600 mg, orally) on responses that occur after interleukin-2 (*IL-2*) administration. Fever, tachycardia, symptoms, and cortisol elaboration were markedly attenuated in the pretreated subjects. (Adapted from [4], with permission)

In a recent clinical study, ibuprofen improved blood pressure and temperature, alleviated respiratory disturbance, and increased the frequency of shock reversal in patients with sepsis syndrome or septic shock [34, 35].

Unwanted Effects

The major concerns with the use of NSAID in the acute catabolic state are the risks of gastrointestinal ulcerations and nephrotoxicity. The NSAID are extensively used in chronic disease, mainly joint disease, which requires high dosages and continued long-term use. In addition, these patients are also often elderly with other chronic organ involvement. The general unwanted effects of NSAID include dyspepsia, nausea, vomiting, and in some patients ulcer of the stomach or small intestine, sometimes complicated by hemorrhage or perforation. This side effect is thought to be a result of the decreased production of PGE_2, which has a protective effect of the gastric mucosa. Recent data indicate that the strongest inhibitors of cyclooxygenase-1 are the NSAID that cause the most gastric damage [36]. The fact that gastric mucosal blood flow often is decreased in acute disease could also add to the possible negative effects of the cyclooxygenase inhibitors. However, this was not the case when investigated in a septic animal model [37]. The gastric mucosal lesions seemed, if anything, to be less pronounced in the indomethacin-treated animals. This might be due to a "shunting phenomenon" [38, 39] in which prostaglandins known to be cytoprotective (PGE_2 and PGE_1) are inhibited by indomethacin, but might be synthesized in excess after the TXA_2 synthetase inhibitor, due to the shunting phenomenon between different prostanoids when one metabolic pathway is blocked. In this study gastric mucosal capillary congestion was a dominant finding in animals given a thromboxane A_2 synthetase inhibitor, but not in the animals given a cyclooxygenase inhibitor.

The nephrotoxicity of the cyclooxygenase inhibitors has lately become a major concern in with for the use of these substances in acutely ill patients [40]. The basis of these renal effects is the inhibition of the biosynthesis of important renal regulatory prostanoids (PGE_2, PGI_2). These prostaglandins are minimally involved in the maintenance of renal microvascular tone and blood flow [41, 42]. Because reduced renal flow is often seen in the acutely ill patient, the reduction in production of PGE_2 and PGI_2 by the NSAID may increase the risk of nephrotoxicity in these patients [43]. However, if adequate hydration is provided in these patients, these deleterious effects can probably be avoided [44, 45].

Therapeutic Recommendations

In elective surgery, pretreatment with NSAID should be considered. Substances with principal effects on cyclooxygenase-2 should be preferred. The use of ibuprofen in dosages of 1200 mg daily divided into two or three doses is probably in the range that is needed in most cases. There are, however, new substances with more specific actions upon the different cyclooxygenases that need to be inhibited in the different situations which should be considered in the future.

References

1. DeWitt DL, Smith WL (1988) Primary structure of prostaglandin G/H synthase from sheep vesicular gland determined from the complementary DNA sequence. Proc Natl Acad Sci USA 85:1412–1416
2. O'Banion MK, Winn VD, Young DA (1922) cDNA cloning and functional activity of a glucocorticoid-regulated inflammatory cyclooxygenase. Proc Natl Acad Sci USA 89:4888–4892
3. Lee SH, Soyoola E, Chanmngam P et al. (1992) Selective expression of mitogen-inducible cyclooxygenase in macrophages stimulated with lipopolysaccharide. J Biol Chem 267:25934–25938
4. Mitchell JA, Akarasereenont P, Thiemermann C, Flower RJ, Vane JR (1994) Selectivity of nonsteroidal antiinflammatory drugs as inhibitors of constitutive and inductible cyclooxygenase. Proc Natl Acad Sci USA 90:11693–11697
5. Vane JR (1971) Inhibition of prostataglandins synthesis as a mechanism of action for asperin-like drugs. Nature New Biology 231:232–239
6. Lands WE (1981) Actions of anti-inflammatory drugs. Trends Pharmacol Sci 2:78-80
7. Dinarello CA (1988) Biology of interleukin-I. FASEB J 2:108–115
8. Rang HP, Dale MM (eds) (1991) Pharmacology, 2nd edn. Churchill Livingstone, London

9. Butler RR Jr, Wise WC, Haluska PV (1983) Gentamicin and indomethacin in the treatment of septic shock: effects on prostacyclin and thromboxane A_2 production. J Pharmacol Exp Ther 225:94–101
10. Jacobs ER, Soulsby ME, Bone RC et al. (1982) Ibuprofen in canine endotoxin shock. J Clin Invest 70:536–541
11. Fletcher JR, Ramwell PW (1980) Indomethacin treatment following baboon endotoxin shock improves survival. Adv Shock Res 4:103–111
12. Zanaboni PB, Bradley JD, Baundendistel LJ et al. (1990) Cyclooxygenase inhibition prevents PMA-induced increases in lung vascular permeability. J Appl Physiol 69:1494–1501
13. Ljungman AG, Grum CM, Deeb GM et al. (1991) Inhibition of cyclooxygenase metabolite production attenuates ischemia-reperfusion lung injury. Am Rev Respir Dis 143:610–617
14. Jacobs ER, Bone RC, Balk RA et al. (1986) Increased survival in bacteremic sheep treated with ibuprofen. J Crit Care 1:142–149
15. Rome LH, Lands WEM (1975) Structural requirements for time-dependent inhibition of prostaglandin biosynthesis by anti-inflammatory drugs. Proc Natl Acad Sci USA 72:4863–4865
16. Evans DA, Jacobs DO, Revhaug A, Wilmore DW (1989) The effects of tumor necrosis factor and their selective inhibition by ibuprofen. Ann Surg 209:312–321
17. Hansbrough J, Peterson V, Zapata-Sirvent RL, Claman HN (1984) Postburn immunosuppression in an animal model. II. Restoration of cell-mediated immunity by immunomodulating drugs. Surgery 95:290
18. Zapata-Sirvent RL, Hansbrough JF (1985) Postburn immunosuppression in an animal model. III. Maintenance of normal splenic helper and suppressor lymphocyte subpopulations by immunomodulating drugs. Surgery 97:721
19. Okusawa S, Gelfand JA, Ikejima T et al. (1988) Interleukin 1 induces a shock-like state in rabbits: Synergism with tumor necrosis factor and the effect of cyclooxygenase inhibition. J Clin Invest 81:1162–1172
20. Fink MP, Rothschild HR, Deniz YF, Wang H, Lee PC, Cohn SM (1989) Systemic and mesenteric O_2 metabolism in endotoxic pigs: effect of ibuprofen and meclofenamate. J Appl Physiol 67:1950–1957
21. Revhaug A, Michie HR, Manson J McK et al. (1988) Inhibition of cyclooxygenase attenuates the metabolic response to endotoxin in humans. Arch Surg 123:162–170
22. Michie HR, Manogue KR, Spriggs DR et al. (1988) Detection of circulating tumor necrosis factor after endotoxin administration. N Engl J Med 318:1481–1486
23. Ganong WF (1986) Neuroendocrine responses to injury. In: Little R, Faryn K (eds) The scientific basis for the care of the critically ill. Manchester University Press, Manchester, pp 45–60
24. Bessey P, Watters J, Aoki T, Wilmore D (1984) Combined hormonal infusion stimulates the metabolic response to injury. Ann Surg 200:264–281
25. Michie HR, Eberlein TJ, Spriggs DR et al. (1988) Interleukin-2 initiates metabolic responses associated with critical illness in humans. Ann Surg 208:493–503
26. Plotsky PM, Cunningham ET, Widmaier EP (1989) Catecholaminergic modulation of corticotropin-releasing factor and adrenocorticotropin secretion. Endocr Rev 10:437–458
27. Michie HR, Majzoub JA, O'Dwyer ST, Revhaug A, Wilmore DW (1990) Both cyclooxygenase-dependent and cyclooxygenase-independent pathways mediate the neuroendocrine response in humans. Surgery 108:254–261
28. Michie HR, Eberlein TJ, Spriggs DR, Manogue KR, Cerami A, Wilmore DW (1988) Interleukin-2 initiates metabolic responses associated with critical illness in humans. Ann Surg 208:493–503
29. Asoh T, Shirasaka C, Uchida I et al. (1987) Effects of indomethacin on endocrine responses and nitrogen loss after surgery. Ann Surg 206:770–777
30. Rodrick ML, Moss NM, Grbic JT et al. (1992) Effects of in vivo endotoxin infusions on in vitro cellular immune responses in humans. J Clin Immunol 12:440–450
31. Faist E, Ertel W, Cohnert T, Huber P, Iknthorn D, Heberer G (1988) Immune protective effects of cyclo-oxygenase inhibition in patients with major surgical trauma. J Trauma 30:8
32. Hyers TM, Tricomi SM, Liao J-J (1992) Inhibition of some human neutrophil functions by the cyclooxygenase inhibitor ketorolac tromethamine. J Leukoc Biol 51:490–495

33. Abrahamson S, Weissmann G (1989) The mechanisms of action of nonsteroidal antiinflammatory drugs. Arthritis Rheum 32:1
34. Bernard GR, Reines HD, Metz CA et al. (1988) Effects of a short course of ibuprofen in patients with severe sepsis. Am Rev Respir Dis 137(4 Part 2):137 (abstr)
35. Bernard GR, Reines HD, Halushka PV et al. (1991) Prostacyclin and thromboxane A_2 formation is increased in human sepsis syndrome. Am Res Respir Dis 144:1095
36. Lanza FL (1989) A review of gastric ulcer and gastroduodenal injury in normal volunteers receiving aspirin and other non-steroidal anti-inflammatory drugs. Scand J Gastroenterol Suppl 163:24–31
37. Svartholm E, Arvidsson S, Fält K, Haglund U (1989) Influence of prostanoids on gastrointestinal mucosal injury in experimental septic shock. AMPIS 97:61–67
38. Ball HA, Parratt JR, Zeitlin IJ (1983) Effect of dazoxiben, a specific inhibitor of thromboxane synthetase, on acute pulmonary responses to E. coli endotoxin in anaesthetized cats. Br J Clin Pharmacol 15:121S–127S
39. Watkins WD, Hüttemeier PC, Kong D, Peterson MB (1982) Thromboxane and pulmonary hypertension following E. coli endotoxin infusion in sheep; effect of an imidazole derivative. Prostaglandins 23:273–285
40. Bennett WM, DeBroe ME (1989) Analgesic nephropathy – a preventable renal disease. New Engl J Med 320:1269–1271
41. Cryer HM, Unger LS, Garrison N, Harris PD (1988) Prostaglandins maintain renal microvascular blood flow during hyperdynamic bacteremia. Circ Shock 26:71
42. DiBona GF (1986) Prostaglandins and nonsteroidal antiinflammatory drugs: effects on renal hemodynamics. Am J Med 80:12
43. Carmichael J, Shankel SW (1985) Effects of nonsteroidal antiinflammatory drugs on prostaglandins and renal function. Am J Med 78:992
44. Hardie EM, Olsen NC (1987) Prostaglandin and thromboxane levels during endotoxin-induced respiratory failure in pigs. Prostaglandins Leuko Med 28:255
45. Harris RH, Zmudka M, Maddox Y, Ramwell PW, Fletcher JR (1980) Relationships of TXB_2 and 6-keto-$PGF_{1\alpha}$ to the hemodynamic changes during baboon endotoxic shock. In: Samuelsson B, Ramwell RW, Paoletti R (eds) Advances prostaglandins thromboxane research, vol 7. Raven, New York, pp 843

Cytokines and the Acute Catabolic State

H. R. Michie

Introduction

Classic studies performed in the early 1980s sought to determine whether the acute catabolic state that occurs after injury or infection could be explained by the altered hormonal milieu. Healthy subjects received counterregulatory hormones such as adrenaline, cortisol and glucagon, alone or in combination [1, 2]. It was found that these hormones, acting in synergy, produced transient alterations in glucose, protein and lipid kinetics that resembled those seen after infection and injury, but the responses were less severe and were not sustained. Furthermore, such hormonal infusions did not replicate the fever, neutrophil alterations or elaboration of acute phase proteins that characterize inflammation. The "holy grail" for investigators in this field became the search for the missing factor accounted for the non-hormonal component of the host response and which explained the basis of neuroendocrine activation.

The characterization, in the last 15 years, of the inflammatory cytokines seemed to offer the hope that the missing link had been found. Certain inflammatory cytokines which were found to be elaborated following injury, inflammation and infection, particularly tumour necrosis factor alpha (TNF-α) [3–6] and interleukin-1β (IL-1β) [7, 8], appeared on the basis of preliminary evidence to have exactly the biological qualities required to explain much of the altered host response. Additionally, they were related to other diseases which are characterized by increased nitrogen loss, e.g. cancer [9], acquired immunodeficiency syndrome (AIDS) [10], rheumatoid arthritis [11] and chronic parasitemias [12]. Such findings held the additional promise that agents which antagonized the effects of such cytokines might reverse the adverse catabolic responses. In 1995 it has to be said that this promise has not, as yet, been fulfilled and many problems exist within the whole field of study of cytokine activity in vivo. The purpose of this chapter is to discuss the problems that persist in the interpretation of available data and in the synthesis of a unifying hypothesis. The situation is made yet more complex by the fact that it must be borne in mind that in most clinical situations, the flow phase of the injury response, which is associated with acute catabolism, is preceded by an ebb phase, in which energy expenditure and substrate turnover are reduced. Many investigators believe that it is during the ebb phase, a short time after the initial inflammatory insult, that mediators are released and alterations occur to tissue that will go on to initiate and sustain the flow phase. It is thus clear that cytokines may play a role in acute catabolism both through direct and indirect effects on host homeostasis.

What Has Been Learned from Infusion of Cytokines into Animals and Human Beings?

Various cytokines have been administered to laboratory animals, healthy humans and patients with advanced malignant disease, by both single bolus injections and by chronic infusions. With regard to TNF-α, the data obtained after single injections are fairly consistent between animals and humans. Low doses of TNF-α induce subclinical alterations such as iron redistribution and neutrophil changes. Intermediate doses evoke fever and acute phase protein synthesis. Higher doses are required before neuroendocrine activation occurs, and such doses also evoke increased energy expenditure with enhanced turnover of glucose and fatty acid pathways. At the highest doses employed, animals die within hours of circulatory collapse and have autopsy findings which are similar to those observed in mammals dying of overwhelming infection [13–16].

A clinical syndrome which resembles the early changes of severe sepsis was also observed in cancer patients receiving the highest doses of TNF-α in phase I/II clinical trials [17]. The comparability of the dose-related effects of TNF-α to those of endotoxin [18] have provided important evidence suggesting that TNF-α is a pivotal mediator of the host response following endotoxemia. This has been further suggested by important studies on transgenic mice deficient for the 55-kDa TNF-α receptor which reveal that such animals are resistant to endotoxic schock [19].

Other cytokines, including IL-1β [7, 8] and IL-2 [20, 21], also induce acute inflammatory and neurohormonal changes, generally in a dose-dependent fashion, although sophisticated studies of substrate turnover, which have been performed in relation to TNF-α, are generally lacking with regard to these mediators. It is interesting to note that the time course of responses differs for these mediators – TNF-α acts rapidly, whereas IL-2 responses take longer to appear and are associated with a different pattern of secondary cytokine mediator generation.

It is clear that the catabolic responses associated with non-lethal doses of these cytokines are short-lived. For this reason investigators have examined the effects of continuous intravenous infusion of cytokines. A 5-day intravenous infusion of TNF-α to rats induced profound anorexia and debilitation, but the nitrogen balance was not different from that of pair-fed controls [22]. These findings have been replicated in humans. TNF-α infusions at certain doses produce a profound anorexia in the absence of abdominal pain or nausea, but nitrogen balance is similar to that of similarly fasted normals [23]. Interestingly, chronic infusion or repeated boluses of TNF-α are associated with marked tachyphyllaxis and also with cross-tolerance to endotoxin. Possible mechanisms explaining this have been discussed elsewhere [24].

Table 1 summarizes the principal recognized properties of the cytokine which are believed to be most important in the inflammatory/catabolic response.

Table 1. The principal cytokines involved in inflammatory/catabolic processes and principal biological responses which have been related to these cytokines

Cytokine	Response
TNF-α	Hypotension
	ARDS
	Coagulopathy
	Anorexia
	Cachexia?
	Neuroendocrine activation
	↑ Hypertriglyceridemia
	↑ Insulin resistance
	↑ Acute phase protein synthesis
	↑ Gluconeogenesis
	↑ Amino acid and fatty acid turnover
	Neutropenia
IL-1β	Hypotension (synergizes with TNF-α)
	Anorexia
	Fever
	Neuroendocrine activation
	CNS depression
	Neutrophilia
IL-2	Appears to be more important in antigenic responses but may have endotoxin-like properties
IL-6	↑ Hepatic acute phase protein synthesis
	Inhibits TNF-α and IL-1β synthesis
IL-8	Neutrophil recruitment into infected sites
IL-10	Inhibits TNF-α and IL-1β synthesis
Interferon-γ	Synergistic with TNF-α and other cytokines

TNF, tumour necrosis factor; ARDS, adult respiratory distress syndrome; IL, interleukin; CNS, central nervous system

What Are the Problems Associated with Studies Involving Administration of Exogenous Cytokines?

Physiology or Pharmacology?

It is clear that the injury response is a fairly stereotyped series of alterations which can be initiated by numerous inflammatory, infective and antigenic causes. The fact that a given cytokine is capable of initiating such alterations can in no way be taken to imply that such observations have any physiological as opposed to pharmacological relevance.

Route of Administration

The vast majority of such studies have involved intravenous administration of cyto-kines. As will be discussed later, there are probably few situations in which the bulk of cytokine elaboration occurs within the circulation. Cytokines generated in dif-ferent fixed tissues may elicit a different series of responses and may have differ-ent effects on key systems such as the gut–liver axis or the hypothalamus. This compartmentalization of the effects of TNF-α was well demonstrated by studies which showed that a TNF-α-secreting tumour in muscle appeared to induce chron-ic cachexia, whereas implantation into the brain principally induced anorexia [25].

Another cytokine, IL-6, has enjoyed a brief period of popularity as a possible mediator of the acute response to injury, but acute injections of recombinant IL-6 to animals appears to be associated with a marked increase in hepatic acute phase protein synthesis but few other stigmata of the classical acute response to injury or infection [26]. Conversely, in a recent paper, Brady and colleagues have provided evidence that the role of IL-6 may be much more subtle. Their data, based on cyto-kine infusions directly into the brain, suggest that sepsis-induced changes may be due to release of IL-6 from the central nervous system through a hypothalamic/pi-tuitary mechanism, and through this mechanism the c-*fos* gene may be activated [27]. This gene appears to be important in transcriptional events during sepsis, in-cluding not only those relating to acute phase synthesis but also the modulation of enzymes that are critical for fatty acid oxidation. A pathway of such complexity could never have been deduced by intravenous administration of IL-6.

Synergy Between Cytokines

The situation is further complicated by the fact that the effects of two or more cytokines acting in synergy are clearly dramatically greater than either acting alone. Perhaps the most impressive demonstratrion of this is the demonstration, in rabbits, that doses of TNF-α and IL-1β (which when given separately induce few demon-strable alteration) given together initiate gross haemodynamic instability [28]. Furthermore, certain cytokines induce other cytokines; TNF-α induces IL-1β and IL-6 [29], whereas IL-2 evokes TNF-α and interferon-γ [20, 21], and interferon-γ markedly up-regulates TNF-α receptor expression [30]. Such complexities at the moment prevent an accurate dissection of the metabolic response to injury.

Synergy may also exist between given cytokines and classical hormones with very complex interrelationships between cytokine induction and neuroendocrine activation [31].

What Has Been Learned from Measuring Cytokines During Catabolic States?

One of the commonest approaches used with the aim of elucidating the role of a given mediator in disease has been to measure, repeatedly over time, the circulating level of that mediator. For classical hormones this approach has proved very successful because, by definition, a hormone must circulate in order to elicit its effects, most hormones are easily measurable in the bloodstream and their biological effects do not long outline their appearance in the circulation. This is not the case with regard to cytokines.

TNF-α can be measured in blood samples taken in patients with early but not established meningococcal septicaemia [32], cerebral malaria [33] and other conditions associated with acute and gross septic consequences. Apart from these examples, the detection of TNF-α in the blood stream of infected or injured patients has been sporadic and inconsistent. The appearance of TNF-α in the blood stream appears to represent an "overspill" phenomenon which heralds dire clinical consequences. Circulating TNF-α can be detected in individuals receiving intravenous endotoxin, but only at the onset of clinical consequences and not when fever and hypermetabolism are at their maximum extent [34, 35]. It appears that this cytokine is released in a pulsatile fashion and the biological effects long outlive the period when it can be detected. With regard to IL-1β, the situation appears to be more complex still, since this cytokine lacks a signal peptide that allows it to be exported from the cell [8]. Most of the biological effects of IL-1β appear to be caused by cell-associated IL-1β, and the mediator can only be detected in the blood stream following cellular necrosis or apoptosis.

Other factors which influence the interpretation of circulating cytokine levels in health and disease have been discussed in detail elsewhere [36] and can be summarized as follows:

1. The normal range for circulating cytokines in health has not been established. These mediators are released in a pulsatile fashion and have short half-lives, and there is no good urinary marker by which we can quantify cytokine elaboration in an integrated fashion.
2. There are binding proteins, including receptor fragments, that bind given cytokines [37]. The bound cytokine may be neutralized, enhanced or unaffected by such binding. Cytokines may up-regulate their own binding proteins. Furthermore, depletion of certain binding proteins may cause exaggerated responses to otherwise harmless levels of a given cytokine in the circulation. The administration of endotoxin to normal subjects is associated with the induction of a potent endogenous inhibitor of IL-1β known as the IL-1 receptor antagonist (IL-1ra) [38]. IL-1β activity cannot be interpreted without also knowing the levels of this natural antagonist.
3. Several cytokines exhibit polymorphism, including TNF-α [39] and IL-1β [7], which means that a given assay may not detect all the different active forms of that cytokine.
4. There remain problems with current assay systems. Enzyme-linked immunosorbent assay (ELISA) systems measure immunoactive moieties but may not reflect bioactivity. Bioassays do measure bioactivity but may not be specific.
5. The knowledge of the circulating concentration of a given cytokine is valueless unless we also know levels of other cytokines with which it may be synergistic, as mentioned previously.

6. Compartmentalized cytokine production (e.g. in the liver, gut or brain) may be associated with systemic effects in the absence of detectable circulating cytokine.

It is clear from the foregoing that we urgently need better methods of measuring whole body cytokine bioactivity if we are to come nearer to establishing associations between given cytokines and particular syndromes such as the acute catabolic state.

What Can Be Learned from Studies in Which a Given Cytokine is Antagonized?

The possibility that antagonism of certain cytokines might reverse many of the most adverse host responses to injury or inflammation has led to an explosion in the biotechnology industry, a host of clinical trials costing overall in excess of $ 10 billion and a very uncertain outcome.

Perhaps the most influential experiment in animals that caused this explosion was that of Tracey and colleagues in which they showed that a monoclonal antibody against TNF-α, when given prophylactically, prevented death following injection of an otherwise invariably lethal dose of live *Escherichia coli* organisms [40]. At the time, this experiment seemed to indicate that the blockade of just one host mediator was sufficient to block a pathophysiological pathway that accounts for more deaths on intensive treatment units than any other in the Western world. It should be emphasized that this study suggested that TNF-α blockade was only beneficial if given *before* the infective insult. Nevertheless, two large clinical trials have been performed in patients with the established sepsis syndrome, largely as a result of this study. One study has shown no difference in survival [41] and the other suggests that blockade of TNF-α is positively harmful (reported in [42]). A detailed discussion of possible explanations for these observations lies outside of the scope of this chapter but some considerations are relevant to studies which may be performed in the future which aim to attenuate the acute catabolic state in humans.

Importance of Dose–Response Relationships

As mentioned above, baboons receiving anti-TNF-α antibodies at doses of 10 mg/kg do not die when subsequently injected with 1.2×10^{11} live *E. coli* organisms intravenously (an otherwise invariably lethal dose). When data are presented in this way the results seem dramatic, but such reports do not answer the key question, which is: *to what extent is the dose–response curve for survival of animals receiving increasing doses of endotoxin/organisms shifted to the right by the presence of a fixed dose of neutralizing antibody?*

Beutler and colleagues investigated such dose–response relationships in mice receiving a fixed and large dose of anti-TNF-α agent and varying doses of endotoxin [43]. The median lethal dose (LD_{50}) of endotoxin was increased by a factor of

2.4, and administration of larger doses of antibody did not further improve survival. Mice receiving more than 480 μg endotoxin died whether they received the TNF-α antagonist or not. This study demonstrates that anti-TNF-α therapy is not protective against severe endotoxemia. It is the author's belief that the importance of these sigmoid dose–response relationships for anti-cytokine therapies cannot be overestimated. If the level of endotoxemia lies outside the range in which TNF-α antagonists are effective, then it is not surprising that no advantage is shown in terms of survival. Such studies also make it clear that in overwhelming endotoxemia sufficient quantities of other noxious mediators are evoked to cause death even when TNF-α has been effectively neutralized.

Site of Infection

In laboratory animals TNF-α antagonists appear to increase survival following a subsequent *intravenous* challenge with endotoxin. Very few common sources of sepsis arise within the circulation. Most are accumulations of infected fluid within body cavities. Echtenacher and colleagues studied the effects of TNF-α antagonism in a mouse model of experimental peritonitis induced by cecal ligation and puncture. Inhibition of TNF-α converted a sub-lethal model into a lethal one [44]. The authors propose that TNF-α may stimulate granulocytes, macrophages and other non-lymphoid cells to ingest bacteria and localize inflammation. This is supported by work in animals that has shown that in infections where granuloma formation is an essential part of the eradication of infection, blockade of TNF-α strongly inhibits the development of granulomas and other aspects of bacterial resistance [45, 46].

Thus, TNF-α clearly evokes beneficial as well as adverse host alterations during sepsis, and the indications for TNF-α antagonism in infected humans remain to be clarified.

Do Neutralizing Antibodies Neutralize?

It appears that even if an anti-cytokine antibody neutralizes a given cytokine *in vitro,* this does not guarantee that the antigen–antibody complex does not have pro-inflammatory effects *in vivo.*.In one recent study in rabbits, animals receiving recombinant human TNF-α who also received an immunoglobulin (Ig)G₄ anti-TNF-α antibody showed a dose-dependent reduction in pyrexia compared with those receiving TNF-α alone. In contrast, rabbits receiving TNF-α with an IgG₁ anti-TNF-α antibody demonstrated a greater fever than was seen with TNF-α alone [47]. The authors related differences between the effects of the IgG₁ and the IgG₄ antibody to the fact that immune complexes containing the former, but not the latter, can generate secondary effector mechanisms including secondary cytokine generation and complement activation via Fc receptor binding.

Finkelman and colleagues have shown than an anti-IL-4 monoclonal antibody that was neutralizing *in vitro* appeared to increase and prolong the biological effects of the cytokine *in vivo*. The authors proposed the intriguing hypothesis that the antibody acts as a "chaperone" to prevent modification of the cytokine's active site and to delay excretion. The cytokine dissociates slowly from the antibody and, overall, the magnitude and duration of the cytokine's activity is prolonged. Such effects were not seen with antibodies which bound to, but did not neutralize IL-4 [48].

These animal studies raise the worrying possibility that in our efforts to neutralize cytokines in critically ill patients we may, in fact, have been inadvertently enhancing their bioactivity.

A further concern relating to cytokine antagonists is that the majority are of high molecular weight (particularly monoclonal antibodies) and therefore may well be confined to the circulation when administered intravenously. It is likely that much cytokine elaboration during infection occurs within fixed tissues which may not be exposed to such antagonists.

How Many Cytokines Must We Neutralize?

In experimental models of endotoxic shock, prophylactic administration of antagonists of TNF-α [40, 43], IL-1β [49], interferon-γ [50] and possibly IL-6 [51] prevented death. However, in phase 111 trials, anti-TNF-α therapy [41, 42] and anti-IL-1β therapy [52] have proved ineffective in reducing the death rate in the sepsis syndrome. It is possible that the agents have been given too late to be effective. It is also possible that in critically ill humans multiple cytokines must be antagonized before an improved outcome is achieved.

Does Anti-Cytokine Therapy Specifically Attenuate the Acute Catabolic State?

The major thrust of anti-cytokine therapy has been in the amelioration of the sepsis syndrome and septic shock, and little work has been performed in human beings specifically addressing the acute catabolic state. A clinical response which resembles the acute catabolic state can be induced in healthy humans by injection of a single intravenous dose of *E. coli* endotoxin [34]. Prophylactic administration of IL-1ra had only minimal effects in attenuating endotoxin-induced responses [53]. Neither the fever nor the neuroendocrine response was attenuated by this therapy. Healthy individuals have also received an anti-TNF-α antibody prior to endotoxin administration. TNF-α antagonism was associated with a delay in the onset of clinical responses, but individuals had a higher fever than those receiving endotoxin alone and the neuroendocrine response, although delayed, was not different in terms of its final magnitude when compared with endotoxin alone (H. R. Michie, manuscript submitted).

Thus, in a relevant human model, blockade of the two cytokines considered of the greatest importance in the acute inflammatory state did not prove effective in diminishing catabolic responses.

Conclusion

The cytokine network is clearly one of enormous complexity. It involves multiple mediators with similar properties, soluble and bound receptors, natural antagonists and has autocrine, paracrine and endocrine components. It is also clear that individuals vary greatly both in the magnitude of the cytokine response to a given stimulus and in end-organ responsiveness. Tracking such a complex network in given catabolic states is not possible with available technology, and most experimental and clinical studies performed to date are probably crude and simplistic.

The view that it is beneficial to block certain cytokines in critical infective illness is now being increasingly challenged in the light of the recent clinical trials. Although cytokine blockade may be of benefit in certain conditions, particularly those involving excessive cytokine generation within the circulation, in other conditions it may be detrimental, as the same cyotkines that, when produced in excess, may mediate shock and catabolism appear also to be vital components of the body's integrated system for localizing and eradicating infection.

A possible alternative approach to antagonizing cytokines such as TNF-α and IL-1β may lie in the administration of other cytokines such as IL-6 [54, 55] and IL-10 [56, 57], which appear to down-regulate production of these cytokines.

Further insights into the role of TNF-α in cachexia may derive from clinical trials of anti-TNF-α therapy in rheumatoid arthritis, a condition associated with marked cachexia and in which blockade of TNF-α appears to be a very promising approach. However, it is likely that we are years, if not decades, away from understanding the exact role of cytokines in the catabolic process. Given the serious reservations that must currently be expressed concerning the safety of cytokine blockade in sepsis, it is by no means easy to see how the role of cytokines in acute catabolism in humans is going to be clarified. Much can be learned from further studies in animals, but there remains the concern that, in the septic and the catabolic state, animal models have not been at all effective in predicting efficacy of new agents in man.

References

1. Bessey P, Watters J, Aoki T, Wilmore D (1984) Combined hormonal infusion stimulates the metabolic response to injury. Ann Surg 200:264–281
2. Watters J, Bessey P, Dinarello C, Wolff S, Wilmore D (1986) Both inflammatory and endocrine mediators stimulate host responses to sepsis. Arch Surg 121:179–190
3. Tracey KJ (1992) TNF and other cytokines in the metabolism of septic shock and cachexia. Clin Nutr 11:1–11
4. Tracey KJ, Cerami A (1994) Tumor necrosis factor: a pleiotropic cytokine and therapeutic target. Ann Rev Med 45:491–503
5. Streiter RM, Kunkel SL, Bone RC (1993) Role of tumor necrosis factor in disease states and inflammation. Crit Care Med 21 [Suppl 10]:S447–S463
6. Beutler B, Krochin N, Milsark I, Luedke C, Cerami A (1986) Control of cachectin (tumor necrosis factor) synthesis: mechanisms of endotoxin resistance. Science 232:977–980
7. Dinarello CA (1994) Interleukin-1. Adv Pharmacol 25:21–51
8. Dinarello C (1988) Biology of interleukin-1. FASEB J 2:108–115
9. Moldawer LL, Rogy MA, Lowry SF (1992) The role of cytokines in cancer cachexia. J Parenter Enteral Nutr 16:43S–49S

10. Grunfeld C, Feingold KR (1992) Metabolic disturbance and wasting in the acquired immuno-deficiency snydrome. N Engl J Med 327:329–337
11. Roubenoff R, Roubenoff RA, Cannon JG et al. (1994) Rheumatoid cachexia: cytokine-driven hypermetabolism accompanying reduced body cell mass in chronic inflammation. J Clin Invest 93:379–386
12. Scuderi P, Lam K, Ryan K et al. (1986) Raised serum levels of tumour necrosis factor in parasitic infections. Lancet ii:1364-1365
13. Michie HR, Spriggs DR, Manogue KR et al. (1988) Tumor necrosis factor and endotoxin induce similar metabolic responses in human beings. Surgery 104:280–286
14. Evans D, Jacobs D, Revhaug A, Wilmore D (1989) The effects of tumor necrosis factor and their selective inhibition by ibuprofen. Ann Surg 209:312–321
15. van der Poll, Romijn JA, Endert E et al. (1991) Tumor necrosis factor mimics the metabolic response to acute infection in healthy humans. Am J Physiol 26:E457–E461
16. Tracey K, Beutler B, Lowry S et al. (1986) Shock and tissue injury induced by recombinant human cachectin. Science 234:470–474
17. Spriggs DR, Sherman ML, Michie HR et al. (1988) Recombinant human tumor necrosis factor administered as a 24 hour continuous infusion. A phase 1 and pharmacologic study. J Clin Oncol 12:128–135
18. Wolff S (1973) Biological effects of bacterial endotoxins in man. In: Wolff S, Kass E (eds) Bacterial lipopolysaccharides. University of Chicago Press, Chicago, pp 251–256
19. Pfeffer K, Matsuyama T, Kundig TM et al. (1993) Mice deficient for the 55 kD tumor necrosis factor receptor are resistant to endotoxin shock yet succumb to L monocytogenes infection. Cell 73:457–467
20. Michie HR, Eberlein TJ, Spriggs DR et al. (1988) Interleukin-2 initiates metabolic responses associated with critical illness in humans. Ann Surg 208:493–503
21. Mier J, Vachino G, Van Meer J et al. (1988) Induction of circulating tumor necrosis factor (TNF) as the mechanism for the febrile response to interleukin-2 (IL-2) in cancer patients. J Clin Immunol 8:426–436
22. Michie H, Spriggs D, Rounds J, Wilmore D (1987) Does cachectin cause cachexia? Surg Forum 37:38–40
23. Michie HR, Sherman ML, Spriggs DR et al. (1989) Chronic TNF infusion causes anorexia but not accelerated nitrogen loss. Ann Surg 209:19–24
24. Zuckerman SH, Evans GF (1992) Endotoxin tolerance: in vivo regulation of tumor necrosis factor and interleukin-1 synthesis is at the transcriptional level. Cell Immunol 140:513–519
25. Tracey KJ, Morgello S, Koplin B et al. (1990) Metabolic effects of cachectin/tumor necrosis factor are modified by site of production. Cachectin/tumor necrosis factor-secreting tumor in skeletal muscle induces chronic cachexia, while implantation in brain induces predominantly anorexia. J Clin Invest 86:2014–2024
26. Kishimoto T, Akira S, Taga T (1992) Interleukin-6 and its receptor: a paradigm for cytokines. Science 258:593
27. Barke RA, Roy S, Chapin R et al. (1994) Sepsis-induced release of interleukin-6 may activate the immediate-early gene program through a hypothalamic-hypophyseal mechanism. Surgery 116:141–149
28. Okusawa S, Gelfand JA, Ikejima T, Connolly RJ, Dinarello CA (1988) Interleukin-1 induces a shock-like state in rabbits. Synergism with tumor necrosis factor and the effects of cyclooxygenase inhibition. J Clin Invest 81:1162–1172
29. Fong YM, Tracey KJ, Moldawer LL et al. (1989) Antibodies to cachectin/TNF reduce interleukin-1β and interleukin-6 appearance during lethal septicemia. J Exp Med 170:162716–162733
30. Ruggiero V, Tavernier J, Fiers W, Baglioni C (1986) Induction of the synthesis of tumor necrosis factor receptors by gamma interferon. J Immunol 136:2445–2450
31. Jones TH, Kennedy RL (1993) Cytokines and hypothalamic-pituitary function. Cytokine 5:531–538
32. Girardin E, Grau G, Dayer J, Roux-Lombard P, The J5 Study Group, Lambert P (1988) Tumor necrosis factor and interleukin-1 in the serum of children with severe infectious purpura. N Engl Med J 319:397–400

33. Graue GE, Taylor TE, Molyneux ME et al. (1989) Tumor necrosis factor and disease severity in children with Falciparum malaria. N Engl J Med 320:1586–1591
34. Michie HR, Manogue KR, Spriggs DR et al. (1988) Detection of circulating tumour necrosis factor after endotoxin administration. N Engl J Med 318:1481–1486
35. Revhaug A, Michie HR, Manson J et al. (1988) Inhibition of cyclooxygenase attenuates the metabolic response to endotoxin in humans. Arch Surg 123:1459–1464
36. Cannon JG, Nerad JL, Poutsiaka DD, Dinarello CA (1993) Measuring cytokine levels. J Appl Physiol 75:1897–1902
37. Aderka D, Engelmann H, Maor Y, Brackebusch C, Wallach D (1992) Stabilization of the bio-activity of tumor necrosis factor by its soluble receptors. J Exp Med 175:323–329
38. Granowitz EV, Santos AA, Poutsiaca DD et al. (1991) Production of interleukin-1 receptor antagonist during experimental endotoxemia. Lancet 338:1423–1424
39. Smith RA, Baglioni C (1987) The active form of tumor necrosis factor is a trimer. J Biol Chem 262:6951–6954
40. Tracey KJ, Fong Y, Hesse DJ et al. (1987) Anti-cachectin/TNF monoclonal antibodies prevent septic shock during lethal bacteremia. Nature 330:662–666
41. Anonymous (1993) New hope for an anti-TNF MAb in sepsis. SCRIP 1868 (October 29) p 29
42. Stone R (1994) Search for sepsis drugs goes on despite past failures. Science 264:365–367
43. Beutler B, Milsark I, Cerami A (1985) Passive immunization against cachectin/tumor necrosis factor protects mice from lethal effect of endotoxin. Science 229:869–871
44. Echtenacher B, Falk W, Mannel DN, Krammer PH (1990) Requirement of endogenous tumor necrosis factor/cachectin for recovery from experimental peritonitis. J Immunol 145:3762–3766
45. Kindler V, Sappino AP, Graue GE, Piguet PF, Lambert PH, Vassali P (1989) The inducing role of tumor necrosis factor in the development of bacterial granulomas during BCG infection. Cell 56:731–740
46. Havell EA (1989) Evidence that tumor necrosis factor has an important role in bacterial resistance. J Immunol 143:2894–2899
47. Suitters AJ, Foulkes R, Opal SM et al. (1994) Differential effect of isotype on efficacy of anti-tumor necrosis factor α chimeric antibodies in experimental septic shock. J Exp Med 179:849–856
48. Finkelman FD, Madden KB, Morris SC et al. (1993) Anti-cytokine antibodies as carrier proteins. J Immunol 151:1235–1244
49. Ohlsson K, Bjork P, Bergenfeldt M, Hageman R, Thompson RC (1990) Interleukin-1 receptor antagonist reduces mortality from endotoxin shock. Nature 348:550–552
50. Silva AT, Cohen J (1992) Role of interferon-γ in experimental gram-negative sepsis. J Infect Dis 166:331–335
51. Starnes HF, Pearce MK, Tewari A, Yim JH, Zou JC, Abrams JS (1990) Anti-IL-6 monoclonal antibodies protect against lethal Escherichia coli infection and lethal tumor necrosis factor-α challenge in mice. J Immunol 45:4185–4191
52. Fischer CJ, Slotman GJ, Opal SM et al. (1994) Initial evaluation of human recombinant interleukin-1 receptor antagonist in the treatment of sepsis syndrome: a randomized, open-label, placebo-controlled multicenter trial. Crit Care Med 22:12–21
53. Granowitz EV, Porat R, Mier JW et al. (1993) Hematologic and immunomodulatory effects of an interleukin-1 receptor antagonist coinfusion during low-dose endotoxaemia in healthy humans. Blood 82:2985–2990
54. Tilg H, Trehu E, Atkins MB, Dinarello CA, Mier JW (1994) Interleukin-6 as an anti-inflammatory cytokine: induction of circulating IL-1 receptor antagonist and soluble tumor necrosis factor receptor p55. Blood 83:113–118
55. Dinarello CA (1992) Blocking cytokines in infective diseases. In: Lamy M, Thijs LG (eds) Mediators of sepsis. Springer, Berlin Heidelberg New York, pp 362–366
56. Cassatella MA, Meda L, Bonora S, Ceska M, Constantin G (1993) Interleukin-10 (IL-10) inhibits the release of proinflammatory cytokines from human polymorphonuclear leukocytes. Evidence for an autocrine role of tumor necrosis factor and IL-1β in mediating the production of IL-8 triggered by lipopolysaccharide. J Exp Med 178:2207–2211
57. Marchant A, Deviere J, Byle B, De Groote D, Vincent JL, Goldman M (1994) Interleukin-10 production during septicaemia. Lancet 343:707–708

Antioxidants and the Acute Catabolic State

J. Kjæve, D. W. Wilmore, and A. Revhaug

Toxic oxygen metabolites have been shown to constitute a major final common pathway of tissue injury in a wide variety of acute disease processes. Accordingly, therapy has aimed to inhibit or dampen the effects of these free radicals. These systems are extremely fast reacting and accordingly of utmost importance in the early phases of an acute disease. This chapter reviews the pathophysiology of some common toxic oxygen metabolites and focuses on how antioxidants may ameliorate the damage of these substances.

Actions of Free Radicals and Other Oxidant Molecules

A free radical is an unstable molecule containing one or more unpaired electrons [1]. By reduction or excitation of molecular oxygen, several oxygen free radicals may be produced [2]. Superoxide is produced in normal cellular metabolism and is derived from mitochondrial, endoplasmic reticular, and nuclear membrane electron transport processes, and from soluble proteins [3, 4]. The hydroxyl radical can be catalyzed by iron complexes [5], and is the most reactive of the free radicals in biological systems [6]. It causes lipid peroxidation and can oxidize sulfhydryl groups, inactivate cytochrome enzymes, and change the membrane transport proteins. Singlet oxygen and perhydroxyl, also radicals produced from oxygen, are probably direct initiators of lipid peroxidation [7].

Different mechanisms of free radical production have been identified in biological systems. In pathological states, these radicals may be derived from different sources, e.g., activated neutrophils, xanthine oxidase metabolism, and endothelial cells [8–10].

There are also toxic nonoxygen products, e.g., the free radicals of lipids, and a free radical of sulphur; this is why cystine is a toxic substance to the body. Moreover, the body has a variety of reactions which take these highly charged radicals down to a more reduced state, but they are generally still toxic products even though not free radicals. For example, hydrogen peroxide is a natural breakdown metabolite of free radical products although it is not a free radical. During the neutrophil respiratory burst, hydrochloric acid (HCl) is also produced.

These oxidants injure cells in three basic ways. The cell membranes which are comprised primarily of lipid substances are attacked, causing lipid peroxidation and the phospholipids within the membrane, which maintain fluidity, are damaged.

The proteins are also subject to free radical mediated denaturation, which leads to structural damage or enzymatic deactivation. Injury to the nucleic acid by the radicals may result in cell mutation or even cell death [11]. Finally, the extracellular tissue components such as hyaluronic acid and collagen may be injured by the toxic oxidants [12].

Nature of Free Radicals and Other Oxidants in the Acute Catabolic State

Ischemia – Reperfusion

During interrupted blood supply to a tissue (ischemia), a sequence of chemical events is initiated leading to cellular dysfunction, interstitial edema, and cell death. During ischemia, the lack of oxygen results in anaerobic metabolism and a local increase in lactic acid. The resulting acidosis will alter the normal enzymatic genetics, and fewer high energy bonds will be created with deficient energy cell supply [13]. So far, no single process has been identified as the critical factor leading to ischemia-induced cell death. The depletion of cellular energy stores results in a failure of cell membrane functions [14]. The plasma membrane changes will in turn lead to a loss of ions, clamping of chromatin, and nuclear pyknosis [15].

After a shorter or longer period of ischemia, reperfusion may take place and a reperfusion injury may originate [16]. This type of injury has been demonstrated in a diversity of experimental models, in several of which it could be prevented by administration of superoxide dismutase or allupurinol at the end of ischemia but be-

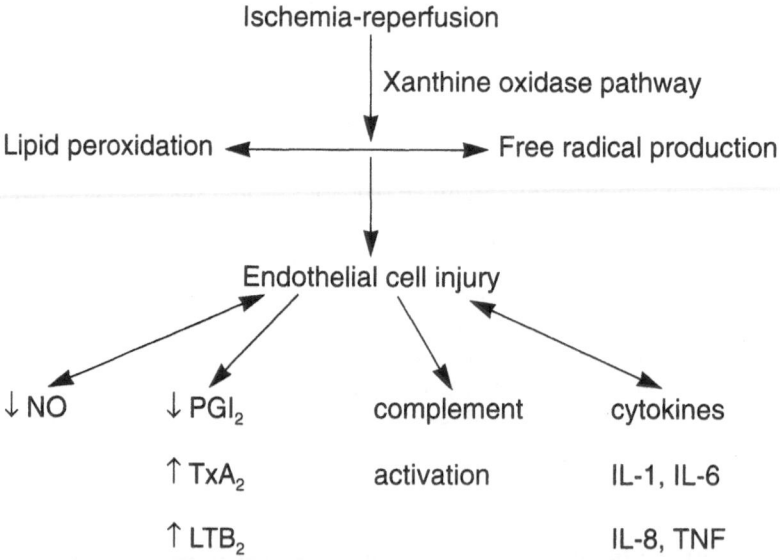

Fig. 1. The endothelial cells in ischemia-reperfusion injury (modified from [64])

fore reperfusion [16, 17]. Thus, oxygen-derived mediators of the reperfusion injury are believed to be important (Fig. 1) [1, 14, 18].

Immune Cells and Free Radicals

The cells of the immune system that are mainly responsible for the production of free radicals and other oxidant molecules are the neutrophils and other phagocytes. The respiratory burst of free radicals and other oxidant molecules from the neutrophils are important during phagocytosis. Activated neutrophils adhere to and migrate across the endothelium causing local destruction by release of free radicals and proteolytic enzymes [19, 20]. The injured endothelial cells may subsequently produce nitric oxide and other free radicals [21, 22].

Interaction Between Free Radicals and the Cytokines

It has recently been demonstrated that cytokines and free radicals enhance each others' production, as is seen when endotoxin-stimulated tumor necrosis factor (TNF) production was enhanced by alloxane, a pro-oxidant drug [23]. This effect could be prevented by administration of an antioxidant or an iron-chelating agent.

The enzymes involved in the metabolism of the superoxide radical and hydrogen peroxide are increased by the actions of interleukin-1 (IL-1) and TNF [24, 25]. Cytokines may also induce changes that minimize free radical production by enhancing the synthesis of hemoglobin and transferrin, thereby limiting the exposure of tissues to iron [26, 27]. IL-1 production from endotoxin-stimulated murine macrophages has been shown to be reduced by probucol, an antioxidant agent [28]. In similar studies it has also been shown that in vitro production of TNF, IL-1, IL-2, and IL-8 is stimulated by hydrogen peroxide [23, 29]. The mechanism for this enhancing effect of free radicals on cytokine production has been supposed to be the ability of the radicals to activate the nuclear transcription factor [30–32]. Accordingly, the up and down regulation of cytokine production is influenced by the free radicals, and vice versa, resulting a delicate balance between the immnune cells, cytokines, and the free radicals.

Antioxidants

Modification of the deleterious effects of free radicals to the tissues can be done at different levels i.e., inhibiting generation of the substances, scavenging oxidants after their generation, and improving the endogenous antioxidant systems. The antioxidants are capable of interrupting peroxidation and thereby preventing tissue damage and further actions of free radicals and/or other toxic mediators.

Two main types of antioxidants can be used in acute injury, i.e., endogenous and exogenous antioxidants (Tables 1, 2). The endogenous antioxidants represent an extremely important defense mechanism that allows organisms based on aerobic

Table 1. Endogenous antioxidants

Enzymatic antioxidants
Cytochrome oxidase
Superoxide dismutase
Catalase
Glutathione peroxidase
Peroxidase
Nonenzymatic antioxidants
α-Tocopherol
β-Carotene
Glutathione
Ascorbic acid
Urate
Cystein
Albumin
Ceruloplasmin
Transferrin
Lactoferrin
Ferritin

Modified after Reilly et al. [34]

Table 2. Exogenous antioxidants

Antioxidants	Mechanism of action
Xantine oxidase inhibitors:	
Allupurinol	Inhibition of superoxide production
Oxypurinol	
SOD	
Native SOD	Catalyze superoxide to hydrogen peroxide
Catalases	Scavenge hydrogen peroxide and superoxide peroxide
NADPH oxidase inhibitors:	
Adneosine	Inhibit superoxide generation by NADPH oxidase in neutrophils
Calcium channel blockers	
NSAIDs	
Nonenzymatic free radical scavengers:	
Mannitol	Scavengers of free radicals
Albumin	
Glutathione	

SOD, superoxide dismutase; NADPH, reduced form of nicotinamide-adenine dinucleotide phosphate; NSAID, nonsteroidal anit-inflammatory drug

metabolism to survive the normal oxidative stress. The body's way of protecting itself against the toxic substances is by cellular compartmentalization; the mitochondrion, lysosome, and cytoplasm are separate micro-environments, all containing free radical generating systems coupled to immediately adjacent antioxidant mechanisms [33] (Fig. 2). The endogenous antioxidants are primarily subdivided in enzymatic or nonenzymatic antioxidants [34].

Naturally occurring antioxidant defense substances are localized throughout the body to protect the cells from the adverse effects of the free radicals. In the circulation and in the cells, antioxidants such as glutathione, deriving from glycine, cysteine and glutamate, and ceruloplasmin are important antioxidants. α-Tocopherol (vitamin E) is located in the cell membrane and within the cell itself. Vitamin C resides within the aqueous part of the cell and also represents an important defense against free radicals in the plasma. An important function of vitamin C is to recirculate vitamin E by absorbing free radicals from the vitamin E molecule. When vitamin E has been used, β-carotene has its most potent antioxidative effect.

In addition to the defense systems capable of directly inactivating the free radicals, there are important indirect systems which can prevent radicals from propagating. The importance of ceruloplasmin in the context is typical as ceruloplasmin can sequester metal ions. Several trace metals like iron and copper, if present in free forms, are capable of catalyzing the transformation of hydrogen peroxide to active hydroxyl radicals. The importance of transition metal ion binding has been demonstrated in several studies [35–37].

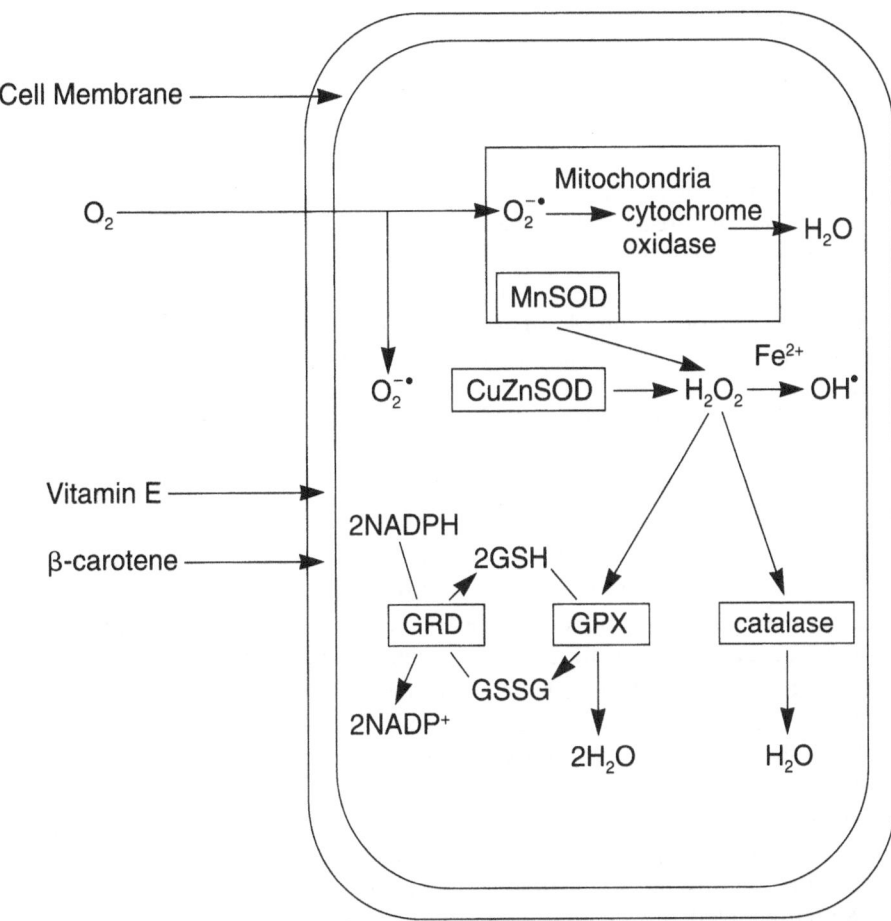

Fig. 2. Antioxidant defense system of a cell. (O_2, superoxide radical; MnSOD, manganese super-oxide dismutase; CuZnSOD, copper-zinc superoxide dismutase; NADP, nicotinamide adenine dinucleotide phosphate; NADPH, NADP (reduced form); GPX, glutathione peroxidase; GRD, glutathione reductase; GSH, reduced glutathione; GSSG, oxidized glutathione; OH, hydroxyl radical. (Reproduced with permission from [65]) (Adapted with permission from the American Journal of Medicine).

Antioxidative State of the Acute Catabolic Patient

Several direct and indirect data indicate that the antioxidative sytems are depleted in the acute catabolic state [38–40]. The combination of ischemia-reperfusion injury with or without an inflammatory component can both utilize the stores of naturally occurring antioxidants and limit the intake and production of these substances. However, it should also be stressed that the antioxidative systems are very robust and highly interactive. In this way when one component is reduced in amount or activity, compensatory changes often occur regarding other components. One such interacitve mechanism can be seen with regard to β-carotine, which functions as an antioxidant under conditions of low oxygen tension [41], and a marked synergistic effect between β-carotene and vitamin E has been described in their ability to reduce free radical damage [42, 43]. Another example is the increased production of ceruloplasmin in response to TNF when the capacity for glutathione synthesis is decreased due to a low protein status [44].

In most acute catabolic states, with the exception of some accidents and acute infections in otherwise healthy persons, the patient suffers from some underlying disease. In most such situations, the levels of naturally occurring antioxidant defense factors will already be depressed before the acute catabolic insult takes place [45]. The addition of the acute catabolic insult will then further depress the antioxidative reserve and, with an almost obligatory deficient supply, the situation will become further compromised. An insufficient protein intake, which often is the situation in an acute catabolic state, reduces the glutathione content in liver and lungs [46, 47].

Clinical Implications

Even though there is a great uncertainty with regard to the importance and mechanisms of action for the possible use of antioxidants to prevent the damage by free radicals during acute catabolic situations, several lines of evidence seem at present to indicate several options for therapeutic antioxidant interventions.

Several factors have to be taken into consideration when planning the use of antioxidants in the acute catabolic state. Therapy aimed at improving the antioxidant defense should involve intra- and extracellular protection against superoxide, hydrogen peroxide, hydroxyl radicals, and membrane lipid peroxidation. Antioxidants may be supplied in various ways, e.g., in the form of endogenous or exogenous antioxidant supplementation or with nutritional aids as a supportive therapy in order to improve the production of endogenous antioxidants.

So far relatively few clinical studies have been reported that explore the different ways of using antioxidants in acute catabolic states. Not surprisingly, the first reports on beneficial effects of antioxidant therapy related to transplant patients. In several large randomized, double-blind, placebo-controlled, clinical studies it has been shown that there was a significant reduction in the incidence of acute renal failure and improved early as well as late graft function in kidneys with medium or long preservation periods when superoxide dismutase was given at the time of reperfusion [48, 49]. As a result of these and other data, commonly used organ preservation solutions such as the University of Wisconsin solution include the antioxidants allupurinol and glutathione. Similar, but not so convincing data have been reported with the use of antioxidants in conjunction with global myocardial ischemia [50, 51].

After manx years of using antioxidants such as vitamin E [52, 53] superoxide dismutase [52, 54], allupurinol [55], and N-acetyl cysteine [56], in experimental animal septic or trauma models with clear indication of positive effects, similar studies have been started in humans. Patients with sepsis-related adult respiratory distress syndrome (ARDS) who were administered N-acetyl cysteine demonstrated increased cardiac output and oxygen delivery [57], and repletion of glutathione [58]. Patients trated with a combinant of ascorbic acid, N-acetyal cysteine and vitamin E showed a marked reduction in mortality [59]. Vitamin E has been shown to improve immune function in AIDS [60], in middle aged and elderly persons [61], and in patients undergoing chemotherapy for malignant diseases (D. W. Wilmore et al., unpublished data). Vitamin C has been shown to decrease the frequency and severity of upper respiratory infections in marathon runners [62]. There has been an increasing focus on nutrients as modulators of the antioxidant defense. The metabolic consequences of an acute catabolic state include an increased demand for protein, specific amino acids, and trace elements. In several experimental studies, Grimble et al. have demonstrated that the intake of sulfhydryl compounds such as cysteine, gluthathione and *N*-acetyl cysteine potentially improves immune functions and antioxidative defense [63]. In a similar way, Wilmore and collaborators have shown that nutritional manipulation with both oral and intravenous gluatmine, which serves as the precursor for glutathione, improves the outcome of patients with drug intoxications and chemotherapy-induced liver diseases.

Major problems with regard to the timing of intervention with antioxidants in the acute catabolic state should, however, not be underestimated. These problems have clearly been demonstrated with regard to the ischemia-reperfusion situation [64]. Ischemia-reperfusion represents only a portion of the problems compared with the diversity of pathophysiological events seen in the acute catabolic situations. On the other hand, the possibilities of achieving clinically important progress in patient outcome require ongoing efforts to elucidate ways of improving antioxidative defense in acute catabolic situations. At this time, the use of antioxidants should probably have a rightful place in clinical medicine. It is our opinion that patients who enter an acute catabolic state need antioxidant repletion at an early stage, vitamins C and E being the most appropriate in the acute situation. It also seems that within a few days after injury the nutritional supplementation of glutamine and other precursors of the endogenous tissue antioxidants is important.

References

1. Halliwell B (1989) Free radicals, reactive oxygen species and human disease: a critical evaluation with special reference to atherosclerosis. Br J Exp Pathol 70:737–757
2. Kukreja RC, Hess ML (1992) The oxygen free radical system: from equations through membrane protein interactions to cardiovascular injury and protection. Cardiovasc Res 26:641–655
3. Chance B, Sies H, Boveris A (1979) Hyperoxide metabolism in mammalian organs. Physiol Rev 59:527–605
4. Freeman BA, Crapo JD (1982) Biology of disease, free radicals and tissue injury. Lab Invest 47:412–426
5. Halliwell B (1987) Oxidants and human disease: some new concepts. FASEB J 1:358–364
6. Perry MO (1991) Skeletal muscle ischemia and revascularization injury. In: Bernhard VM, Towne JB (eds) Complications in vascular surgery. Quality Medical Publishing, St Louis, Missouri, pp 330–335
7. Svingen AS, O'Neal FO, Aust SD (1978) The role of superoxide and singlet oxygen in lipid peroxidation. Photochem Photobiol 28:803–809
8. McCord JM (1987) Oxygen-derived radicals: a link between reperfusion injury and inflammation. Fed Proc 46:2402–2406
9. Chambers DE, Parks DA, Patterson G et al. (1985) Xanthine oxidase as a source of free radical damage in myocardial ischemia. J Mol Cell Cardiol 17:145–152

10. Beckman JS, Beckman TW, Chen J, Marshall PA, Freeman BA (1990) Apparent hydroxyl radical production by peroxynitrite: implications for endothelial injury from nitric oxide and superoxide. Proc Natl Acad Sci USA 87:1620–1624
11. Imlay JA, Linn S (1988) DNA damage and oxygen radical toxicity. Science 240:1302
12. Greenwald RA, Moy WW (1979) Inhibition of collagen gelation by action of the superoxide radical. Arthritis Rheum 22:251
13. Rhodes RS, DePalma RG (1989) Mitochondrial dysfunction of the liver and hypoglycemia in hemorrhagic shock. Surg Gynecol Obstet 150:347–352
14. McCord JM (1985) Oxygen-derived free radicals in postischemic tissue injury. N Engl J Med 312:159–163
15. Sandritter W, Reid UN (1975) Morphology of liver cell necrosis. In: Keppler D (ed) Pathogenesis and mechanisms of liver cell necrosis. MTP Press, Lancaster, pp 1–14
16. Granger DN, Rutilli G, McCord JM (1981) Superoxide radicals in feline intestinal ischemia. Gastroenterology 81:22
17. Parks DA, Bulkley GB, Granger DN et al. (1982) Ischemic injury in the cat small intestine: role of superoxide radicals. Gastroenterology 82–89
18. Morris JB, Bulkley GB, Haglund U, Cadenas E, Sies H (1987) The direct real-time demonstration of oxygen free radical generation at re-perfusion following ischemia in rat small intestine. Gastroenterology 92:1541
19. Welbourn CRB, Goldman G, Paterson IS, Valeri CR, Shepro D, Hechtman HB (1991) Pathophysiology of ischemia-reperfusion injury: central role of the neutrophil. Br J Surg 78:651–655
20. Windsor ACJ, Mullen PG, Fowler AA, Sugerman HJ (1993) Role of the neutrophil in adult respiratory distress syndrome. Br J Surg 80:10–17
21. Matsubara T, Ziff M (1986) Superoxide anion release by human endothelial cells: Synergism between a phorbol ester and a talcum ionophore. J Cell Physiol 127:207–210
22. Ochoa JB, Udekwu AO, Billiar TR et al. (1991) Nitrogen oxide levels in patients after trauma and during sepsis. Ann Surg 214:621–616
23. Chaudhri G, Clar IA (1989) Reactive oxygen species facilitate the in vitro and in vivo lipopolysaccharide-induced release of tumor necrosis factor. J Immunol 143:1290–1294
24. Visner GA, Dougall WC, Wilson JM et al. (1990) Regulation of manganese superoxide dismutase by lipopolysaccharide, interleukin 1, and tumor necrosis factor. Role in the acute inflammatory response. J Biol Chem 265:2856–2864
25. Wong GHL, Goeddel DV (1988) Induction of manganous superoxide dismutase by tumor necrosis factor: Possible protective mechanisms. Science 242:941–944
26. Barber EF, Cousins RJ (1988) Interleukin-1-stimulated induction of ceruloplasmin synthesis in normal and copper deficient rats. J Nutr 118:375–381
27. Heinrich PC, Castell JV, Andus T (1990) Interleukin 6 and the acute phase response. Biochem J 265:621–636
28. Ku G, Doherty NS, Schmidt LF et al. (1990) Ex vivo lipopolysaccharide-induced interleukin-1 secretion from murine peritoneal macrophages by probucol, a hypocholesterolemic agent with antioxidant properties. FASEB J 4:1645–1653
29. De Forge LE, Fantone JC, Kenney JS (1992) Oxygen radical scavengers selectively inhibit IL8 production in human whole blood. J Clin Invest 90:2123–2129
30. Peristeris P, Clark BD, Gatti S et al. (1992) N-acetyl cysteine and glutathione as inhibitors of tumor necrosis factor production. Cell Immunol 140:390–399
31. Pfizenmaier K, Himmler A, Schutze S et al. (1992) TNF receptors and TNF signal transduction. In: Beutler B (ed) Tumor necrosis factors. The molecules and their emerging role in medicine. Raven, New York, pp 439–472
32. Schreck R, Rieber P, Baeurerle PA (1991) Reactive oxygen intermediates as apparently widely used messengers in the activation of NFκB transcription factor and HIV-1. EMBO J 10:2247–2256
33. Rangan U, Bulkley GB (1993) Prospects for treatment of free radical-mediated tissue injury. Br Med Bull 49:700–718
34. Reilly PM, Schiller HJ, Bulkley GB (1991) Reactive oxygen metabolites in shock, chap. 8. In: Wilmore DW, Carpentier YA (eds) Care of the surgical patient. Scientific American, New York, pp 1–30

35. Fairburn K, Grootveld M, Ward RS et al. (1992) α-tocopherol, lipids and lipoproteins in knee joint synovial fluid and serum from patients with imflammatory joint disease. Clin Sci 83:657–664

36. Bast A, Haenen GRMM, Doelman CJA (1991) Oxidants and antioxidants: State of the art. Am J Med 91 [Suppl 3C]:2S–13S

37. Ogino T, Kawabala T, Awai M (1989) Stimulation of glutathione synthesis in iron-loaded mice. Biochem Biophys Acta 1006:131–135

38. Richard C, Lemonnier F, Thibault M et al. (1990) Vitamin E deficiency and lipoperoxidation during adult respiratory distress syndrome. Crit Care Med 18:4–9

39. Bertrand Y, Pincemail J, Hanique G et al. (1989) Differences in tocopherol-lipid ratios in ARDS and non-ARDS patients. Intensive Care Med 15:87–93

40. Louw J, Werbeck A, Louw M et al. (1992) Blood vitamin concentration during the acute phase response. Crit Care Med 20:934–940

41. Krinsky NI (1989) Antioxidant functions of carotenoids. Free Rad Biol Med 7:617–635

42. Palozza P, Moualla S, Krinsky NI (1992) Effects of beta carotene and alpha tocopherol on radical-initiated peroxidation of microsomes. Free Rad Biol Med 13:127–136

43. Palozza P, Krinsky NI (1992) Beta carotene and alpha tocopherol are synergistic antioxidants. Arch Biochem Biophys 297:184–187

44. Grimble RF, Jackson AA, Wride MJ et al. (1992) Cysteine and glycine supplementation modify the metabolic response to tumor necrosis factor alpha in rats fed a low protein diet. J Nutr 122:2066–2073

45. Losowsky MS, Walker BE, Kelleher J (1974) Malabsorption in clinical practice. Churchill Livingstone, London

46. Deneke SM, Fanburg BL (1989) Regulation of cellular glutathione. Am J Physiol 257:L163–L173

47. Pathirana C, Grimble RF (1992) Taurine and serine supplementation modulates the metabolic response to tumor necrosis factor α in rats fed a low protein diet. J Nutr 122:1369–1375

48. Schneeberger H, Schleibner S, Schilling M et al. (1990) Prevention of acute renal failure after kidney transplantation by treatment with rh-SOD: interin analysis of a double-blind placebo-controlled trial. Transplant Proc 22:2224

49. Schneeberger H, Schleibner S, Illner WD et al. (1992) Kidney transplantation in the cyclosporine era – the Munich experience. Transplant Proc 24:78

50. Johnson WD, Kayser KL, Brenowitz JB, Saedi SF (1991) A randomized controlled trial of allupurinol in coronary bypass surgery. Am Heart J 121:20

51. Rashid MA, William-Olsson G (1991) Influence of allopurinol on cardiac complications in open heart operations. Ann Thorac Surg 52:127

52. Kunimoto F, Morita T, Ogawa R et al. (1987) Inhibition of lipid peroxidation improves survival rate of endotoxemic rats. Circ Shock 21:15–22

53. Powell RJ, Machiedo GW, Rush BF Jr et al. (1991) Effect of oxygen free radical scavengers on survival in sepsis. Am Surg 57:86–88

54. Warner BW, Hasselgren P-O, Fischer JE (1986) Effect of allopurinol and superoxide dismutase on survival rate in rats with sepsis. Curr Surg 43:292–293

55. Allan G, Cambridge D, Lee-Tsang-Tan L et al. (1986) The protective action of allopurinol in an experimental model of hemorrhagic shock and reperfusion. Br J Pharmacol 89:149–155

56. Bernard GR (1990) Potential of n-acetyl cysteine as treatment for the adult respiratory distress syndrome. Eur Resp J 11 [Suppl]:496S–498S

57. Bernard GR (1991) N-acetyl cysteine in experimental and clinical acute lung injury. Am J Med 92 [Suppl 3C]:54S–59S

58. Bernard GR, Swindell BB, Meredith MJ et al. (1989) Glutathione repletion by n-acetyl cysteine in patients with adult respiratory distress syndrome. Am Rev Resp Dis 139:A221 (abstract)

59. Sawyer MAJ, Mike JJ, Chavin K et al. (1989) Antioxidant therapy and survival in ARDS. Crit Care Med 17:S153 (abstract)

60. Odelys O, Watson RR (1991) The potential role of vitamin E in the treatment of immunologic abnormalities during acquired immune deficiency syndrome. Prog Food Nutr Sci 15:1–19

61. Meydani SK, Hayek M, Coleman L (1992) Influence of vitamins E and B_6 on immune responses. Ann N Y Acad Sci 669:125–140
62. Peters EM, Goetzsche JM, Grobbelaar B et al. (1993) Vitamin C supplementation reduces the incidence of postrace upper-respiratory-tract infection in ultramarathon runners. Am J Clin Nutr 57:170–174
63. Grimble RF (1993) The maintenance of antioxidant defenses during inflammation. In: Wilmore DW, Carpentier YA (eds) Metabolic support of the critically ill patient. Springer, Berlin, Heidelberg, New York, pp 347–352. Update in intensive care and emergency medicine vol 17
64. Grace PA (1994) Ischemia-reperfusion injury. J Surg 81:637–647
65. Ferrari R, Ceconi C, Curello S et al. (1991) Oxygen free radicals and myocardial damage: protective role of thiol-containing agents. Am J Med 91 [Suppl 3C]:95S–105S

Effects of Amino Acid Therapy on Skeletal Muscle in the Acute Catabolic State

J. Wernerman

Following trauma and sepsis, body protein losses emanate almost exclusively from skeletal muscle. This is in contrast to the tissue losses seen during starvation, when the protein losses are equally distributed among all organs excluding the central nervous system. This implies that the speed of the muscle tissue loss is much higher in the acute catabolic state than in starvation, due to the elevated need of substrates in combination with muscle being the only tissue to supply virtually all other tissues with substrates. Conventional nutritional therapy can only partly attenuate this pattern. A hypercaloric support of energy may improve nitrogen balance marginally, but at the expense of lipogenesis, resulting in a gain of adipose tissue during critical illness [1]. Furthermore, a higher than necessary supply of amino acids or proteins will not improve whole body nitrogen economy beyond what is achieved with a nutritional support designed to meet the measured resting energy expenditure combined with a nitrogen supply of 0.15 g N/kg body weight per day [2].

The depletion of skeletal muscle proteins following trauma and sepsis is accompanied by a very low concentration of free glutamine intracellulary [3]. This decline in glutamine concentration is profound, and it occurs early during critical illness. It seems not to be influenced by whether the condition of the patient improves or detoriates, and furthermore the depletion seems to remain relatively unaltered over time [4]. Glutamine is shown to be the major constituent of the amino acid export from peripheral tissues to the splanchnic area. This transfer of amino acids is augmented manifold in the acute catabolic state [5]. During long-standing critical illness, such as multiple organ failure or burns, a reduction of the glutamine flux has been reported [6, 7]. Enterocytes and immunocompetent cells in the splanchnic area are pointed out as the main consumers of glutamine [8, 9]. These are rapidly dividing cells which exhibit elevated metabolic needs in acutely stressed states. The underlying rationale is thought to be an improved metabolic regulation, which enables a rapid increase in nucleotide synthesis, necessary for cell division. Enterocytes as well as lymphocytes are shown to prefer glutamine as an oxidative fuel, and this preference is even more pronounced during metabolic stress. Consequently, these cells have a comparatively low intracellular level of glutamine [10, 11], but simultaneously the concentrations of glutamate and aspartate are higher. The gradient of glutamine between the extracellular and intracellular spaces is thus low compared to muscle. This is probably the result of the high activity of glutaminase, which converts glutamine to glutamate. The activity of glutamine synthetase, on the other hand, which is very high in muscle, is not detectable. Glutamate is then converted into α-ketoglutarate through deamination producing ammonia or trans-amination producing aspartate and alanine. α-Ketoglutarate can directly be used in the tricarboxylic acid (TCA) cycle localized on the inner membrane of the mi-tochondrion, thus directly and effectively providing an energy substrate to the cells [12]. In contrast to the dramatic changes in skeletal muscle [3, 13, 14], short-term starvation [15], elective surgery [16], and acute critically illness [17] do not chan-ge the gradient between glutamine and glutamate in the duodenal mucosa. Al-though marginal in absolute terms, the concentration of glutamine is actually in-creased following elective surgery and in acute critical illness as compared to the basal state. Not surprisingly, the concentrations of aspartate and alanine are elevat-ed in the intestinal mucosa of intensive care unit (ICU) patients [16, 17].

To summarize, the need for glutamine as a metabolic substrate in the intestinal mucosa and in immunocompetent cells during acute catabolic illness is well estab-lished. Nature itself provides large amounts of glutamine by export from skeletal muscle, at least in the acute state of critical illness. Furthermore, we know that fol-lowing elective abdominal surgery provision of extra glutamine intravenously at-tenuates the reduction of free glutamine and of protein synthesis in skeletal muscle, together with a reduction of whole body nitrogen losses [18, 19]. Therefore, the use of glutamine supplementation to nutrition of patients in the acute catabolic state seems justified. The following discussion will deal with the scientific rationale and clinical documentation for such a therapy.

Conventional intravenous nutrition does not contain glutamine, as glutamine is un-stable in aqueous solution. However, the stability is sufficient to allow the prepara-tion of solutions for immediate use or for short-term storage in refrigerators. Initial-ly, a supplementation of 20 g glutamine/day was chosen [18, 19]. The rationale for this quantity was that a 40% decrease of muscle-free glutamine on the third day fol-lowing surgery corresponds to approximately 60 g glutamine in a male subject with normal muscle mass. Consequently, the original clinical studies were designed to compensate for this loss. We know that 20 g glutamine/day during 3 days attenuates the decline of muscle-free glutamine by 50%–90%. However, when patients were studied for 30 days postoperatively, a delayed decrease in muscle glutamine was seen when the patients received their habitual food intake orally [20]. Although ordinary dietary proteins contain 5%–10% glutamine, this supply was quite ineffective to maintain the effect that 20 g glutamine given intravenously for 3 days postoperative-ly had (Fig. 1). This may be explained by an insufficient amount of glutamine or by the inefficiency of the enteral route when glutamine is provided. Nevertheless, the glutamine depletion seen on the tenth day following surgery is astonishing, as the pa-tients had normal muscle glutamine levels when they left the hospital on the third postoperative day and were eating normal food in adequate quantities after that.

Animal experiments have suggested that muscle glutamine concentration and muscle protein synthesis may be related. The basis for this hypothesis is the finding of a statistical correlation between the two variables in endotoxemic rats suffering from a variable degree of malnutrition [21]. A similar observation is also reported in man following open cholecystectomy, where a weak but statistically significant cor-relation exists between the decrease in muscle glutamine and the decrease in muscle

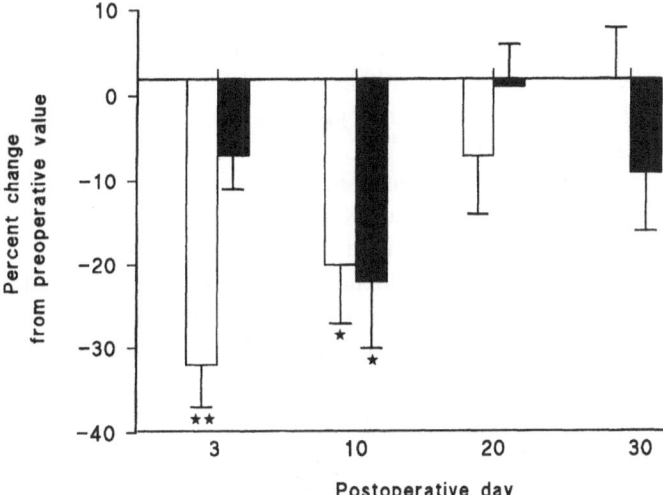

Fig. 1. The concentration of free glutamine in skeletal muscle of patients undergoing open cholecystectomy during 30 days postoperatively. In patients receiving total parenteral nutrition (TPN) for 3 days postoperatively (*open bars; n=9*) and thereafter their habitual oral intake, a 30% decrease in muscle glutamine was seen on the third postoperative day, still decreased by 20% on the tenth postoperative day, and thereafter normalized in most individuals. These patients were mobilized as soon as possible and they left hospital on the third or fourth postoperative day. Another group of patients were randomized to receive TPN containing 20 g glutamine during 3 days immediately following surgery (*filled bars; n=8*). There was no significant decrease of muscle glutamine on the third postoperative day, but on the tenth postoperative day a similar 20% decrease as in the control group was seen. This happened although those patients had an oral diet containing a normal amount of glutamine [20]

polyribosomes, reflecting muscle protein synthesis [12]. Muscle protein synthesis, as assessed by the ribosome concentration and the size distribution of ribosomes, has a parallel pattern to muscle free glutamine concentration during postoperative glutamine supplementation. On the third postoperative day, the decrease otherwise seen was prevented by 20 g glutamine daily, but when i.v. glutamine is discontinued a delayed decline of the ribosomes is seen [22]. However, in the convalescence period after open cholecystectomy, muscle glutamine is restituted back to the preoperative level in the majority of patients [20], while the polyribosome concentration is still low on day 30 postoperatively [22]. Thus, the postulated relation between glutamine concentration and muscle protein synthesis was not supported during the restoration phase, which on the contrary gave evidence against a causal relationship.

So far the beneficial effects of extra glutamine postoperatively have been demonstrated when glutamine was given as a constituent of total parenteral nutrition (TPN). However, also when given together with hypocaloric glucose, 20 g glutamine prevented a decrease in muscle glutamine [23] and muscle polyribosomes [24]. This is shown on the first postoperative day in patients undergoing hip replacement surgery. Elective orthopedic surgery as a human model of trauma is less established than open cholecystectomy or hysterectomy. The advantage of this model is a large number of patients undergoing a significant trauma, while the disadvantage is that many patients are old and have other disorders of possible metabolic significance. In addition, i.v. nutrition is not possible postoperatively; furthermore, the majority of patients prefer regional anesthesia. The result is a larger patient scatter, requiring larger groups of patients to reach statistical significance concerning the results.

Very little has been published so far on the results of administering glutamine to critically ill patients. Patients given 20–40 g/day during 5 days showed marginal increases in muscle free glutamine [25]. When 60 g glutamine/day was given, a clear effect was seen in two patients [26]. A dose of glutamine of this magnitude contains more then 10 g nitrogen, and the documentation for supplying patients with such large amounts of glutamine and nitrogen are presently non-existing. When given 20 g glutamine/day, ICU patients did not show any detectable elevation of muscle glutamine (unpublished results). Together these observations indicate that i.v. glutamine may prevent the decrease of muscle glutamine, when provided immediately after elective surgical trauma. However, when muscle glutamine depletion is established, very large amounts of glutamine are required to influence the muscle glutamine level. This is, of course, of no relevance in forming an opinion of whether exogenous glutamine is of any benefit for enterocytes and lymphocytes in the same patients.

Very soon commercial products containing glutamine will appear on the market. Glutamine in the form of a dipeptide will then be included in amino acid solutions. Such dipeptides as alanyl glutamine or glycyl glutamine are rapidly hydrolyzed to the constituent amino acids when infused intravenously [27]. An alternative way is of course to have the glutamine solution prepared by the hospital pharmacy very soon before its administration. One disadvantage is the limited solubility of glutamine in water, which limits the concentrations to 12–15 g/l. Dipeptides have a much greater solubility, avoiding the potential volume problem. Such a dipeptide solution to be added to other nutritional products may be an ideal way of giving glutamine to ICU patients on an individual basis. Another way of providing glutamine would be to support the production and export of glutamine from skeletal muscle. α-Ketoglutarate is the carbon skeletal of glutamine, and it is transported easily across membranes. In muscle it may be utilized for the production of glutamine or for energy production. In the enterocytes and in immunocompetent cells, α-ketoglutarate may also be used directly. In dogs, α-ketoglutarate is consumed in all tissues [28] and in particular is used in the production of glutamine from the muscle. In the postoperative state, glutamine, the dipeptides, or α-ketoglutarate in isomolar amounts have similar effects upon muscle free glutamine and muscle ribosome content [19, 20, 22, 29, 30].

Furthermore, glutamine and α-ketoglutarate are equally effective in maintaining muscle glutamine and muscle polyribosomes when supplemented to hypocaloric glucose following hip replacement surgery [23, 24]. In ICU patients, α-ketoglutarate may have an advantage over glutamine in restituting muscle glutamine concentration [31]. As compared to 20 g glutamine [25], 20 g α-ketoglutarate resulted in a 70% increase of muscle glutamine in a group of ICU patients (Fig. 2). There is at present no documentation concerning enteral glutamine support in man as far as its effects upon muscle tissue are concerned.

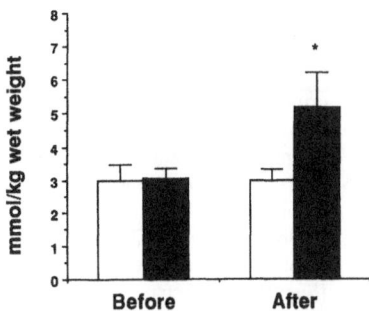

Fig. 2. Critically ill patients in the intensive care unit (ICU) were randomized to receive total parenteral nutrition (TPN) with or without α-ketoglutarate supplementation (20 g/day). Controls (*open bars; n*=9) showed an unaltered muscle glutamine concentration on the 5 days, while α-ketoglutarate-treated patients (*filled bars; n*=5) showed a 70% increase of muscle glutamine. Thus in this small pilot study, a clear beneficial effect was seen of α-ketoglutarate upon muscle-free glutamine in critically ill patients [31]

In conclusion, evidence exists that glutamine supplementation reduces nitrogen losses following elective surgery by preventing a decrease in muscle-free glutamine concentration together with a more or less maintained muscle protein synthesis. It is still debatable whether or not this limited effect is of sufficient importance to motivate a higher cost for the nutritional products in a group of patients in which the use of intravenous nutrition as such is questioned. However, there may be beneficial effects of glutamine supplementation postoperatively on the gut or on the immune system; so far the only documentation available in man is for skeletal muscle. Following bone marrow transplantation, on the other hand, a beneficial effect upon immunological parameters has been demonstrated [32], and in gastroenterological patients on i.v. nutrition beneficial effects in the intestinal mucosa are reported [33]. The most convincing theoretical rationale for glutamine supplementation is in patients with an acute critical illness of long duration, i.e., patients that stay in the ICU for more than 1 week. Evidence exists that endogenous glutamine production and export is impaired concomitantly with high demands for substrates in tissues that prefer glutamine as an oxidative substrate. Clinical documentation of glutamine supplementation is, however, so far not convincing in this patient group. Unfortunately, the pharmaceutical industry does not see any large profits around the corner in connection with glutamine-containing nutritional products. Consequently, the lack of an economic sponsor is the main obstacle to a large, multicenter outcome trial being carried out. The glutamine discussion has been around for several years now, but unfortunately no definite recommendations can be made for or against its use in clinical nutrition.

References

1. Streat SJ, Beddoe AH, Hill GL (1987) Aggressive nutritional support does not prevent protein loss despite fat gain in septic intensive care patients. J Trauma 27:262–266
2. Larsson J, Lennmarken C, Mårtensson J et al. (1990) Nitrogen requirements in severely injured patients. Br J Surg 77:413–416

254   J. Wernerman

3. Roth E, Funovics J, Mühlbacher F et al. (1982) Metabolic disorders in severe abdominal sepsis: glutamine deficiency in skeletal muscle. Clin Nutr 1:25–42
4. Gamrin L, Wernerman J, Vinnars E (1992) The free amino acid pattern in skeletal muscle of critically ill patients does not change over time. Clin Nutr 11 [Suppl]:48 (abstr)
5. Clowes GHA, Randell HT, Cha C-J (1980) Amino acid and energy metabolism in septic and traumatized patients. JPEN 4:195–203
6. Pearl HR, M.D., Clowes GHA, Hirsch EF et al. (1985) Prognosis and survival as determined by visceral amino acid clearance in severe trauma. J Trauma 25:777–781
7. Biolo G, Maggi SP, Fleming DY et al. (1994) Glutamine kinetics in skeletal muscle of severely burned patients: transmembrane transport and intracellular de novo snythesis. JPEN 18 [Suppl]:17S (abstr)
8. Souba WW, Herskowitz K, Klimberg SV et al. (1990) The effects of sepsis and endotoxemia on gut glutamine metabolism. Ann Surg 211:543–551
9. Newsholme EA, Crabtree B, Ardawi SM (1985) Glutamine metabolism in lymphocytes: its biochemical, physiological and clinical importance. Q J Exp Physiol 70:473–489
10. Ahlman B, Leijonmarck C-E, Wernerman J (1993) The content of free amino acids in the human duodenal mucosa. Clin Nutr 12:266–271
11. Januszkiewicz A, Essén P, Sang XT et al. (1994) The pattern of free amino acids in human peripheral blood lymphocytes. Clin Nutr 13 [Suppl]:20 (abstr)
12. Wernerman J, Hammarqvist F, Vinnars E (1990) Alpha-ketoglutarate and postoperative muscle catabolism. Lancet 335:701–703
13. Andersson K, Luo J, Hammarqvist F, Wernerman J (1994) The effect of fasting on muscle glutathione levels. Clin Nutr 13 [Suppl]:4 (abstr)
14. Vinnars E, Bergström J, Fürst P (1975) Influence of the postoperative state on the intracellular free amino acids in human muscle tissue. Ann Surg 182:665
15. Ahlman B, Andersson K, Leijonmarck C-E et al. (1994) Short-term starvation alters free amino acid content of the human intestinal mucosa. Clin Sci (in press)
16. Ahlman B, Andersson K, Ljungqvist O et al. (1995) Elective abdominal operations alter the free amino acid content of the human intestinal mucosa. Eur J Surg 161:595–603
17. Ahlman B, Ljungqvist O, Persson B et al. (1995) Intestinal amino acid content in critically ill patients. JPEN 19:272–278
18. Stehle P, Mertes N, Puchstein C et al. (1989) Effect of parenteral glutamine peptide supplements on muscle glutamine loss and nitrogen balance after major surgery. Lancet 1:231–233
19. Hammarqvist F, Wernerman J, Ali MR et al. (1989) Addition of glutamine to total parenteral nutrition after elective abdominal surgery spares free glutamine in muscle, counteracts the fall in muscle protein synthesis, and improves nitrogen balance. Ann Surg 209:455–461
20. Petersson B, Waller S-O, Vinnars E, Wernerman J (1994) Long-term effect of glycyl-glutamine after elective surgery on muscle free amino acids. JPEN 18:320–325
21. Jepson MM, Bates PC, Broadbent P et al. (1988) Relationship between glutamine concentration and protein synthesis in rat skeletal muscle. Am J Physiol 255:E166–E172
22. Petersson B, von der Decken A, Vinnars E, Wernerman J (1994) Long-term effect of postoperative TPN supplemented with gylcyl-glutamine on subjective fatigue and muscle protein synthesis, as assessed by ribosome analysis. Br J Surg 81:1520–1523
23. Blomqvist BI, Hammarqvist F, von der Decken A, Wernerman J (1993) Glutamine and alpha-ketoglutarate attenuate the fall in muscle free glutamine concentration after total hip replacement. Clin Nutr 12 [Suppl]:12 (abstr)
24. Blomqvist BI, Hammarqvist F, Wernerman J, von der Decken A (1994) Glutamine alpha-ketoglutarate attenuate the postoperative decline protein synthesis in skeletal muscle after total hip replacement. Clin Nutr 13 [Suppl]:89 (abstr)
25. Karner J, Roth E (1990) Alanyl-glutamine infusions to patients with acute pancreatitis. Clin Nutr 9:43–44
26. Roth E, Winkler S, Hölzengein T et al. (1992) High load of alanylglutamine in two patients with acute pancreatitis. Clin Nutr 11 [Suppl]:99 (abstr)
27. Albers S, Wernerman J, Stehle P et al. (1988) Availability of amino acids supplied intravenously in healthy man as synthetic dipeptides: kinetic evaluation of L-ananyl-L-glutamine and glycyl-L-tyrosine. Clin Sci 75:463–468

28. Roth-Merten A, Karner J, Winkler S et al. (1990) Influence of alpha-ketoglutarate infusion on glutamate and glutamine metabolism. Clin Nutr 9:46–47
29. Hammarqvist F, Wernerman J, von der Decken A et al. (1990) Alanylglutamine counteracts the depletion of free glutamine and the decline in protein synthesis postoperatively in skeletal muscle. Ann Surg 212:637–644
30. Hammarqvist F, Wernerman J, von der Decken A et al. (1991) An addition of alpha-ketoglutarate to total parenteral nutrition given following elective abdominal surgery improves nitrogen balance, counteracts the fall in protein synthesis and spares intracellular free glutamine in skeletal muscle. Surgery 109:28–36
31. Petersson B, Gamrin L, Hammarqvist F et al. (1992) Alpha-ketoglutarate given together with TPN improves the free glutamine levels in glutamine-depleted intensive care patients. Clin Nutr 11 [Suppl]:56 (abstr)
32. Ziegler TR, Young LS, Benfell K et al. (1992) Clinical and metabolic efficacy of glutamine-supplemented parenteral nutrition after bone marrow transplantation: a randomized, double-blind, controlled study. Ann Intern Med 116:821–828
33. Van der Hulst RRWJ, van Kreel BK, von Meyenfeldt MF et al. (1993) Glutamine and the preservation of gut integrity. Lancet 341:1363–1365

Nutrition in the Acute Catabolic State

A. Revhaug and J. Kjæve

Introduction

The acute catabolic state represents a major metabolic challenge to the organism. In recent decades major progress has been achieved in understanding the underlying processes which control these changes. There has also been a tremendous increase in the knowledge of nutritional needs and ways of supporting these demands in the diseased states.

The acute catabolic state may be induced in a great diversity of pathological states, including trauma, operation, and infection. The overall therapeutic guidelines have so far concentrated on stabilizating the patient with regard to circulatory and respiratory functions. To us, this has become increasingly frustrating. In our opinion, more emphasis should be placed on the nutritional preparation of a patient in connection with the acute catabolic situation. In all other situations when the body is subjected to a physical challenge, such as in physical work and sports, a major impact on results is achieved by nutritional intervention. An athlete is nutritionally prepared before a sports competition. Is there any reason why nutritional preparation should not have a major influence on the physical impact that a trauma or an operation represents? Accordingly, in any situation when an acute catabolic response might be foreseen, for example, an operative procedure or a possible infectious contamination, it is our hypothesis that the individual should be nutritionally prepared. Likewise, during an especially after physical exercise it is well known that specific nutritional and fluid requirements are important for the proper and efficient recovery of the body functions. Why should this be different after medically relevant acute catabolic states?

This chapter focuses on the current knowledge in the field of nutritional requirements for the acute catabolic patient. As the needs for nutrition and fluids depend on the kind of healthy physical acitivity, there are also different needs in the diseased states depending on the magnitude and etiology of the acute catabolic state.

Typical Acute Catabolic Situations and Nutritional Needs

There are principally two conditions in which a patient is encountered in the acute catabolic state. First, a foreseen situation, is before a surgical procedure or when an infectious complication can be expected to occur. Second, the acute catabolic state can be initiated without any previous knowledge, for example, trauma and acute infection. Obviously, precatabolic nutritional preparation can be achieved only in the former situation. In the latter, nutritional intervention is necessary at some stage in the acute catabolic response.

Typical features of the catabolic response are related to the etiology of the acute catabolic state. Acute infections may be very different in respect to the magnitude of the response which is generated, depending on the infectious agents' qualities. Similarly, the acute catabolic response differs depending on whether the body is subjected to a controlled trauma situation during an operation in anesthesia or, for example, to a multitrauma traffic accident or a severe gastrointestinal hemorrhage. The metabolic changes differ in all these situations both qualitatively and quantitatively.

An important quality which must be considered when the patient enters the acute catabolic state is the current nutritional state of the individual. A depleted or otherwise malnourished patient has other nutritional needs in connection with the acute catabolic state than the well-nourished individual. In this context, the obese nontrained individual probably has other needs than the physically well-trained individual. The host response also differs depending on other qualities of the host. Age, accompanying diseases, medications, and other factors influence the ability of the host to respond to an agent.

To summarize, predictable acute catabolic states include: (a) planned operative procedure, (b) expected postoperative infection, and (c) expected combined infected or metabolic complication. Unpredictable acute catabolic states include (a) unexpected trauma to bones or soft tissues, hemorrhage, (b) multiple trauma, (c) hemorrhage with or without other trauma, and (d) acute infections with or without shock state. Factors which may influence the metabolic response in the acute catabolic state include the etiology of the acute catabolic state: (a) trauma, simple or multiple, (b) infection, (c) hemorrhage, (d) operation; and the metabolic state of the host: (a) malnutrition , (b) medication, (c) age, and (d) accompanying disease.

Experimental Data and Nutrition in the Acute Catabolic State

There is a huge body of evidence from experimental data that nutrition and thereby metabolic modification can alter the responses and especially the outcome of various acute catabolic states.

As early as 1877 Claude Bernard demonstrated a hyperglycemic response to hemorrhage [1]. This hyperglycemic response is important for the maintenance of intravascular volume during hemorrhage. In the 1970s Jährhult demonstrated in various animal models that the nutritional status of an animal predicts the glycemic response in hemorrhage [2, 3] and is thereby important for the outcome. Starvation for 24 h was shown by Ljungquist [4] to alter negatively the hormonal response to hemorrhagic hypotension. Ljungqvist et al. later showed that even shorter periods of fasting reduce the defense that a hyperglycemic response to hemorrhage represents [5]. These animal and human studies indicate that glycogen reserves are totally consumed in approximately 24 h [6, 7] and are reduced by more than half by

12h of fasting, and are further reduced by an operation [8]. Accordingly, there is strong evidence that blood and fluid losses are handled less well in a fasted individual than in a fed one. The effects of feeding versus fasting on the outcome of endotoxemic challenges have been more controversial in experimental studies, as gluconeogenic enzyme induction can be favored by fasting [9, 10]. However, recent data clearly indicate that fasting is also associated with higher mortality in septic models, partly by reducing the glycogen reserves [11].

The quality of the nutrients has recently been suggested to be of importance. Among several nutrients investigated are the lipids. The use of dietary ω-3 fatty acids during stress has been studied extensively by Alexander et al. [12, 13] and shown to improve outcome of burn injury in guinea pig models. Improved survival has also been obtained in endotoxin models [14, 15]. The ust of ω6-polyunsaturated fatty acid, which is found in fish oils, improved survival to endotoxemia in guinea pigs [16]. However, Gielen et al. found no such beneficial results with respect to prevention of multiple organ failure in a mice model with diets enriched by fish oils [17].

Glutamine supplementation has been proposed to preserve the gut mucosal barrier which might afford protection to septic stress [18–23]. In a rat model bacterial translocation showed reduction by glutamine supplementation [24]. Similar studies in a radiation model demonstrated improved intestinal integrity [20]. Improved survival to *Escherichia coli* induced peritonitis has been demonstrated by addition of glutamine to rats [25].

Vitamin depletion has long been known for its negative influence on the outcome of infectious diseases [26]. Vitamin A increases survival in experimental peritonitis [27] and endotoxemia [28]. Among other effects, vitamin A treatment increases the speed of the elimination of endotoxin from the circulation [29]. The antioxidative effects of vitamins A, C, and E have been shown in several models to influence positively the outcome in septic and other acute shock models when administered in doses ten- to a hundredfold the daily recommended dosages [39].

Nutritional Support of the Catabolic Patient

In the preparation for a surgical procedure it seems of utmost importance to maintain a daily diet as complete as possible until the moment of operation. This can probably be achieved by oral nutrients in the majority of patients until a few hours before the operation. The common clinical situation of an often long fasting period due to preoperative examinations should be avoided. Hospital routines should be scrutinized to prevent unnecessary fasting.

There is no indication for a longer period of preoperative feeding in situations with acute surgical diseases [31]. Eliminating the active catabolic drive represented by the disease process should clearly be of first priority. However, a nutritional support that can restore glycogen deposits, vitamins, and deficits which can be restored over 1–2 days, should be instituted if the disease process does not demand an acute intervention. The chronically malnourished patient (loss of >10% of usual body weight over 3 months) should be given special attention from the day of hospitalization as the nutritional stores are deficient already before the operation.

Accordingly, it is our practice to feed the patient until a few hours before an elective surgical procedure if possible. In the same manner, as most surgical patients can resume some oral food intake already from the first postoperative day, they should be offered food as soon as they want it. The most important reason why patients do not eat postoperatively is that they are not offered food or permitted to eat because of old, scientifically unproved routines. All patients should be allowed an encouraged to drink and eat postoperatively from the day of surgery if it cannot be proven that doing so will impair healing or recovery. This hypothesis obviously also applies to states of trauma and medically acute diseases.

The accepted guidelines for the time to start additional nutritional support to the acute catabolic patient have until recently been as follows [32]:

- When the patient has been without nutrition for 5 days. During this period most patients will either have eaten some food, or in the unconscious patient been administered some calories with intravenous glucose infusions. When this period has passed, nutritional support must be started to supply the patient with necessary substrates.
- When the duration of the catabolic state and nonsatisfactory nutrient intake is expected to last longer than 1 week. In these patients (trauma with injury score >15, major burns, and others) a nutritional deficit of importance for the recovery appears. Nutritional support should therefore be initiated as soon as possible.
- When the patient is already malnourished. In these individuals nutritional support is started immediately. The major callenges to the clinicians are to realize that the patient is malnourished at admission and to start the replacement. However, recent data indicate that early enteral nutrition significantly improves morbidity and mortality in the severely ill patients [33, 34].

The Nutritional Needs in the Acute Catabolic State

The nutritional needs in the early acute catabolic state have been difficult to determine. It has also become a general recommendation that priority should be given to cardiovascular and respiratory resuscitation in the unstable patient. The optimal nutrient metabolism is considered to require adequate tissue circulation and oxygenation. However, it may be that other nutrients than the ones used now or in other administration formulas can be of equal importance in the future.

Energy Requirements

The classic means for calculating the energy needs is according to the Harris-Benedict formulas [35]:

- Males: BMR (kcal/day)=66+[13.7×weight (kg)]+[5×height (cm)]−[6.8×age (years)]
- Females: BMR (kcal/day)=65+[9.6×weight (kg)]+[1.7×height (cm)]−[4.7×age (years)]

Table 1. Alterations in metabolic rate

Patient condition	Basal metabolic rate
No postoperative complications	Normal
Fistula without infection	
Mild peritonitis	25% above normal
Long bone fracture or mild to moderate injury	
Severe injury or infection in ICU patient	50% above normal
Multiorgan failure	
Burn of 40%–100% of total body surface	100% above normal

However, in the acute catabolic state the basic metabolic rate (BMR) is increased depending on the magnitude of the catabolic injury (Table 1). The BMR also varies according to the mobility of the patient, for example, a patient on a ventilator or walking about has a different BMR. With modern ventilators the BMR can be determined relatively easily for a specific individual, and the current nutritional needs be tailored to each patient in such critical condition. It must be emphasized however, that the measurement of energy expenditure (EE) with modern indirect calorimeters is subject to many pitfalls in the critically ill patient, and careful interpretation of the results in the situation must therefore be emphasized [36]. It is generally accepted that the energy needs should be met by administering a mixture of glucose and fat. The amount of fat recommended in the acute catabolic state is, however, under constant debate. A general recommendation usually given by most European clinicians is to supply approximately 30%–40% of energy needs as fat. Although the amounts of both calories and protein required to meet the metabolic demands in this state are increased, relatively more protein than calories is required [37]. Thus, the optimal nonprotein calorie: nitrogen ratio is lower in the critically ill patient (100: 1) than in healthy individuals (150: 1), and the amount of protein to administer on a daily basis is higher (approx. 2.0 g/kg per day).

Lipids

In recent years there has been major interest not only in the quantities but also in the quality of lipids which should be administered to the acute catabolic patient. Lipids do not only represent a source of energy but are increasingly becoming potential candidates in modulating all cell membrane functions and ultimately organ functions. It is apparent that further investigations with different lipids, including structured triglycerides, fish oil triglycerids, and medium-chain trigylcerides, are very much needed. The possibilities for modifying the cell membrane composition and thereby the regulation of important mediators are exciting and can only be achieved by basal and clinical research [38–40].

Proteins

Protein requirements are in the order of 1.0 g protein/kg b.w. per day in most patients. The major catabolic states may require approximately the double amount.

This amount of protein supplied to a catabolic patient reduces the losses of lean body mass. However, a positive N-balance is not achieved in the acute catabolic patient with nutritional support alone.

On the basis of currently available knoweldge there is no indication that any one special mixture of proteins or amino acids is more efficient in the acute catabolic state than others. Recently the amino acid glutamine has been claimed to be of particular value. Glutamine is a necessary component for nucleotide and protein synthesis. Glutamine has been shown to be an important substrate for all rapidly dividing cells, for example, enterocytes, alveolar cells of the lung, and white blood cells [41–46]. These tissues use glutamine in increased amounts during catabolic stress. Glutamine is oxidized via the Krebs cycle and yields 30 mmol ADP per mole of glutamine. Until intravenous amino acid solutions with glutamine or glutamine dipeptide compounds are commercially available, the clinical use of this amino acid is limited to enteral use. For enteral use L-glutamine powder can be added to the oral diets. Daily doses of 10–20 g have been recommended for enteral use. However, the actual role of this amino acid in the acute catabolic state still needs further clinical investigation.

Increased amounts of branched-chain amino acids (leucine, isoleucine, and valine) during acute stress can support the energy needs of the skeletal muscle without glucose or fat intolerance. Accordingly, some authors have recommended their use during maximal stress [47, 48]. Especially in the comporimised liver disease their use may be beneficial in these patients when under extreme stress.

Arginine has become a possibly important amino acid in reducing protein catabolism during stress [49, 50]. Arginine is a major source of nitrous and nitric oxides and has been shown to stimulate various immunological functions. T-cell mediated immunity has particularly proven to be positively influenced by the amino acid in experimental work [51–53]. Further controlled clinical investigations are also needed for this amino acid before general recommendations of its clinical use can be made.

Vitamins

Vitamin supplementation to the acute catabolic patient has become an important issue in recent years. Several years ago it was generally accepted that it is not important to supplement vitamins during the first days of an acute catabolic state. Recent investigations have shown that a great diversity of vitamin deficiencies are encountered in the catabolic patients. These deficiencies are thought to be of importance for the optimal acitivty of the immune system. The use of vitamins as antioxidants in acute inflammatory states has also increasingly become a focus of attention. Vitamin C represents a first-line defense in plasma against free radicals liberated from activated leukocytes, etc. Vitamin C also recirculates vitamin E by absorbing free radicals bound to the vitamin E molecule. Vitamin E inhibits the production of lipid peroxides in addition to its direct antioxidative effects. However, the specific vitamin requirements of acute catabolic patients have not been scientifically determined. The general recommendation of vitamins to the healthy individual has been

Table 2. Recommended daily vitamin dose ranges for prevention and treatment of various diseases

Vitamin		Prevention of vitamin deficiency	Treatment of vitamin deficiency
Vitamin A	(IU)	250–2500	5000–10000
Vitamin D	(IU)	400[a]	400–5000
Calcifediol	(μg)	–	–
Calcitriol[b]	(μg)	–	–
Vitamin E	(IU)	6–30[c]	–
Vitamin K	(mg)	–	1[d]
Ascorbic acid (vitamin C)	(mg)	50–100	250–500
Thiamine	(mg)	1–2	5–25
Riboflavin	(mg)	1–2	5–25
Niacin	(mg)	10–20	25–50
Vitamin B_6	(mg)	1.5–2.5	5–25
Pantothenic acid	(mg)	5–20[c]	5–20
Biotin	(mg)	–	0.15–0.30
Folic acid	(mg)	0.1–0.4	1.0
Vitamin B_{12}	(μg)	3–10	–

[a] For infants and children; 200 IU/day for adults.
[b] 1.25-Dihydroxyviatmin D
[c] To be usd only in conjunction with multivitamin mixtures
[d] To be used parenterally as needed

determined by the United States National Research Council (Table 2). The needs of the catabolic patients are higher, but must nevertheless be kept under the recommended safety levels [54, 55]:
- At least 50–100 times recommended daily allowance: vitamin B_1, vitamin B_2, niacin, vitamin C, vitamin E, biotin, folic acid, pantothenic acid
- Ten times recommended daily allowance: vitamin A, vitamin B_6, vitamin D, vitamin K.

The Route of Nutrient Administration

The normal way in which humans are supported with nutrients is through the oral and enteral route. Therefore it is no surprise that as long as the oral or enteral route can be used, this is the best way to make use of the nutrients by the body. However obvious this may be, for several reasons it seems to have been forgotten over a period of several decades. Among the factors which explain this, the most important is probably the common belief that most critical ill patients are not able to use the gastrointestinal tract. The reason for this is the phenomenon of gastric paresis in the critically ill patient. Another factor is that the way of administering nutrients to the intestine in an unconscious patient was almost forgotten when the practice of intravenous nutrition became available in the 1970's. Intravenous administration of nutrients may also be an easier way for the nursing staff to administer nutrition than an individual support of oral nutrients.

Over the past two decades new knowledge has clearly demonstrated that the route of nutrient administration influences the response to injury. It has become clear that the intestine, even in the acute diseased state, usually absorbs nutrients very well, and that this way of administrating nutrients supports the maintenance of an effective barrier against intraluminal toxins and bacteria. Enteral feeding preserves gut mass [56] as well as providing positive effects on the metabolic, hormonal [57], immunological [58], and visceral response to injury [59–61). Enteral support of nutrients may also be of benefit for the function of the gastrointestinal tract itself. The importance of the metabolic activity of the gut has, as pointed out by Page [62], been hampered by the fact that the whole splancnic bed has usually been studied as a whole. Important work in the 1980s demonstrated that the gut and liver certainly have very different activity [63,–66]. Apart from the metabolically favorable results with enteral feeding, maintaining gut integrity by administrating nutrients to the gastointestinal tract has been hypothesized to be of importance in avoiding the development of the multiple organ failure syndrome [67–70).

Several human studies have recently demonstrated the efficacy of enteral nutrition in the trauma situation. The majority of these studies have investigated the metabolic, septic, and other trauma-related complications when administering nutrients in the trauma situation by jejunostomy [71–75]. The clear indication is that enteral administration of nutrients not only is economically favorable and technically feasible but also metablically and otherwise favorable. The oral or enteral route should therefore be used whenever possible in the acute catabolic state.

Summary

Any patient who may be thought to enter a catabolic state should be maintained nutritionally as completely as possible. The oral or enteral route should be preferred if possible. Addition of vitamins to the classical nutritional formulas is recommended.

References

1. Bernard C (1877) Leçcons sur le diabetic et la glycogénès animale. Baillière, Paris
2. Järhult J (1973) Osmotic fluid transfer from tissue to blood during haemorrhagic hypotension. Acta Physiol Scand 89:213–226
3. Järhult (1975) Osmolar control of the circulation in haemorrhagic hypotension. Acta Physiol Scand 423:1–84
4. Ljungqvist O, Efendic S, Eneroth P, Hamberger B, Nylander G, Ware J (1986) Nutritional status and endocrine response to hemorrhage. Can J Physiol Pharmacol 64:1185–1188
5. Ljungqvist O, Alibegovic A (1994) Hyperglycaemia and survival after haemorrhage. Eur J Surg 160:465–469
6. Nilsson Hänson L, Hultman E (1973) Liver glycogen in man – the effect to total starvation and a carbohydrate-poor diet followed by carbohydrate refeeding. Scand J Clin Lab Invest 32:325–330
7. Sunzel H (1963) Effects of surgical trauma on the livers glycogen in fasting and in glucose fed patients. Acta Chir Scand 125:118–128

8. Rothman DL, Magnusson I, Katz LD, Schulmann RG, Schulman GI (1991) Quantification of hepatic glucogenolysis and gluconeogenesis in fasting humans with 13C-NMR. Science 254:573–576
9. Filkins JP, Cornell RP (1974) Depression of hepatic gluconeogenesis and the hypoglycemia of endotoxin shock. Am J Physiol 227:778–781
10. Filkins JP (1979) Adrenergic blockade and glucoregulation in endotoxin shock. Circ Shock 9:99–197
11. Esahili AH, Boija PO, Ljungqvist O, Rubio C, Ware J (1991) Twenty-four hour fasting increases endotoxin lethality in the rat. Eur J Surg 157:89–95
12. Alexander JW, Saito H, Ogle CK, Trocki O (1986) The importance of lipid type in the diet after burn injury. Ann Surg 204:1–8
13. Trocki O, Heyd TJ, Waymack JP, Alexander JW (1987) Effects of fish oil on postburn metabolism and immunity. IPEN J Parenter Enteral Nutr 11:521–528
14. Mascioli E, Leader L, Flores E et al. (1988) Enhanced survival to endotoxin in guinea pigs fed IV fish oil emulsion. Lipids 623–625
15. Mascioli EA, Iwasa Y, Trimbo S et al. (1989) Endotoxin challenge after menhaden oil diet: effects on survival of guinea pigs. Am J Clin Nutr 49:277–282
16. Blackburn GL (1992) Nutrition and inflammatory events: highly unsaturated fatty acids (ω-3 vs ω-6) in surgical injury. Proc Soc Exp Biol Med 200:183–188
17. Gielen CJM, As AB van, Goris RJA (1993) Diets enriched with oil prevent multiple organ failure in mice? Eur J Surg 159:609–612
18. Wilmore DW, Smith RJ, O'Dwyer ST et al. (1988) The gut: a central organ after surgical stress. Surgery 104:917–923
19. Grant JP, Snyder PJ (1988) Use of L-glutamine in total parenteral nutrition. J Surg Res 1988:44:506–513
20. Souba WW, Klimberg VS, Hautamaki RD et al. (1990) Oral glutamine reduces bacterial translocation following abdominal radiation. J Surg Res 48:1–5
21. Souba WW, Klimberg VS, Plumley DA et al. (1990) The role of glutamine in maintaining a healthy gut and supporting the metabolic response to injury and infection. J Surg Res 48:383–391
22. Alverdy JA, Aoys E, Weiss-Carrington P, Burke DA (1992) The effect of glutamine-enriched TPN on gut immune cellularity. J Surg Res 52:34–38
23. Carrico CJ, Meakins JL, Marshall JC et al. (1986) Multiple-organ-failure syndrome. Arch Surg 121:198–208
24. Burke DJ, Alverdy JC, Aoys E, Moss GS (1989) Glutamine-supplemented total parenteral nutrition improves gut immune function. Arch Surg 124:1396–1399
25. Inoue Y, Grant JP, Snyder PJ (1993) Effect of glutamine-supplemented intravenous nutrition on survival after Escherichia coli-induced peritonitis. JPEN J Parenter Enteral Nutr 17:41–46
26. Robertson EC, Tisdall FF (1939) Nutrition and resistance to disease. Can Med Assoc J 40:282–284
27. Demetriou AA, Franco I, Baark S, Rettura G, Seifter E, Levenson SM (1984) Effects of vitamin A and beta carotene on intra-abdominal sepsis. Arch Surg 199:161–165
28. Drott PW (1991) Effects of vitamin A on endotoxaemia in rats. Eur J Surg 157:565–569
29. Henriks HFJ, Horan MA, Durham SK et al. (1987) Endotoxin-induced liver injury in aged and subacutely hypervitaminotic A rats. Mech Ageing Dev 41:241–250
30. Marks J (1989) The safety of vitamins: an overview. Int J Vitam Nutr Res 30 [Suppl]:12
31. The Veteran Affairs Total Parenteral Nutrition Cooperative Study Group (1991) Perioperative total parenteral nutrition in surgical patients. N Engl J Med 325:525–532
32. Rombeau JL, Rolandelli RH, Wilmore DW (1994) Nutritional support. In: Wilmore DW, Brennan M, Harken H, Holcroft J, Meakins J.L. (eds) Care of the surgical patient, chap 10. Scientific American, New York
33. Hadley MN, Grahm TW, Harrington T et al. (1986) Nutritional support in neurotrauma: a critical review of early nutrition in 45 acute head injury patients. Neurosurgery 19:367
34. Herndon DN, Barrow RE, Stein M et al. (1989) Increased mortality with intravenous supplemental feeding in severely burned patients. J Burn Care Rehabil 10:309–313
35. Wilmore DW (1977) Metabolic management of the critically ill. Plenum, New York

36. Bursztein S, Elwyn DH, Askanazi J, Kinney JM (1989) Energy metabolism, indirect calorimetry, and nutrition. Williams and Wilkins, Baltimore
37. Bessey PQ (1990) Nutritional support in critical illness. In: Deitch EA (ed) Multiple organ failure: pathophysiology and basic concepts in therapy. Thieme, New York, pp 104–125
38. Carpentier YA (1993) Are present fat emulsions appropriate? In: Wilmore DW, Carpentier YA (eds) Update in intensive care and emergency medicine 17. Springer, Berlin Heidelberg New York, pp 157–171
39. Rössle C, Carpentier YA, Richelle M et al. (1990) Medium chain triglyceride hydrolysis of soy vs fish oil LCT emulsions. Clin Nutr 11 [Suppl]:44
40. Gollaher CJ, Swenson ES, Mascioli EA, Babayan VK, Blackburn GL, Bistrain BR (1992) Dietary fat level as determinant of protein-sparing actions of structured triglycerides. Nutrition 8:348–353
41. Ardawi MSM (1988) Glutamine and glucose metabolism in human peripheral lymphocytes. Metabolism 37:99–103
42. Fong Y, Minei J, Marano MA et al. (1991) Cellular injury and decreased mRNA for myofibrillar proteins: potential role of intracellular glutamine as mediator. Surg Forum 42:21–23
43. Newsholme EA, Crabtree B, Ardawi MSM (1985) Glutamine metabolism in lymphocytes: its biochemical, physiological and clinical importace. Q J Exp Physiol 70:473–489
44. Souba WW, Herskowitz K, Salloum RM et al. (1990) Gut glutamine metabolism. JPEN J Parenter Enteral Nutr 14:45S–50S
45. Souba WW, Herskowitz K, Salloum RM et al. (1990) Gut glutamine metabolism. JPEN J Parenter Enteral Nutr 14 [Suppl]:45S–50S
46. Windmueller HG, Spaeth AE (1974) Uptake and metabolism of plasma glutamine by the small intestine. J Biol Chem 249:5070–5079
47. Jimenez FJ, Leyba CO, Mendez SM et al. (1991) Prospective study on the efficacy of branched-chain amino acids in septic patients. JPEN J Parenter Enteral Nutr 15:252–261
48. Gimmon Z, Freund HR, Fischer JF (1985) The optimal branched-chain to total amino acid ratio in the injury-adapted amino acid formulation. JPEN J Parenter Enteral Nutr 9:133–138
49. Sitren HS, Fisher H (1977) Nitrogen retention in rats fed on diets enriched with arginine and glycine. Improved N retention after trauma. Br J Nutr 37:195–208
50. Barbul A, Wasserkrug HL, Yoshimura N et al. (1984) High arginine levels in intravenous hyperalimentation abrogate post-traumatic immune suppression. J Surg Res 36:620–624
51. Reynolds JV, Daly JM, Zhang S et al. (1988) Immunomodulatory mechanisms of arginine. Surgery 104:142–151
52. Nirgiotis JG, Hennessy PJ, Andrassy RJ (1991) The effects of an arginine-free enteral diet on wound healing and immune function in the postsurgical rat. J Pediatr Surg 26:936–941
53. Barbul A, Wasserkrug HL, Seifter E et al. (1980) Immunostimulatory effects of arginine in normal and injured rats. J Surg Res 29:228–235
54. Council on Scientific Affairs (1987) Vitamin preparations as dietary supplements and as therapeutic agents. JAMA 257:1929
55. Marks J (1989) The safety of vitamins: an overview. Int J Vitam Nutr Res 30 [Suppl]:12
56. Levine GN, Derin JJ, Steiger E, Zinno R (1974) Role of oral intake and maintainence of gut mass and disaccharide activity. Gastroenterology 67:975–982
57. Saito H, Trocki O, Alexander JW et al. (1987) The effect of route of nutrient administration on the nutritional state, catabolic hormone secretion and gut mucosal integrity after burn injury. JPEN 11:1–7
58. Alverdy JC, Aoy SE, Moss GS (1988) Total parentral nutrition promotes bacterial translocation form the gut. Surgery 104:185–190
59. Peterson VM, Moore EE, Jones TN et al. (1988) Total enteral nutrition vs. total parenteral nutrition after major turso injury: attenuation of hepatic protein reprioritization. Surgery 104:199–207
60. Rowlands BJ, Giddings AEB, Johnston AOB, Hindmarsh JT, Clark RG (1977) Nitrogen-sparing effect of different feedings regimes in patients after operation. Br J Anaesth 49:781–787
61. Hulten L, Andersson H, Bosaeus I et al. (1980) Enteral elimentation in the early postoperative course. JPEN 4:455–459
62. Page CP (1989) The surgeon and gut maintenance. Am J Surg 158:485–490

63. Wilmore DW, Smith RJ, O'Dwyer ST et al. (1988) The gut: a central organ after surgical stress. Surgery 104:917–923
64. Windmueller HG, Spaeth AE (1978) Identification of ketone bodies and glutamine as major respiratory fuels in vivo of postabsorptive rat small intestine. J Biol Chem 253:69–76
65. Windmueller HG (1982) Glutamine utilization by the small intestine. Adv Enzymol 53:201–237
66. Roediger WEW (1982) Utilization of nutrients by isolated epithelial cells of the rat colon. Gastroenterology 83:424–429
67. Rush BF (1989) Irreversibility in hemorrhagic shock is caused by sepsis. Am Surg 55:204–208
68. Wells CL, Rotstein OR, Pruett TL, Simmons RL (1986) Intestinal bacteria translocate into experimental intra-abdominal abscesses. Arch Surg 121:102–107
69. Alexander JW, Boyce ST, Babcock GF et al. (1990) The process of microbial translocation. Ann Surg 212:496–512
70. Deitch EA (1990) Bacterial translocation of the gut flora. J Trauma 30:184–189
71. Adams S, Dellinger EP, Wetz MJ, Oreskovich MR, Simonowitz D, Johansen K (1986) Enteral versus parenteral nutritional support following laparotomy for trauma: a randomized prospective trial. J Trauma 26:882–891
72. Peterson VM, Moore EE, Jones TN et al. (1988) Total enteral nutrition versus total parenteral nutrition after major torso injury: attenuation of hepatic protein reprioritization. Surgery 104:199–207
73. Moore FA, Moore EE, Jones TN, McCroskey BL, Peterson VM (1989) TEN versus TPN following major abdominal trauma – reduced septic morbidity. J Trauma 29:916–923
74. Kudsk KA, Croce MA, Fabian TC et al. (1992) Enteral versus parenteral feeding: effects on septic morbidity after blunt and penetrating abdominal trauma. Ann Surg 215:503–513
75. Moore FA, Feliciano DV, Andrassy RJ et al. (1992) Early enteral feeding, compared with partenteral, reduces postoperative septic complications. The results of a metaanalysis. Ann Surg 216:172–183

Growth Hormone

M. Mjaaland, K. Unneberg, and A. Revhaug

Introduction

Wasting of skeletal muscle is a hallmark of the catabolic state. Sir David Cuthbertson was the first to show not only that this state was associated with net whole body nitrogen loss, but also that pituitary extracts could reduce this loss [1,2].

After surgical stress, several metabolic changes take place. Energy expenditure is increased, generally in proportion to the trauma size [3,4]. There is a shift to fat oxidation for energy requirements [3]. At the same time, there is also increased carbohydrate oxidation [5]. There is a net protein breakdown resulting in net whole body nitrogen losses proportional to the trauma size [6]. In skeletal muscle, there is a synthesis of alanine and glutamine from branched-chain amino acids [7,8]. Glucose taken up by the muscle is glycolyzed to lactate and pyruvate. These substances, together with other amino acids and glycerol from triglycerides, are taken to the liver and act as precursors for gluconeogenesis [5, 9, 10].

These responses obviously supply the organism with necessary substrates at a time of increased needs and are thus in general protective. However, they do have disadvantages: peripheral tissue is sacrificed, in particular skeletal muscle, which is important for movement and for respiration. However, the supplementation of these substrates as parenteral nutrition does not prevent the degradation of the body's own tissue, regardless of the amounts of substrates given. Rowlands et al. showed that in spite of increasing energy levels in parenteral nutrition given to patients after abdominal surgery, the patients continued to lose whole body nitrogen [11]. Streat et al. determined changes in body composition in ten intensive care patients after 10 days of total parenteral nutrition. They found that in spite of the nutrition given, the patients continued to lose weight and proteins. Their only gain was in fat [12].

Apparently there are mechanisms preventing the organism from utilizing nutrition after surgical stress. This inability to utilize nutrition was our basis for studying growth hormone.

Growth Hormone

Pituitary growth hormone was detected in the early 1930s [13,14]. it has been detected in the pituitary glands of representatives of all vertebrae classes and is one of the principal factors regulating somatic growth in vertebrates. Chemically, growth hormone molecules from different vertebrates are not identical, but they are closely related [15].

Human growth hormone or somatotropin is a polypeptide consisting of 191 amino acids with two disulfide bridges. It has a molecular mass of 21 500 Da and its secretion is controlled by hormonal, neurogenic, and metabolic mechanisms. The release of growth hormone is stimulated by the release of growth hormone releasing hormone (GHRH). The main inhibitor of growth hormone secretion is somatostatin, which is synthesized in several tissues in the body as well as in the hypothalamus. The secretion of growth hormone is pulsatile, with huge diurnal variations during a 24-h-period. Human studies indicate that the growth hormone pulse amplitudes are increased during slow-wave sleep so that most growth hormone secretion occurs during the night [16, 17].

Human growth hormone circulates in the blood partially bound to each of two different growth hormone-binding proteins (GHBP), one with low capacity and high affinity and another with lower affinity [18, 19]. In the tissue, growth hormone binds to transmembrane glycoprotein receptors [20]. The high-affinity, low-capacity GHBP may represent the extracellular binding domain of the growth hormone receptor [21, 22]. Laron dwarfs lacking GHBP do not respond to growth hormone treatment [23].

Insulin-like growth factor-I (IFG I) is growth hormone's most important mediator. It is mainly synthesized in the liver, but also in other tissues. Circulating IGF-I is bound to several distinct IGF-I-binding proteins (IGFBP) the two major ones being IFGBP-1 and IGFBP-3. Nutritional status has an important influence on the growth hormone/IGF I axis. Fasting results in increased growth hormone pulsatility and secretion and decreased IGF-I levels [24]. Decreased IGF-I levels have also been seen after surgery [25] and sepsis [26] and in other critically ill patients [27]. This has been interpreted as a growth hormone resistance in these states. However, several aspects of the growth hormone/IGF-I interactions remain unclarified. It is still not known in detail which of the metabolic effects seen after growth hormone treatment is due to growth hormone itself, which are induced by IGF-I, and which are caused by the combination of the two [28]. In addition, IGF-I has autocrine and paracrine as well as endocrine actions, and the first two are believed to be the most important [29], which means the the circulating levels, which are what has been measured in the studies mentioned, reflect only a minor part of the picture.

Growth hormone plays an important role in regulating normal growth and development in childhood by stimulating proliferation of bone and muscle [30]. Body growth is not exclusively stimulated by growth hormone. Growth hormone is the major determinant for growth only from the second year of life until puberty. During the first year of life, growth is mainly determined by nutrition [31]. During puberty, sex hormones become important determinants [32].

Growth hormone deficiency during childhood causes retarded growth, and such children have successfully been treated with growth hormone for years [33]. There are indications that even children with growth retardation from other causes may benefit from growth hormone treatment. Turner's syndrome being one of those [33]. However, this depends on normal levels of GHBP. Possible beneficial effects of growth hormone treatment in growth hormone-deficient adults are presently being studied, also during the naturally occurring low levels seen in old age [34].

This way of utilizing growth hormone, as a substitution in growth hormone deficiency, has been the traditional indication for growth hormone therapy. Our interest in growth hormone is based on a quite different apporach. We have given growth hormone as supplementation therapy in large doses to utilize the metabolic effects of growth hormone in patients after surgical stress.

Growth Hormone Effects on Carbohydrate and Lipid Metabolism

Adipose tissue has long been recognized as a target for the action of growth hormone. More than 50 years ago, Lee and Schaffer reported that treatment with pituitary extracts resulted in a relative decrease in carcass fat in rats [14], something that was confirmed later by Greenbaum [35].

Growth hormone has also for a long time been known to influence carbohydrate metabolism. Both insulin-like and anti-insulin-like effects of growth hormone have been described [36, 37]. The insulin-like influences upon both carbohydrate and fat metabolism, with increased uptake of glucose, conversion of glucose to glycogen in the liver and lipids in adipose tissue, and a resulting hypoglycemia and hypolipidemia, appear to occur during the first hour after the tissue has been exposed to growth hormone. Glucose oxidation is increased [37]. However, during the second hour of exposure, this effects wears off, and a refractoriness to this action occurs, lasting for several hours. Then an anti-insulin-like effect occurs, with hyperglycemia, lipolysis with increased plasma free fatty acids and glycerol, and increased fat oxidation relative to the carbohydrate oxidation. No refractoriness to this effect occurs [37].

Growth Hormone Effects on Protein Metabolism

In 1950 Greenbaum reported that rats treated with growth hormone not only increased in weight, but that this was due mostly to an increase in protein compartments, in particular skeletal muscle [38]. Later, it was shown that growth hormone stimulates protein synthesis in a variety of tissues: skeletal muscle [39], liver [40], and heart muscle [41]. Although often following an increased amino acid uptake, there is also evidence that this may occur as an independent phenomenon [42].

Growth hormone's particular effect on skeletal muscle morphology was studied by Dudley et al. In a study in human growth hormone transgenic rats, body weight and weight of the soleus muscle were increased compared to nontransgenic littermates, and type I and type II fibers had increased their size [43]. In fasted rats, Lanz et al. showed that there was an atrophy of both fibers in the diaphragma, most pronounced in the fast fibers (type II), and that all fibers were restored to normal size when refeeding was supplemented with growth hormone treatment [44]. In hypophysectomized rats, Ayling et al. found that 11 days of growth hormone treatment increased the proportion of type 1 fibers in skeletal muscle [45]. No effect on muscle strength was found after growth hormone treatment in young males in a study performed by Deyssig et al. [46]. On the other hand, growth hormone treatment increased muscle grip force in patients after abdominal surgery [47] and increased the maximum inspiratory force in patients with chronic pulmonary disease [48]. In growth hormone-deficient adults, strength in some muscles, but not all, was improved by growth hormone treatment [49], as was exercixe performance [50], but no effects on fiber size were detected [51].

Growth Hormone and the Catabolic Surgical Patient

After Cuthbertsen demonstrated that pituitary extracts could reduce the nitrogen loss after injury [2], growth hormone treatment was tried in various clinical settings in the 1960s and 1970s. Liljedahl et al. found decreased nitrogen excretion in five post-burn patients and also noted that there was a favorable tendency toward improved healing of the wounds [52]. Wilmore et al. also gave growth hormone to patients with burn injury. Their nine patients were on oral intake, but the diet was fixed. They also found reduced nitrogen losses (in all but one patient) and potassium retention at ratio of 3:1, approximating the relationship between these substances found in muscle. They found increased insulin levels and a slight increase in blood glucose and observed that the glucose tolerance curves plateaued at an increased level [53].

Only human growth hormone produces reliable effects in humans. The production of human growth hormone by recombinant DNA technique from the mid 1980s on made growth hormone both more pure and more available, starting a new era of research. Manson et al. gave growth hormone to hypocaloric-fed volunteers, inducing improved nitrogen balance [54] and increased protein synthesis and fat oxidation [55]. Interesting as those findings were, in our opinion they do not apply to the stress-induced catabolic state. There may be a problem in recognizing starvation in surgical patients, but, once recognized, this condition is no problem to treat.

We set ourselves the task of discovering how patients undergoing surgical stress could be made to improve their utilization of exogenous nutrition. We investigated patients undergoing elective, abdominal surgery as a fairly reproducible model of surgical stress. Our main objektive was to see whether growth hormone treatment in this situation would improve the utilization of nutrition. We therefore gave the patients nutrition designed to cover their basic needs (daily amount, 6 g nitrogen/m^2 body surface area; energy 125% of basal metabolic rate, BMR, 50% as glucose and 50% as fat). Nineteen patients were randomized to treatment with growth hormone (Genotropin; 24 IU i.m.) or placebo in a double-blind fashion. The treatment was given each morning for the first 5 postoperative days. Perioperatively, they all received epidural analgesia with local anesthetics in addition to general anesthesia, which partially blocks the catabolic response [56]. The epidural catheter was kept in place for the whole study period for the administration of opioids to secure a standardized pain relief regimen. Preoperatively and on the second and

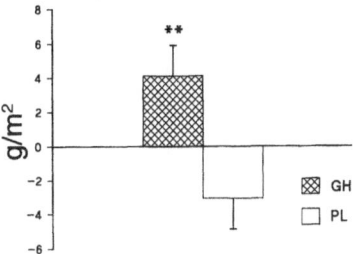

Fig. 1. Cumulative nitrogen balance in patients treated with growth hormone (*GH*) and placebo (*PL*) on the first 5 postoperative days. **$p<0.01$. Published with permission from European Journal of Surgery [57]

fourth postoperative days, forearm substrate fluxes were performed at 12 noon, 4 h after the growth hormone injection. Indirect calorimetry was performed each morning just before the growth hormone injection was given and at 4 P.M. Daily nitrogen balances were recorded.

The growth hormone-treated patients had a net cumulative nitrogen retention, whereas the placebo-treated patients excreted nitrogen (Fig. 1) [57]. They had increased energy expenditure, increased fat oxidation, and decreased carbohydrate oxidation, calculated from the indirect calorimetry (Fig. 2) [58]. Increased levels of free fatty acids in the growth hormone-treated patients supported the increased fat oxidation found by the indirect calorimetry, whereas the increased glycerol levels were indications of increased lipolysis (Fig. 3). Improved nitrogen balance was found postoperatively with a hypocaloric dextrose infusion only by Ward et al. [59] and on a higher energy level by Ponting et al. [60]. Ward et al. also demonstrated increased fat oxidation [59]. Douglas et al. found increased fat oxidation in the postabsorptive septic and traumatized patients, but this could not be detected in similart patients who were given nutrition parenterally [61]. In these studies no changes in carbohydrate oxidation was demonstrated. However, Gore et al. found decreased carbohydrate oxidation in patients given growth hormone after burn injury [62].

In our study β-hydroxybutyrate levels were increased (Fig. 3). Manson et al. found increased excretion of ketones in the fasting volunteers given growth hormone [54], and Fleming et al. demonstrated increased levels of β-hydroxybutyrate in burn patients given growth hormone [63]. Ketogenesis and oxidation of ketones instead of glucose in the brain is a normal response during prolonged starvation, supposed to be responsible fot the "adaptive" protein sparing seen with time during starvation [64]. This is normally not seen during stress-induced catabolic states [65]. Considering its role in protein sparing during starvation, ketogenesis may be connected to the protein sparing seen during growth hormone treatment.

On the second postoperative day of our study, forearm release of amino acid nitrogen was attenuated by growth hormone treatment [66]. Amino acid release from skeletal muscle after stress consists mainly of glutamine and alanine [67]. The reduction in amino acid release in the present study was due mainly to reduced release of glutamine and alanine (Fig. 4). Jiang et al. also found decreased arteriove-

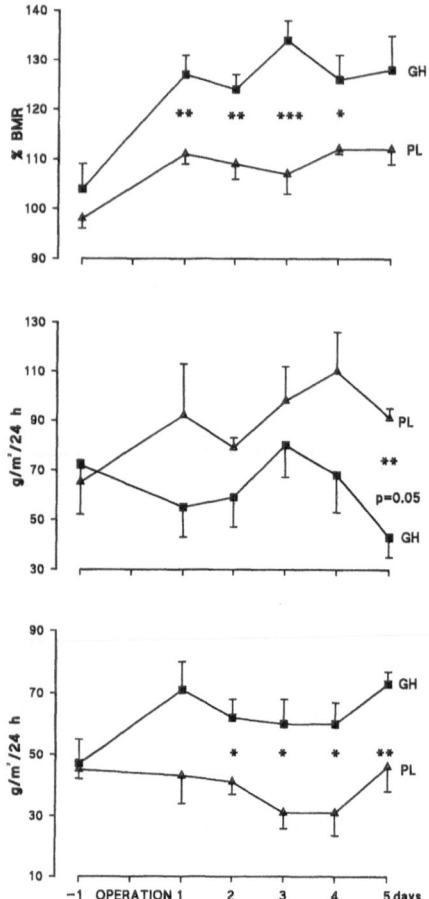

Fig. 2. Resting energy expenditure (*top*), carbohydrate oxidation (*middle*), and fat oxidation (*bottom*) at 4 P.M. preoperatively and on the first 5 postoperative days in patients treated with growth hormone (*GH, closed squares*) or placebo (*PL, open triangles*). *p<0.05, **p<0.01, ***p<0.001. *BMR*, basal metabolic rate. Published with permission from Metabolism [58]

nous differences in amino acids over forearm tissue in postoperative patients on hypocaloric nutrition; in particular, the release of glutamine was reduced [47]. Hammarqvist et al. demonstrated that the decrease in net glutamine loss from skeletal muscle was associated with a decreased loss of intracellular glutamine and a maintained protein synthesis in skeletal muscle [68]. In our study, release of 3-methylhistidine from forearm tissue was also attenuated (Fig. 5) [66]. 3-Methylhistidine is a breakdown product from contractile protein which is not metabolized further. This finding thus indicates decreased breakdown of contractile protein in skeletal muscle [69].

In the overwhelming majority of studies performed with growth hormone treatment in humans, an improved nitrogen balance has been demonstrated, both in the postoperative or post-traumatic [59–61] and in the fasting catabolic state [54]. Consistently, protein synthesis measured by isotope tracers has been elevated [55,

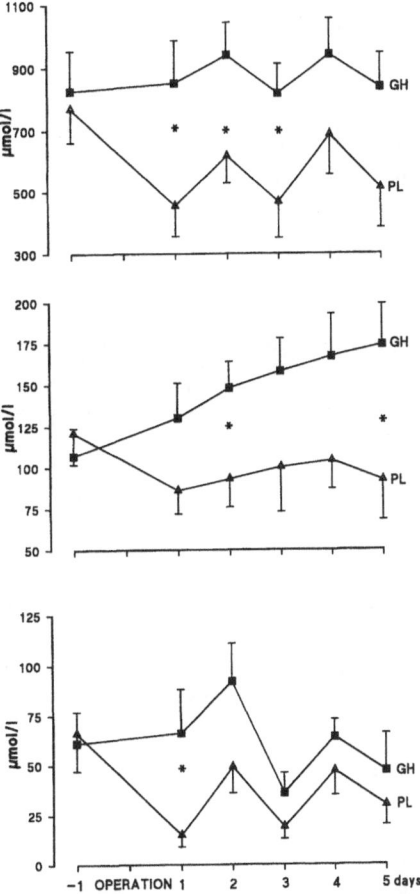

Fig. 3. Free fatty acids (*top*), glycerol (*middle*), and β-hydroxybutyrate at 12 noon preoperatively and on the first 5 postoperative days in patients treated with growth hormone (*GH, closed circles*) or placebo (*PL, open circles*). *$p<0.05$, ***$p<0.001$. Published with permission from Metabolism [58].

59–61], whereas data regarding protein breakdown have varied [59, 61]. Fong ct al. found muscle myosin heavy-chain mRNA accumulation and amino acid accrual, but unchanged whole body leucine oxidation after 6 h of growth hormone infusion in nutritionally depleted humans during intravenous refeeding [70]. Fryberg et al. found that an acute arterial growth hormone infusion stimulated forearm protein synthesis after 6 h in humans [71].

We found increased levels of growth hormone, and towards the end of the study levels of IGF-I also increased (Fig. 6). The reason for the late rise in IGF-I may be the so-called growth hormone resistance present in stress-induced catabolic states [27]. However, it should be noted that in our study the effect on the forearm amino acid fluxes was most pronounced on the second postoperative day, before the increase in serum levels of IGF-I was detected. This may indicate that the influence of forearm amino acid release was a direct growth hormone effect.

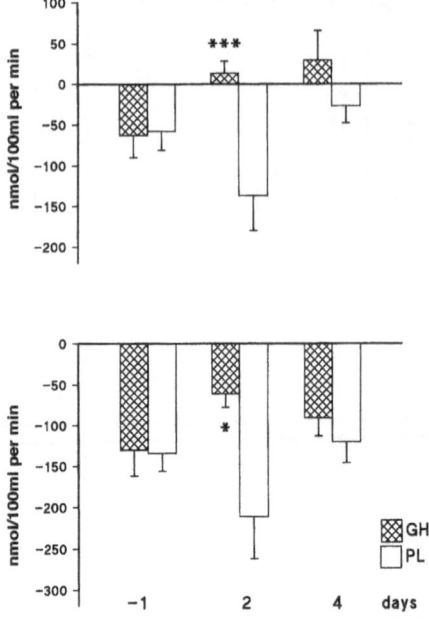

Fig. 4. Forearm release of glutamine (GLN, *top*) and alanine (ALA, *bottom*) preoperatively and on the second and fourth postoperative days in patients treated with growth hormone (*GH*) or placebo (*PL*). *$p<0.05$, ***$p<0.001$. Published with permission from Annals of Surgery [66]

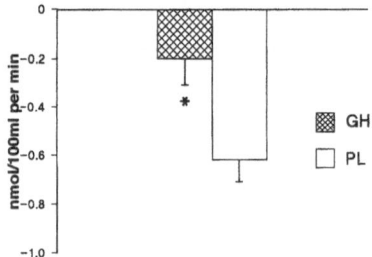

Fig. 5. Forearm release of 3-methylhistidine preoperatively on the second postoperative days in patients treated with growth hormone (*GH*) or placebo (*PL*). *$p<0.05$. Published with permission from Annals of Surgery [66]

Alternatively, it may be that the tissue levels of IGF-I, which we were unable to measure, where elevated [28]. In our study, insulin levels were slightly increased. Glucagon levels were markedly increased in patients treated with growth hormone (Fig. 6); this was also found by Fleming at al., who in addition found increased levels of catecholamines in patients treated with growth hormone after burn injury [63].

Our patients had a weight gain on the third postoperative day, which was normalized by the fifth postoperative day [57]. This transient fluid retention is well known. In hemodynamically unstable patients, this may be an important adverse effect of growth hormone treatment.

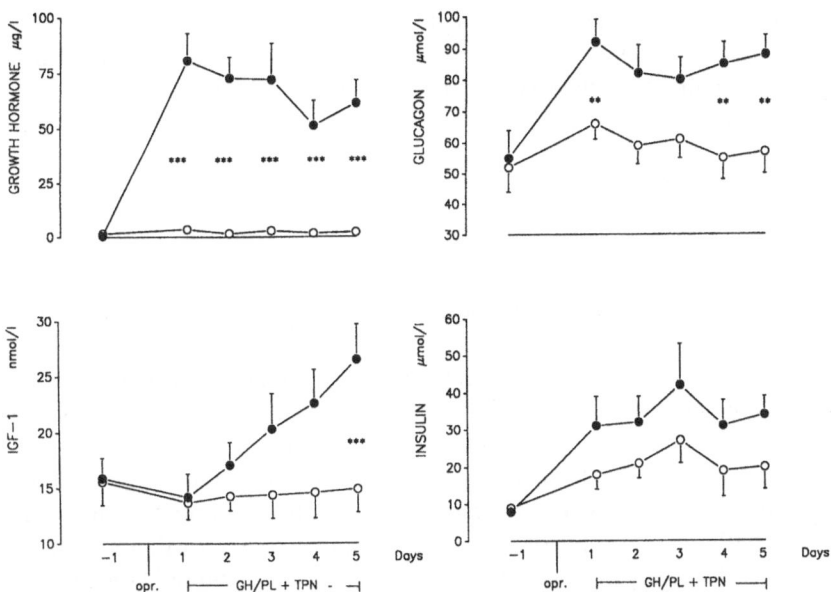

Fig. 6. Growth hormone (*GH*), insulin-like growth factor (*IGF*)-I insulin, and glucagon at 12 noon preoperatively and on the first 5 postoperative days in patients treated with growth hormone (*closed circles*) or placebo (*PL*, open circles). **$p<0.05$, ***$p<0.001$. Published with permission from Metabolism [58]

In more severe catabolic states, such as sepsis and burn injury, the effect of growth hormone has been questioned because of growth hormone resistance [25–27]. Dahn et al. found decreased levels of IGF-I in their septic patients and suggested that this was the cause of the lack of response to growth hormone treatment [26]. However, Voerman et al. recently found that growth hormone improved nitrogen economy in patients recovering from septic shock [72], and Gore et al. found that growth hormone induced nitrogen sparing in severe burn injury [62].

Regenerative and Healing Effects of Growth Hormone

Growth hormone treatment has been found to improve healing of grafting sites of skin transplantation after burn injury in adults [73] and children [74]. In animal experiments, tensile strength in abdominal wounds [75] and colonic anastomoses improved [76], and healing of both fractures [77] and leg ulcers [78] appeared to be promoted by growth hormone treatment.

Immunostimulatory Effects of Growth Hormone

Growth hormone may also have immunostimulatory effects. Growth hormone deficiency has been associated with an impairment in natural killer cell activity [79],

278   M. Mjaaland, K. Unneberg, and A. Revhaug

and Christ et al. found increased natural killer cell activity when exogenous growth hormone was given to growth hormone-deficient women [80]. Growth hormone may also stimulate superoxide production of granulocytes and macrophages [81].

Conclusion

Growth hormone treatment induces metabolic patterns in the surgical catabolic patient which are believed to be favorable and improves the utilization of exogenous nutrition. In addition, growth hormone has regenerative and healing effects which may benefit the surgical patient.

However, before this drug can be utilized generally in patient treatment, some questions regarding growth hormone therapy should be elucidated. Growth hormone's effect in severely catabolic patients has not been clarified. Part of this uncertainty is linked to the depression of IFG-I production in severe catabolic states. The metabolic role of IGF-I versus the direct growth hormone effect is not clarified. Preliminary studies suggest that, in combination, growth hormone and IGF-I may act additively or even synergistically [82]. The acute fluid retention seen during growth hormone therapy must be monitored in the hemodynamically unstable patient. Will the effects of growth hormone combined with specific substrates such as glutamine or perhaps other amino acids such as arginine or ornithine improve the results? With regard to lipids, it could be that the endogenous mobilization of fat is sufficient, or, on the other hand, the increased fat oxidation might indicate that lipids will be particularly efficiently handled metabolically when given concomitantly with growth hormone. So far there are no indications that growth hormone therapy on a short-term basis represents a danger in patients with malignant diseases, but more conclusive knowledge is needed in this matter. With these limitions, growth hormone must be regarded as a promising agent in the therapy of the acutely catabolic patient.

References

1. Cuthbertson DP (1930) The disturbance of metabolism produced by bony and nonbony injury, with notes on certain abnormal conditions of bone. Biochem J 24:1244–1263
2. Cuthbertson DP, Shaw GB, Young FG (1941) The anterior pituitary gland and protein metabolism. II. The influence of anterior pituitary extract on the metabolic response of the rat to injury. J Endocrinol 2:468–474
3. Kinney JM, Duke JH, Long CL, Gump FE (1970) Tissue fuel and weight loss after injury. J Clin Pathol 23:65–72
4. Megiud MM, Brennan MF, Aoki TT, Muller WA, Ball MR, Moore FD (1974) Hormone-substrate interrelationship following trauma. Arch Surg 109:776–783
5. Wolfe RR, Durkot MJ, Allsop JR, Burke JF (1979) Glucose metabolism in severly burned patients. Metabolism 28:1031–1039
6. Kien CL, Young VR, Rohrbaugh DK, Burke JF (1978) Increased rates of whole body protein synthesis and breakdown in children recovering from burns. Ann Surg 187:393–391
7. Ruderman NB, Berger M (1974) The formation of glutamine and alanine in skeletal muscle. J Biol Chem 249:5500–5506
8. Garber AJ, Karl IE, Kipnis DM (1976) Alanine and glutamine synthesis and release from skeletal muscle. J Biol Chem 251:836–843

 9. Randle PJ, Garland PB, Hales CN, Newsholme EA (1963) The glucose fatty-acid cycle. Its role in insulin sensitivity and the metabolic disturbance of diabetes mellitus. Lancet 1:785–789
10. Imamura M, Clowes GHA, Blackburn GL, O'Donnell TF, Trerice M, Bhimjee Y, Ryan NT (1975) Liver metabolism and glucogenesis in trauma and sepsis. Surgery 77:868–880
11. Rowlands BJ, Giddings AEB, Johnston AOB, Hindmarsch JT, Clark RG (1977) Nitrogen-sparing effect of different feeding regimes in patients after operation. Br J Anaesth 49:781–787
12. Streat SJ, Beddoe AH, Hill GL (1987) Aggressive nutritional support does not prevent protein loss despite fat gain in septic intensive care patients. J Trauma 27:262–266
13. Riddle OR, Bates RW, Dykshorn SW (1932) New hormone of anterior pituitary. Proc Soc Exp Biol Med 29:1211–1212
14. Lee MO, Schaffer NK (1934) Anterior pituitary growth hormone and the composition of growth. J Nutr 7:337–363
15. Kostyo JL, Regan CR (1976) The biology of growth hormone. Pharmacol Ther 2:591–604
16. Winer LM, Shaw MA, Bauman G (1990) Basal plasma growth hormone levels in man: new evidence for rhythmicity of growth hormone secretion. J Clin Endocrinol Metab 70:1678–1686
17. Hochberg Z, Amit T, Zadik Z (1991) Twenty-four-hour profile of plasma growth hormone-binding protein. J Clin Endocrinol Metab 72:236–239
18. Bauman G, Stalor WM, Armburn K, Barsano CP, DeVries BC (1986) A specific growth hormone-binding protein in human plasma: initial characterization. J Clin Endocrinol Metab 62:134–141
19. Bauman G, Shaw MA (1990) A second lower affinity growth hormone-binding protein in human plasma. J Clin Endocrinol Metab 70:680–686
20. Isaksson OGP, Edén S, Jansson JO (1985) Mode of action of pituitary growth hormone on target cells. Annu Rev Physiol 47:483–499
21. Hochberg Z, Bick T, Amit T, Barkey RJ, Youdim MBH (1990) Regulation of growth hormone receptor turnover by growth hormone. Acta Paediatr Scand Suppl 367:148–152
22. DeVos AM, Utsch M, Kossiakoff AA (1992) Human growth hormone and extracellular domain of its receptor: crystal structure of the complex. Science 25:306–312
23. Daughaday WH, Trivedi B (1987) Absence of serum growth hormone binding proteins in patients with growth hormone receptor defiency [Laron dwarfism]. Proc Natl Acad Sci USA 84:4636–4640
24. Clemmons DR, Underwood LE (1991) Nutritional regulation of IGF-1 and IGF binding proteins. Annu Rev Nutr 11:393–412
25. Frayn KN, Price DA, Maycock PF, Carrol SM (1984) Plasma somatomedin activity after injury in man and its relationship to other hormonal and metabolic changes. Clin Endocrinol 20:179–187
26. Dahn MS, Lange P, Jacobs LA (1988) Insulinlike growth factor 1 production is inhibited in human sepsis. Arch Surg 123:1409–1414
27. Ross RJM, Miell JP, Freeman E, Jones J, Mathews D, Preece M, Buchanan C (1991) Critically ill patients have high basal growth hormone concentrations with low concentrations of insulin-like growth factor I. Clin Endocrinol 35:47–54
28. Pell JM, Bates PC (1992) Differential actions of growth hormone and insulin-like growth factor-I on tissue protein metabolism in dwarf mice. Endocrinology 130:1942–1950
29. D'Ercole JA, Stiles AD, Underwood LE (1984) Tissue concentrations of somatemedin C: further evidence for multiple sites of synthesis and paracrine of autocrine mechanisms or action. Proc Natl Acad Sci USA 81:935–939
30. Isaksson OG, Lindahl, A, Nilsson A, Isgaard J (1988) Action of growth hormone: current views. Acta Paediatr Scand 343:12–18
31. Karlberg J (1990) The infancy-childhood growth spurt. Acta Paediatr Scand Suppl 367:111–118
32. Tanaka T, Suwa S, Yokoya S, Hibi I (1988) Analysis of linear growth during puberty. Acta Paediatr Scand Suppl 347:25–29
33. Tanner JM, Whitehouse RH, Hughes PCR, Vince FP (1971) Effect of human growth hormone treatment for 1 to 7 years on growth of 100 children, with growth hormone deficiency, low

birthweight, inherited smallness, Turner's syndrome, and other complaints. Arch Dis Child 46:745–782

34. Cuneo RC, Salamon F, McGauley GA, Sönsken PH (1992) The growth hormone deficiency syndrome in adults. Clin Endocrinol 37:397–397

35. Greenbaum AL (1953) Changes in body composition and respiratory quotient of adult female rats treated with purified growth hormone. Biochem J 45:400–407

36. Fineberg SE, Merimee TJ (1974) Acute metabolic effects of human growth hormone. Diabetes 23:499–504

37. Goodman HM, Gorin E, Schwartz Y, Tai L-R, Chipkin SR, Honeyman TW, Frick GP, Yamaguchi H (1991) Cellular effects of growth hormone on adipocytes. Chin J Physiol 34:27–44

38. Greenbaum AL, Young FG (1950) Distribution of protein in the tissues of rats treated with anterior-pituitary growth-hormone. Nature 165:521–523

39. Dreskin SC, Kostyo JL (1980) Acute effects of growth hormone on the function of the ribosomes of the rat skeletal muscle. Horm Metab Res 12:60–66

40. Korner A (1960) The effect of hypophysectomy of the rat and the treatment with growth hormone on the incorporation in vivo of radioactive amino acids into proteins of the subcellular fractions of rat liver. Biochem J 74:462–471

41. Prysor-Jones RA, Jenkins JS (1980) Effect of excessive secretion of growth hormone on tissues of the rat, with particular reference to the heart and skeletal muscle. J Endocrinol 85:75–82

42. Kostyo JL (1964) Separation of the effects of growth hormone on muscle amino acid transport and protein synthesis. Endocrinology 75:113–119

43. Dudley GA, Portanova R (1987) Histochemical characteristics of soleus muscle in growth hormone transgenic mice [42561]. Proc Soc Exp Biol Med 185:403–408

44. Lanz JK Jr, Donahoe M, Rogers RM, Ontell M (1992) Effects of growth hormone on diaphragmatic recovery from malnutrition. J Appl Physiol 73:801–805

45. Ayling CM, Moreland BH, Zanelli JM, Schulster D (1989) Human growth hormone treatment of hypophysectomized rats increases the proportion of type-1 fibres in skeletal muscle. J Endocrinol 123:429–435

46. Deyssig R, Frisch H, Blum WF, Waldhör (1993) Effect of growth hormone treatment on hormonal parameters, body composition and strenght in athletes. Acta Endocrinol 128:313–318

47. Jiang Z-M, He G-Z, Zhang S-Y, Wang X-R, Yang N-F, Zhu Y, Wilmore DW (1989) Low-dose growth hormone and hypocaloric nutrition attenuate the protein-caloric response after major operation. Ann Surg 210:513–525

48. Pape GS, Friedman M, Underwood LE, Clemmons DR (1991) The effects of growth hormone on weight gain and pulmonary function in patients with chronic obstructive lung disease. Chest 99:1495–1500

49. Cuneo RC, Salamon F, Wiles CM, Hesp R, Sönsken PH (1991) Growth hormone treatment in growth hormone-deficient adults. I. Effects on muscle mass and strength. J Appl Physiol 70:688–694

50. Cuneo RC, Salamon F, Wiles CM, Hesp R, Sönsken PH (1991) Growth hormone treatment in growth hormone-dificient adults. II. Effects on exercise performance. J Appl Physiol 70:695–700

51. Cuneo RC, Salamon F, Wiles CM, Round JM, Jones D, Hesp R, Sönsken PH (1992) Histology of skeletal muscle in adults with growth hormone deficiency: comparison with normal muscle and response to growth hormone treatment. Horm Res 37:23–28

52. Liljedahl S-O, Gemzell C-A, Plantin L-O, Birke G (1961) Effect of growth hormone in patients with severe burns. Acta Chir Scand 122:1–14

53. Wilmore DW, Moylan JA, Bristow BF, Mason AD, Pruitt BA Jr (1974) Anabolic effects of human growth hormone and high caloric feedings following thermal injury. Surg Gynecol Obstet 139:875–884

54. Manson J McK, Wilmore DW (1986) Positive nitrogen balance with human growth hormone and hypocaloric intravenous feeding. Surgery 100:188–197

55. Manson J McK, Smith RJ, Wilmore DW (1988) Growth hormone stimulates protein synthesis during hypocaloric parenteral nutrition. Ann Surg 208:136–42

56. Kehlet H (1988) The stress response to surgery: release mechanisms and the modifying effect of pain relief. Acta Chir Scand 550:22–28
57. Mjaaland M, Unneberg K, Hotvedt R, Revhaug A (1991) Nitrogen retention caused by growth hormone in patients undergoing gastrointestinal surgery with epidural analgesia and parenteral nutrition. Eur J Surg 157:21–27
58. Mjaaland M, Unneberg K, Bjøro T, Revhaug A (1993) Growth hormone treatment after abdominal surgery decreased carbohydrate oxidation and increased fat oxidation in patients with total parenteral nutrition. Metabolism 42:185–190
59. Ward HC, Halliday D, Sim AJW (1987) Protein and energy metabolism with biosynthetic human growth hormone after gastrointestinal surgery. Ann Surg 206:56–61
60. Ponting GA, Halliday D, Teale JD, Sim AJW (1988) Postoperative positive nitrogen balance with intravenous hyponutrition and growth hormone. Lancet 27:439–440
61. Douglas RG, Humberstone DA, Haystead A, Shaw JHF (1990) Metabolic effects of recombinant human growth hormone: isotopic studies in the postabsorptive state and during parenteral nutrition. Br J Surg 77:785–790
62. Gore DC, Honeycutt D, Jahoor F, Rutan T, Wolfe RR, Herndon DN (1991) Effect of growth hormone on glucose utilization in burn patients. J Surg Res 51:518–523
63. Fleming RYD, Rutan RL, Jahoor F, Barrow RE, Wolfe RR, Herndon DN (1992) Effect of human growth hormone on catabolic hormones and free fatty acids following thermal injury. J Trauma 32:698–703
64. Owen OE, Morgan AP, Kemp HG, Sullivan JM, Herrera MG, Cahill GF (1967) Brain metabolism during fasting. J Clin Invest 46:1589–1595
65. Beisel WR, Wannemacher RW (1980) Gluconeogenesis, ureagenesis, and ketogenesis during sepsis. JPEN J Parenter Enteral Nutr 4:277–285
66. Mjaaland M, Unneberg K, Larsson J, Nilsson L, Revhaug A (1993) Growth hormone after abdominal surgery attenuated forearm glutamine, alanine, 3-methylhistidine and total amino acid efflux in patients receiving total parenteral nutrition. Ann Surg 217:413–422
67. Aulick LH, Wilmore DW (1979) Increased peripheral amino acid release following burn injury. Surgery 85:560–565
68. Hammarqvist F, Strømberg C, von der Decken A, Vinnars E, Wernerman J (1992) Biosynthetic human growth hormone preserves both muscle protein synthesis and the decrease in muscle free glutamine and improves whole body nitrogen economy after operation. Ann Surgery 216:184–191
69. Sjölin J, Stjernström H, Henneberg S, Andersson E, Måtrtenmsson J, Friman G, Larsson J (1989) Splanchnic and peripheral release of 3-methylhistidine in relation to its urinary excretion in human infection. Metabolism 39:23–29
70. Fong Y, Rosenbaum M, Tracey KJ, Raman G, Hesse DG, Matthews DE, Leibel RL, Gertner JM, Fischman DA, Lowry SF (1989) Recombinant growth hormone enhances muscle myosin heavy-chain mRNA accumulation and amino acid accrual in humans. Proc Natl Acad Sci USA 86:3371–3374
71. Fryburg DA, Gelfand RA, Barrett EJ (1991) Growth hormone acutely stimulates forearm muscle protein synthesis in normal humans. Am J Physiol 23:260:E499–E504
72. Voerman HJ, Strack van Schijndel RJM, Groenenveld ABJ, de Boer H, Nauta JP, van der Veen EA, Thijs LG (1992) Effects of recombinant human growth hormone in patients with severe sepsis. Ann Surg 216:648–655
73. Shernan SK, Demling RH, Lalonde C, Lowe DK, Eriksson E, Wilmore DW (1989) Growth hormone enhances reepithelialization of human split-thickness skin graft donor sites. Surg Forum 40:37–39
74. Herndon DN, Barrow RE, Kunkel KR, Broemeling L, Rutan RL (1990) Effects of recombinant human growth hormone on donor site healing in severely burned children. Ann Surg 212:423–431
75. Zaizen Y, Ford EG, Costin G, Atkinson JB (1990) The effects of perioperative exogenous growth hormone on wound bursting strength in normal and malnourished rats. J Pediatr Surg 25:70–74
76. Christensen H, Oxlund H, Laurberg S (1990) Growth hormone increases the bursting strength of colonic anastomoses. An experimental study in the rat. Int J Colorectal Dis 5:130–134

77. Bak B, Jørgensen PH, Andreassen TT (1990) Increased mechanical strength of healing rat tibial fractures treated with biosynthetic human growth hormone. Bone 11:233–239
78. Rasmussen LH, Karlsmark T, Avntorp C, Peters K, Jensen LT, Jørgensen M (1991) Topical human growth hormone treament of chronic leg ulcers. Phlebology 6:23–30
79. Saxena QB, Saxena RK, Adler WH (1982) Regulation of natural killer activity in vivo. Int Arch Allergy Appl Immunol 67:169–174
80. Crist DM, Peake GT, Mackinnon LT, Sibbitt WL, Kraner JC (1987) Exogenous growth hormone treatment alters body composition and increases natural killer cell activity in women with impaired endogenous growth hormone secretion. Metabolism 36:1115–1117
81. Fu Y-K, Arkins S, Wang BS, Kelley KW (1991) A novel role of growth hormone and insulin-like growth factor-I. Priming neutrophils for superoxide anion secretion. J Immunol 146:1602–1608
82. Kupfer SR, Underwood LE, Baxter RC, Clemmons DR (1993) Enhancement of the anabolic effects of growth hormone and insulin-like growth factor I by use of both agents simultaneously. J Clin Invest 91:391–396

The Growth Hormone/Insulin-Like Growth Factor I Axis During Surgical Stress and Critical Illness

R. J. M. Ross and A. M. Cotterill

Introduction

Acquired growth hormone (GH) resistance is found in patients who have malnutrition and protein catabolism in common, such as post-surgical and critically ill patients and patients with organ failure [1]. GH resistance is the finding of high GH levels with low levels of the somatomedin insulin-like growth factor I (IGF I), which mediates the anabolic actions of GH. This may be primary, as in patients with Laron syndrome or acquired GH resistance [2]. There is now a body of evidence to suggest that the changes in the GH/IGF I axis are permissive to protein catabolism and that treatment with either GH and/or IGF I may improve the nutritional state of some patient groups [3].

GH is secreted in a pulsatile fashion from the anterior pituitary and circulates bound to two proteins. The predominant binding protein has an identical sequence to the extracellular portion of the GH receptor (GHR) and is thought to be derived from the receptor by proteolytic cleavage. The GHR is found in many tissues and is a member of the cytokine superfamily of receptors which have a single transmembrane domain. Binding of a single GH molecule results in dimerisation of the GHR. The GHR then associates with the kinase JAK-2, which autophosphorylates and phosphorylates the GHR. There is subsequent phosphorylation of other proteins which transmit the signal to the nucleus, leading to expression of the transcription factors fos and jun and ultimately IGF I. The majority of the anabolic actions of GH appear to be mediated by IGF I, but GH also has direct actions which are predominantly anti-insulin, as illustrated in Fig. 1.

Most of the circulating IGF I is derived from the liver, and the metabolic action of IGF I is modulated by a number of different binding proteins [4]. The main circulating IGF-binding proteins are IGFBP-1, -2 and -3. IGFBP-1 is an inhibitor of IGF's actions in most bioassays, shows an inverse relationship with circulating insulin and may inhibit the actions of IGF I when there is low substrate availability [5, 6]. IGFBP-2 levels rise during situations of stress, and it is a predominant carrier of IGF II [7]. IGFBP-3 carries 80%–85% of circulating IGF I and appears to act as an intravascular store for IGF I [8].

Thus, there are many potential sites for the development of acquired GH resistance, as illustrated in Fig. 2. In this paper we describe the changes in the GH/IGF I axis in a number of different patient groups. We have studied patients with chronic liver disease, as they provide a model for acquired GH resistance in which we

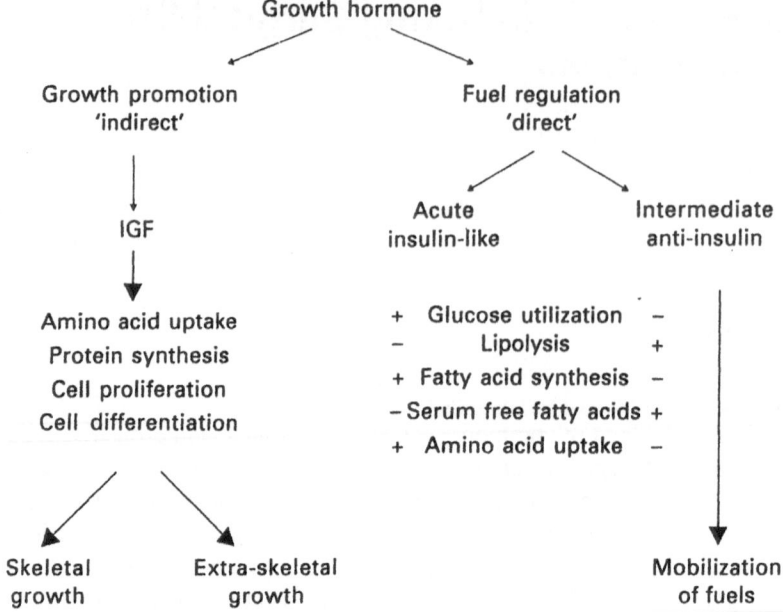

Fig. 1. Actions of growth hormone (GH). The growth-promoting effects are mediated predominantly through generation of insulin-like growth factor (*IGF*) I. Acute insulin-like effects have been demonstrated within 2 h of GH administration, before tissues become refractory to further GH exposure. The major impact of GH on fat and carbohydrate metabolism is, however, to antagonise the actions of insulin. (Reproduced with permission from [26])

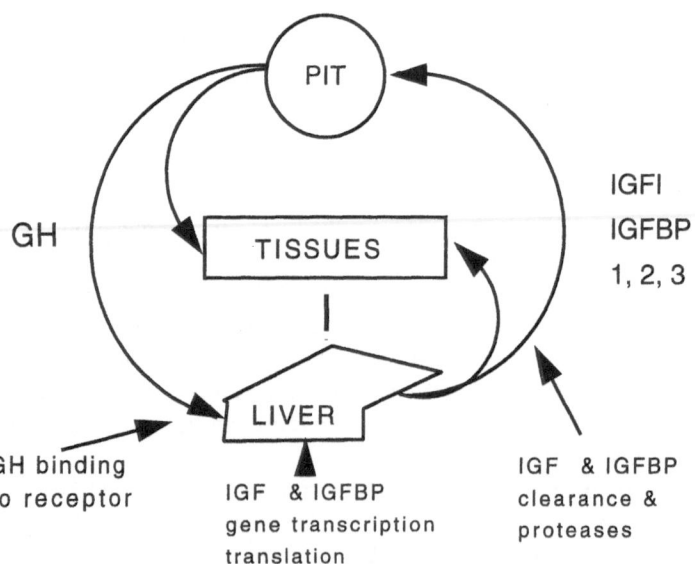

Fig. 2. Sites of potential resistance to the anabolic actions of growth hormone (*GH*). *PIT*, pituitary; *IGF*, insulin-like growth factor; *IGFBP*, IGF-binding protein

can study gene expression. We present evidence to support the hypothesis that acquired GH resistance is permissive to protein catabolism and make some tentative suggestions for the molecular basis of acquired GH resistance.

The Critically Ill

We have studied in detail the changes in the GH/IGF I axis in six critially ill patients in the Intensive Care Unit [9, 10]. All patients had undergone major abdominal surgery, had become septic and required ventilation and parenteral nutrition. They were studied before and then during parenteral nutrition and matched to a group of age-, sex-, height- and weight-matched controls. Fasting in the normal controls resulted in an increase in GH levels. This has previously been well documented, and Ho et al. [11] found this was predominantly due to an increase in GH pulse amplitude. The critically ill patients had raised GH levels similar to fasted controls but with a very distinct pattern. In particular, the patients had raised interpulse or baseline GH levels which never became undetectable. IGF I levels were very low and in the hypopituitary range for all patients and did not increase on parenteral feeding. The patients had high levels of IGFBP-1 and low level of IGFBP-3. Using western ligand blotting, we have found that they have a specific protease for IGFBP-3 which reduces the affinity of IGF I for IGFBP-3 similar to that seen in pregnancy [12, 13]. The critically ill patient therefore has high GH levels due to an increase in basal GH secretion, low IGF I levels, low IGFBP-3 levels with a reduced affinity for IGF I due to protease activity, and high IGFBP-1 levels. The critically ill represent a very heterogeneous population and are therefore difficult to classify. They also receive multiple therapeutic interventions, including dopamine infusions. Recent data have shown that low-dose dopamine infusions suppress GH levels in critically ill patients [14].

Post-surgical Patients

Post-surgical patients provide a much more reproducible model of stress than the critically ill. We have looked at changes in the GH/IGF I axis in 12 adults undergoing major abdominal surgery [15]. Patients were studied before premedication, at the end of surgery and up to 6 weeks after recovery. There were very distinct changes in the hormone levels. IGF I fell rapidly during surgery to reach a nadir at 4 days and did not recover to the pre-operative level until 6 weeks after surgery. IGFBP-3 showed a similar pattern with a nadir at day 2 following surgery. During surgery, IGFBP-1 levels rose, despite an increase in insulin levels, and fell back to basal values at 6 h. In contrast, IGFBP-2 levels fell during surgery and then rose at 6 h and remained elevated for 7 days. It is of interest that the changes in IGF I and IGFBP-3 levels parallel those that were reported 60 years ago in urinary nitrogen excretion by Cuthbertson [16]. There was induction of IGFBP-3 protease activity which appeared between days 1 and 4 following surgery. Thus, there is a complex change in the IGF-binding proteins, the physiological significance of which remains to be established. The data clearly demonstrate the prolonged change in the IGF I levels following acute surgical stress.

Chronic Liver Disease

Patients with chronic liver disease suffer severe protein calorie malnutrition which predicts mortality and outcome from hepatic transplantation. These patients provide an interesting group because we can access liver tissue to study. We have found that they show similar changes in the GH/IGF I axis to other patient groups with acquired GH resistance. In particular, they have high GH levels, low IGF I levels, high IGFBP-1 levels and low IGFBP-3 levels [17]. Their IGFBP-1 levels were high despite high insulin levels, a finding that has only previously been reported in post-surgical patients, as discussed above. It has previously been considered that the low binding protein and IGF I levels in patients with chronic liver disease are due to a specific effect of liver cell damage. However, our results suggest this is not the case. For instance IGF I levels do not relate to severity of liver disease, but rather correlate with markers of nutritional status, a finding that has previously been reported [18].

We looked at the expression of the IGF genes in normal and cirrhotic liver. We found expression of the GHR, IGF I and IGFBP-1–3 genes in both cirrhotic and normal liver [19, 20]. IGFBP-1 expression was still highly expressed in cirrhotic liver despite high insulin levels, and in situ hybridisation localised the expression to the regenerating hepatocytes rather than fibrotic tissue. IGFBP-2 and IGFBP-3 expression appeared to be higher in the cirrhotic liver compared to normal liver. It appears that in these patients the liver remains capable of transcribing the IGF genes and that GH resistance may be a non-specific effect of nutrition rather than an effect specific to liver disease.

Conclusions and Hypothesis

We have presented data from three different patient groups. They all show distinct, yet similar changes in the GH/IGF I axis. There appears to be a switch in the metabolic actions of GH from its indirect IGF I-mediated anabolic actions to a direct counter-regulation effect. This may result in mobilisation of circulating fuels as the direct effects are anti-insulin, therefore reducing glucose uptake and increasing lipolysis. This might have been an advantage from an evolutionary perspective when nutrition was not available. However, it may no longer appear an advantage in the context of modern intensive care. The evidence presented so far is circumstantial. However, there are two lines of thought to directly implicate these changes in protein catabolism. Firstly, if you take out IGF I by administering IGF I antibodies, there is increased net protein catabolism [21]. The second line of evidence comes from the many studies now published demonstrating that supraphysiological doses of GH can overcome GH resistance in many patient groups [22].

We have looked at all levels of the GH/IGF I axis in various patient groups. In the patients with chronic liver disease, there is transcription of the IGF genes and increased expression of IGFBP-3. We have found that GH administration to this patient group results in an increase in IGF I levels. Therefore, these patients remain capable of responding to GH and transcribing the IGF I gene. We would like to make the tentative hypothesis that some of the acquired GH resistance is due to a post-translation effect, perhaps due to IGFBP protease activity. We know that protease activity appears in many patient groups; this protease reduces the affinity of IGFBP-3 for IGF I and therefore may increase clearance of both proteins, which could result in a fall in IGF I and IGFBP-3 levels. There are some preliminary data to support this hypothesis in that patients who have undergone major surgery have a short half-life for IGF I [23]. This change is IGF I binding may increase the bioavailability of IGF I, perhaps in an attempt to counteract increased catabolism [24, 25].

An endocrine therapy which could improve substrate uptake in critically ill patients would provide a major advance in the therapy of these patients. Provisional data suggest GH and IGF I either alone or together can provide such treatment. However, it is clear from the above discussion that the control of GH and IGF I is complex and requires further elucidation before we can maximise the benefits of any therapeutic intervention.

Acknowledgements. This work was supported by the Joint Research Board of St. Bartholomew's Hospital. We are grateful to Pharmacia for both their intellectual and financial support.

References

1. Ross RJM, Miell JP, Buchanan CR (1991) Avoiding autocannibalism: consider growth hormone and insulin-like growth factor-I. BMJ 303:1147–1148
2. Laron Z, Blum WF, Chatelain PG et al. (1993) Classification of growth hormone insensitivity syndrome. J Pediatr 122:241
3. Clemmons DR (1992) Role of insulin like growth factor-I in reversing catabolism. J Clin Endocrinol Metab 75:1183–1185
4. Rosenfeld RG, Lamson G, Pham H et al. (1993) Insulin-like growth factor-binding proteins. Recent Prog Horm Res 46:99–163
5. Taylor AM, Dunger ADB, Preece MA et al. (1990) The growth hormone independent insulin-like growth factor-binding protein BP-28 is associated with serum insulin-like growth factor-I inhibitory bioactivity in adolescent insulin-dependent diabetics. Clin Endocrinol (Oxf) 32:229–239
6. Lewitt MS, Denyer GS, Conney GJ, Baxter RC (1991) Insulin-like growth factor binding protein-1 modulates blood glucose levels. Endocrinology 129:2254–2256
7. Blum WF, Horn N, Kratzsch J et al. (1993) Clinical studies of IGFBP-2 by radioimmunoassay. Growth Regul 3:100–104
8. Blum WF, Ranke MB (1991) Plasma IGFBP-3 levels as clinical indicators. In: Spencer EM (ed) Modern concepts of insulin-like growth factors. Elsevier, New York, pp 381–393
9. Ross RJM, Freeman E, Jones J, Matthews DR, Preece MA, Buchanan CR (1991) Critically ill patients have high basal growth hormone levels with attenuated oscillatory activity associated with low levels of insulin-like growth factor-1. Clin Endocrinol (Oxf) 35:47–54
10. Ross RJM, Miell JP, Holly JMP, Maheshware H, Norman M, Abdulla AF, Buchanan CR (1991) Levels of GH, IGF binding proteins, insulin, blood glucose and cortisol in intensive care patients. Clin Endocrinol (Oxf) 35:361–367

11. Ho KY, Veldhuis JD, Johnson ML et al. (1988) Fasting enhance growth hormone secretion and amplifies the complex rhythms of growth hormone secretion in man. J Clin Invest 81:968–975
12. Davies SC, Wass JAH, Ross RJM et al. (1991) The induction of a specific protease for insulin-like growth factor binding protein-3 in the circulation during severe illness. J Endocrinol 130:469–473
13. Lassarre C, Binoux M (1994) Insulin-like growth factor binding protein-3 is functionally altered in pregnancy plasma. Endocrinology 134:1254–1262
14. Van Den Berghe G (1994) Dopamine and pituitary hormones in critical illness. Leuven University Press, Leuven
15. Cotterill AM, Mendel P, Holly JMP et al. (1995) The differential regulation of the circulating levels of the insulin-like growth factors and their binding proteins (IGFBP) 1, 2 and 3 after elective abdominal surgery. Clin Endocrinol (Oxf) (Submitted)
16. Cuthbertson DP (1931) Observations on the disturbance of metabolism produced by injury to the limbs. Q J Med 2:233–246
17. Donaghy A, Ross RJM, Gimson AE, Hughes SC, Holly J, Williams R (1995) Growth hormone, insulin-like growth factor-I and insulin-like growth factor binding proteins 1 and 3 in chronic liver disease. Hepatology 21: 680–688
18. Mendenhall CL, Chernhausek SD, Ray MB et al. (1989) The interactions of insulin-like growth factor-I (IGF-I) with protein-calorie malnutrition in patients with alcoholic liver disease. V.A. Cooperative study on alcoholic hepatitis. Alcohol Alcohol 24:319–329
19. Ross RJM, Rodriguez-Arnao J, Donaghy A et al. (1994) Expression of IGFBP-1 in normal and cirrhotic human livers. J Endocrinol 141:377–382
20. Ross RJM, Rodriguez-Arnao J, Wraight CJ, Clark AJL (1994) Expression of IGF-I, IGFBP-1, 2, 3, and GH receptor (GHR) genes in normal liver and cirrhosis. J Endocrinol 140:111
21. Koea JB, Gallaher BW, Breier BH et al. (1992) Passive immunization against circulating insulin-like growth factor-I (IGF-I) increases protein catabolism in lambs: evidence for a physiological role for circulating IGF-I. J Endocrinol 135:279–284
22. Wilmore DW (1991) Catabolic illness, strategies for enhancing recovery. N Engl J Med 325:695–702
23. Miell JP, Taylor AM, Jones J et al. (1992) Administration of recombinant insulin-like growth factor-I to patients following major gastrointestinal surgery. Clin Endocrinol (Oxf) 37:542–551
24. Blat C, Villaudy J, Bihoux M (1994) In vivo proteolysis of serum insulin-like growth factor (IGF) binding protein-3 results in increased availability of IGF to target cells. J Clin Invest 93:2296–2290
25. Holly JMP, Claffey P, Cwyfan Hughes SC, Frost VJ, Yateman ME (1993) Proteases acting on IGFBPs: their occurrence and physiological significance. Growth Regul 3:88–91
26. Ross RJM, Buchanan CR (1990) Growth hormone secretion: its regulation and the influence of nutritional factors. Nutrition Res Rev 3:143–162

Therapeutic Recommendations and Future Research

A. Revhaug, J. Wernerman, and B. Vonen

The principal objective of this book has been to focus on the very early changes that take place in an organism exposed to an acute catabolic insult. In this context, "early" means within minutes and until a few days after the initial processes have started during a catabolic situation. Another objective of the volume has been to illustrate that, even though a large number of the body's responses in these situations are general in nature, there are also some typical organ-specific changes and responses which in their turn influence the body's general responses as well as those of the specific organ. The body's response to an acute catabolic injury involves a complex and interactive set of responses among a large number of hormones, neurotransmitters, cytokines, cell types, and organs. The first insult that produces the catabolic state may be very different from situation to situation; some can be anticipated such as with a planned surgical procedure, while others are true emergencies such as trauma accidents.

The various chapters have shown clearly that the different organs respond in a specific way to acute catabolic situations. All the knowledge gathered on systemic and interorgan responses indicates that there are several possible ways of intervening in the acute catabolic response. This evidence should be used in a systematic manner when preparing preventive as well as therapeutic measures in these patients. It must, however, not be forgotten that an important part of the response should not necessarily be prevented. There are in fact many situations in which parts of the response are obviously beneficial and obligatory for a positive recovery. Thus, a combination of measures, some reducing and others stimulating the catabolic responses, must be used to ensure a profitable patient recovery.

Therapeutic recommendations

Measures in Foreseeable Acute Catabolic States

When the acute catabolic state can be foreseen, e.g., before a surgical procedure, there is a set of possible measures which can and should be undertaken (Tables 1–3). These measures involve the psychological and physical preparation of the patient and a diversity of actions to be planned and performed by the surgical team.

Over the past years, changes in surgical techniques and modern technology have made it possible for patients, to withstand a procedure much better than previous-

Table 1. Preoperative measures to avoid negative catabolism

Psychological preparation of the patient	Understanding the procedure Preparation for the procedure Ambient acquaintance
Physical preparation of the patient	Estimate physical status Choose technique accordingly Pulmonary training Ascertain adequate nutrition
Preoperative antibiotics	Follow recommendations
Anti-thrombosis prophylaxis	Low-molecular heparin Additional measures in high-risk patients

Table 2. Intraoperative measures

Decrease neuroendocrine stress	Neural blockade Pain- and stress-free anesthesia Maintain normovolemia Maintain body temperature
Decrease trauma stress	Atraumatic technique Avoid blood losses Minimal surgery

Table 3. Postoperative measures

Pain control	No pain! Epidural analgesia Peripherally acting analgesics
Early mobilization	Conscious patients should walk Unconscious patients need passive mobilization
Early administration of enteral nutrition	Preferably oral, "normal" food Always some enteral nutrition
Additional supplementation for the critically ill	Consider early supplementation of vitamins, hormones, and specific nutrients

ly. Procedures which just a few years ago required several days of hospitalization can now be performed on an outpatient basis. Less tissue injury and shorter operating times when performing minimally invasive surgery are typical examples of how the magnitude of the catabolic response can be significantly reduced [1, 2]. The systematic introduction and use of prophylactic antibiotics in abdominal and other types of surgery has also lowered the surgical complication rate and thereby the stress response [3, 4]. Modern use of anesthesia and perioperative analgesia represents another major factor leading to a much lower catabolic response to surgery [5–7]. The systematic use of intraoperative epidural analgesia, as described earlier in this volume, should be standard for all patients undergoing medium or major surgery.

The recent advances in molecular biology and biotechnology have substantially increased our knowledge of the host response to injury. The same advances have also made available via recombinant DNA technology a rapidly increased number of naturally occurring substances which have the potential of stimulating and/or inhibiting host responses. Tumor necrosis factor (TNF) and the interleukins, their soluble receptors, and antibodies against them, or their receptors are typical examples of the substances which have become available for therapeutic interventions over the past few years [8–10]. However, it must be emphasized that so far the knowledge of how and when to use these substances is still far from being standard clinical use. Other substances which have become available as a result of modern biotechnology include several anabolic or growth-stimulating factors [11, 12].

It is typical, though, that the only substance which seems ready for limited clinical use in some acute catabolic situations is one of the "old" hormones, i.e., growth hormone. The start of investigational use of this substances dates back several decades, but it is hardly a surprise that new knowledge needs more than just a few years before clinical use can be expected.

Specialized enteral and parenteral nutrition are now standard care components in acute catabolic patients. The use of these therapeutic interventions corrects and prevents nutrient deficits, attenuates the loss of body protein, and improves clinical outcome in malnourished patients [13–15]. New strategies have evolved over the past years regarding how and what should be used as nutritional support in acute catabolic patients. One of the major impacts on the clinical practice of nutrition in acute and critical care is the use of enteral feeding in these patients [16–19]. The conditionally essential amino acid glutamin in the acute catabolic situation will probably be of importance in major patient groups in the near future. The use of specialized lipids and antioxidants has a similar potential.

Until recently it was considered that in the early phases of an acute catabolic state the supplementation of hormones such as thyroid hormone was not indicated, even though their circulating levels may often be far below normal. Recent data question this practice [20, 21] and reasonably so: Why should suboptimal levels of thyroideal and other important hormones be beneficial when the body is at maximal stress?

Measures in Unforeseeable Acute Catabolic States

A large number of patients will suffer from an acute catabolic disease process which cannot be foreseen or even anticipated (Table 4). Many acute infectious diseases appear suddenly and without any warning in otherwise healthy individuals. Other such situations include accidents, acute hepatic and renal failure, and other acute destructive processes. In these situations there is obviously no possibility of intervening before the insult, and the measures have to be initiated once the processes have started.

In such situations, patients are in need of specific therapeutic interventions or therapies such as ABC resuscitation, fracture and trauma care, drainage if there is a localizable infectious focus, and antibiotics. Once initial therapy has been effectuated, the various elements of the above-mentioned therapeutic measures for the intra- and post-injury period should be followed, as described earlier (Tables 2, 3).

Table 4. Measures in nonpreventable situations[a]

Trauma and burns	ABC resuscitation
	Maximal attention to definitive procedures
Sepsis	Identify and drain focus
	Circulatory therapy
	Antibiotic therapy

[a] The measures listed here should be supplemented by those in Tables 2 and 3.

Few acute catabolic states have received such a great amount of interest and research as sepsis and septic shock [22–25]. Accordingly, the current state of knowledge of the pathophysiological events has increased substantially over the past few years in this field. The demonstration of TNF and other mediators that are important in the development of the septic processes has led to the hope that possible specific therapies based on modern biotechnology might improve the outcome of such diseases. Until now, however, no such important therapy has come through. The use of anti-endotoxin, TNF antibodies and the like is still at the stage of experimental medicine. Even the use of corticosteroids, which have important regulatory actions on cytokines and other mediator substances important for the propagation of the septic process, has not been established. The fact that it has been so hard to establish the right use of steroids in septic shock is probably an indication of how important the timing of the intervention is. This is hardly a big surprise considering the interactive and intricate up-and-down regulation of the defense system [26, 27]. Further research and clinical experiments will probably sort out when and how to intervene with these agents.

When evaluating the results of modern therapy in sepsis, the effects and results of modern intensive care should not be underestimated. The combination of the use of modern ventilators, different circulatory assisting or filtering devices with modern antibiotics, and circulatory active agents have changed the prognosis of severe infections markedly. It is, however, interesting and important to focus on the fact that most serious infections are also accompanied by a severe degree of catabolism [28].

The focus on therapy aimed at reducing the effects of catabolism has mainly been carried out by scientists and clinicians involved in surgical and trauma-related catabolism. It is important to focus on the same elements when the patient is suffering from acute catabolism induced by infections or other nontrauma-induced diseases as in the trauma situations. The need for nutritional support is as imperative in these situations as in trauma, and the importance of enteral nutrition is probably not reduced in such occasions. The effectiveness of immunomodulatory nutrients also needs to be further explored in sepsis. The need for physical and mental activity is often less focused upon than drug interventions, but must not be forgotten in these situations either.

Another phenomenon which need to be addressed is the *second-hit* concept. It has become relatively clear that the body is in a different state of defense awareness some days after a *first hit,* as represented by a trauma or infection [29, 30]. In these situations, which at the first-hit situation were unforeseeable, an insult occurring later such as an abscess should be treated in the same way as the foreseeable ones. This could be the difference that decides whether a patient will later develop multiple organ failure or not. There are several possibilities of recuding the negative effects of the acute catabolic state, as already described, and these require knowledge and interest in the pathophysiology of these states. An integrated support is necessary and possible at present.

Future Research

Even though it may seem difficult to understand at the moment and in our own time, we must keep in mind that the currently gathered knowledge in the field of the acute catabolic state is only a scratch on the surface of the amount of mechanisms governing these processes. The ongoing research in basic and applied medical research will eventually set these facts straight and those who come after us will be able to use this in the best interest of their patients. Now, how do we proceed to achieve this progress?

The initiating events that take place in the body when the acute catabolic process starts must be clarified. The immediate changes which occur in the cells, the interstitium, and later in the organs and finally the whole body response need to be studied. Another major challenge to future development is to learn how these changes develop over time. Thus we must follow the changes as the processes develop in the sames systems. Establishing a possible interaction with the processes in terms of inhibiting negative responses and stimulating positive responses requires an enormous amount of systematically achieved information based on different kinds of research. Future research in this field must be based on results from basic research in biochemistry and biotechnology along with experimental and clinical research before final clinical achievements can be reached.

A major problem with regard to research in the field of the acute catabolic state is the difficulty of having an adequate acute catabolic model which can be standardized. An acute catabolic model must be characterized by a period of tissue destruc-

Table 5. Acute catabolic animal models

Infectious and inflammatory models	Endotoxins Live bacteria Zymosan
Trauma models	Fractures Soft tissue injury Burns Hemorrhage
Hormonal and mediator stimulations	Single or several hormones Regulatory cytokines
Combination models	Combining several models at the same time or sequentially

Table 6. Acute catabolic human models

Infectious and inflammatory models	Infectious diseases occurring naturally
	Innoculations
	Inflammatory inductors
	    ☐ Lipopolysaccharides
	    ☐ Cytokines
	    ☐ Others

Standardized surgical procedures	Gastrectomies Hip replacement Other procedures with different catabolic drive Cardiopulmonary bypass
Organ failure	Kidney failure Cardiac failure Hepatic failure Other organ failure
Hormonal infusions	Glucocorticosteroids Multiple hormonal infusions
Other catabolic inductors	E.g., Cytostatic regimes

Table 7. Investigational techniques

Biomolecular	Nucleic acids Receptors Others
Biochemical	Qualitative and quantitative substance determinations Isotopes
Morphological	Light and electron microscopy Other structural determinations
Functional	Specific organ function tests Organism outcome

tion due to some active process. This requirement excludes the mere starvation models which often have been used. Both animal and human models can and must be used in this reasearch. A considerable limitation on animal models is that they have to be conducted with the animal under anesthesia. For some questions, this is a major inconvenience, but for others it may be most relevant, as clinical situations very often occur in patients who are under heavy sedation. The most relevant animal models are summarized in Table 5 and serve as an indicator of the variety of situations leading to the acute catabolic state. The specific problems or advantages of these models are beyond the scope of this work. Suffice it to focus on the great variability in these models, the difficulty of standardizing even within the same species, similar problems with the inductory agents, and the differences in host responses.

With the obvious deficiencies of in vitro or animal models, there is always a need for relevant human models. Some possible human models are represented by a diversity of disease states, interventional therapeutic models as well as experimen-

Table 8. Metabolic methods

Whole body studies	Magnetic resonance imaging
	Isotope studies
Whole organ studies	In vivo models
	In vivo isolated models
	In vitro organ models
	Microdialysis
Organ flux studies	Arteriovenous substrate concentrations
	Isotopes
Tissue slice studies	Substrate concentrations
Isolated cell studies	Substrate metabolism
Cell culture studies	Ultrastructure
Cell organelle studies	Mitochondria
	Membranes
	Others

tal human models (Table 6). Once it has been decided which of the models should be used as the investigational model, a diversity of different variables can be evaluated. In general, a combination of different investigational techniques should be used since only a combination of biochemical, morphological and functional results is sufficient to prove or disprove completely the proposed hypothesis (Table 7). As the majority of the changes in the acute catabolic state are originally metabolic changes, they can be investigated systematically, as shown in Table 8. Combinations of these models must be used, and the results evaluated in clinical studies. The interventional experiments must then be performed in the same diversity of model systems. In the future we will then be able to explore the effects of stimulation and modulation of the many important regulatory systems, as described earlier in this book.

The problem with timing the different interventions according to the phase of the catabolic state is a major challenge. However, the most important obstacle to progress is the steadily more restrictive research funding for this type of medical research granted by most official authorities.

References

1. Hill AG, Finn P, Schroeder D (1993) Postoperative fatigue after laparoscopic surgery. Aust N Z J Surg 63:946–951
2. Mealy K, Gallagher H, Barry M, Lennon F, Traynor O, Hyland J (1992) Physiological and metabolic responses to open and laparoscopic cholecystectomy. Br J Surg 79:1061–1064
3. Kaiser AB (1986) Antimicrobial prophylaxis in surgery. N Engl J Med 315
4. Giercksky KE, Danielsen S, Garberg O et al. (1982) A single dose tinidazole and doxycycline prophylaxis in elective surgery of the colon and rectum. Ann Surg 195:227–231
5. Brandt MR, Fernandes A, Mordhorst R, Kehlet H (1978) Epidural analgesia improves postoperative nitrogen balance. Br Med J I:1106–1108
6. Kehlet H (1979) Stress free anaesthesia and surgery. Acta Anaesthesiol Scand 23:503–504
7. Keleth H (1994) Postoperative pain relief – what is the issue? Br J Anaesth 72:375–378

8. Zamir O, Hasselgren PO, Allmen D von, Fischer JE (1991) The effect of interleukin-1a and the glucocorticoid receptor blocker RU 38486 on total and myofibrillar protein breakdown in skeletal muscle. J Surg Res 50:579–583
9. Svoboda P, Kantorova I, Ochmann J (1994) Dynamics of interleukin 1, 2, and 6 and tumor necrosis factor alpha in multiple trauma patients. J Trauma 36:336–340
10. Wenzel RP (1992) Anti-endotoxin monoclonal antibodies – a second look. N Engl M Med 326:1151–1153
11. Revhaug A, Mjaaland M (1993) Growth hormone and surgery. Horm Res 40:99–101
12. Hammarqvist F, Wernerman J, Ali R, Decken A von der, Vinnars E (1989) Addition of glutamine to total parenteral nutrition after elective abdominal surgery spares free glutamine in muscle, counteracts the fall in muscle protein synthesis, and improves nitrogen balance. Ann Surg 209:455–461
13. Zigler TR, Young LS, Manson JM et al. (1988) Metabolic effects of recombinant human growth hormone in patients receiving parenteral nutrition. Ann Surg 208:6–16
14. Herndon DN, Barrow RE, Kunkle KR et al. (1990) Effects of recombinant human growth hormone on donor site healing in severely burned children. Ann Surg 212:424–429
15. Mjaaland M, Unneberg K, Hotvedt R, Revhaug A (1991) Nitrogen retention caused by growth hormone in patients undergoing gastrointestinal surgery with epidural analgesia and parenteral nutrition. Eur J Surg 157:21–27
16. Kudsk KA, Croce MA, Fabian TC et al. (1992) Enteral versus parenteral feeding. Ann Surg 215:503–507
17. Moore FA, Feleciano DV, Andreassy RJ (1992) Early enteral feeding, compared with parenteral, reduces postoperative septic complications. Ann Surg 216:172–176
18. Moore FA, Moore EE, Kudsk KA et al. (1994) Clinical benefits of an immune-enhancing diet for early postinjury enteral feeding. J Trauma 37:607–611
19. Moore EE, Moore FA (1991) Immediate enteral feeding following multisystem trauma – a decade experience. J Am Coll Nutr 33:633–638
20. Berghe GV, Zegher F, Lauwers P (1994) Growth hormone secretion in critical illness: effect of dopamine. J Clin Endocrinol Metab 79:1141–1146
21. Berghe GV, Zegher F, Lauwers P (1994) Dopamine and the sick euthyroid syndrome in critical illness. Clin Endocrinol 41:731–737
22. Beutler B, Mahoney J, Trang NL, Pekala P, Cerami A (1985) Purification of cachectin, a lipoprotein lipase suppressing hormone secreted by endotoxin-induced RAW 264.7 cells. J Exp Med 161:984–995
23. Tracey KJ, Beutler B, Lowry SJ et al. (1986) Shock and tissue injury induced by recombinant human cachectin. Science 234:470–474
24. Michie H, Spriggs D, Manogue K, Sherman M, Revhaug A et al. (1988) Tumor necrosis factor and endotoxin induce similar metabolic responses in human beings. Surgery 104:280–286
25. Revhaug A, Michie H, Manson J et al. (1988) Inhibition of cyclooxygenase attenuates the metabolic response to endotoxin in humans. Arch Surg 123:162–170
26. Granowitz EV, Porat R, Mier JW et al. (1993) Intravenous endotoxin suppresses the cytokine response of periferal blood mononuclear cells of healthy humans. J Immunol 151:1637–1645
27. Warren HS, Danner RL, Munford RS (1992) Anti-endotoxin monoclonal antibodies. N Engl J Med 326:1153–1157
28. Watters JM, Bessey PQ, Dinarello CA, Wolff SM, Wilmore DW (1986) Both inflammatory and endocrine mediators stimulate host responses to sepsis. Arch Surg 121:179–190
29. Røkke O, Giercksky K-E, Revhaug A (1989) Depression of plasma endotoxin levels during Gram-negative septicemia subsequent to moderate trauma. Acta Chir Scand 155:145–149
30. Moore FA, Moore EE (1995) Evolving concepts in the pathogenesis of postinjury multiple organ failure. Surg Clinics 75:257–277

Subject Index